Massimo Lombardi • Carlo Bartolozzi

MRI of the Heart and Vessels

Foreword by

Luigi Donato

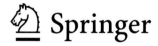 Springer

MASSIMO LOMBARDI
MRI Laboratory
CNR, Institute of Clinical Physiology
Pisa, Italy

CARLO BARTOLOZZI
Diagnostic and Interventional Radiology
University, AOUP
Pisa, Italy

Originally published as:
Risonanza Magnetica del Cuore e dei Vasi
a cura di Massimo Lombardi e Carlo Bartolozzi
© 2004 Springer-Verlag Italia, Milan
All Rights Reserved

Translation by Manuella Walker

Library of Congress Control Number: 2004117794

ISBN 88-470-0306-7 Springer Milan Berlin Heidelberg New York

Springer is a part of Springer Science+Business Media
springeronline.com
© Springer-Verlag Italia 2005
Printed in Italy

Cover design: Simona Colombo, Milan, Italy
Typesetting: ITG, Torino, Italy
Printing: Grafiche Porpora Srl, Cernusco S/N, Italy

Foreword

This reference book on the use of Magnetic Resonance in the study of the heart and vessels by Massimo Lombardi and Carlo Bartolozzi represents an excellent opportunity for meditation and discussion on some of the present trends in clinical medicine.

The first consideration cannot but concern the rapid and continuing evolution of diagnostic technologies, and particularly of those in the field of imaging: a topic that only ten years ago would never have even been considered as a subject for a book of this type, but that today clearly offers evidence of a concrete and relevant contribution, in some cases exclusive, to many applications of cardiovascular diagnostics. From this point of view, the authors deserve particular recognition for having put together a synthesis and a critical presentation of the many applications in the field of Magnetic Resonance Imaging: a contribution that will be of sure interest to the consultants and specialists of imaging techniques and of medical and surgical cardiovascular disciplines.

The second consideration concerns the fundamental importance of the integration of medical and non-medical competencies in the development and management of new technologies in medicine. In sectors such as MRI the collaboration between physicists and engineers not only provides a promise for the correct exploitation of the techniques but also, and perhaps especially, a basis for the very same development of the clinical applications in a sector in which the boundaries between development and application are far from established and indeed in continuous evolution.

The third consideration concerns the importance of the collaboration between the Institute of Clinical Physiology and the departments of University hospitals: the first institution being deeply characterized by the mission of performing clinical research through a broad multi-disciplinarian basis, closely integrated with on-field clinical applications, which validate innovations providing the drive for further research; the second institution characterized by the important task of specialized training and assistance, the quality of which must necessarily be guaranteed and renewed on the basis of the progress of technological knowledge.

My last consideration addresses the importance in the management of continuously evolving technological innovations, through a sound relationship between industrial companies and research institutions that goes far beyond bare commercial aims.

For all the considerations above, this book represents a precious and very significant example, which I am very glad to present.

Finally, I wish to express my particular appreciation to Massimo Lombardi and the entire medical and non-medical staff, nursing, technical and administrative personnel of the Magnetic Resonance laboratory of the IFC-CNR, who have, in less than four years of intense activity – often in difficult working conditions – developed an idea into a consolidated reliable, reality, and have especially demonstrated the ability of the laboratory to be at the cutting age of this developing field.

Pisa, December 2004   **Luigi Donato**
                                                       Head of CNR
                              Institute of Clinical Physiology, Pisa

Preface

The study of the heart and vessels by Magnetic Resonance Imaging represents a relatively new field of application, especially if one considers the large-scale diagnostic use of the technique in the neurological and muscular fields.

The explanation of the delayed application in the cardiovascular field can be sought in the methodological complexity linked to the study of moving anatomical structures.

Due to the important developments in terms of hardware and software seen in recent years, we can now choose a dedicated approach for the study of the heart and vessels that allows us to achieve all that morphological and functional information that otherwise could not have been obtained by means of other imaging techniques.

This monographic text origins from the collaboration of two disciplines that have historically covered specific interests in clinical-diagnostic and technical-applicative settings: Cardiology and Radiology.

The heart and vessels, which have often represented a battle ground, have been for our Groups, fertile ground for development of competencies, driven by our firma belief that a multidisciplinary approach represents the most efficient way to exploit technological resources to the best and respond in the best manner to clinical needs.

Although this is a subject in continuous and rapid evolution, we wanted to dedicate the first part of this text to some particular methodological/technical aspects concerning the techniques of fast acquisition finalized toward the achievement of morphological, functional, and flow related information. The same section deals with contrast agents that nowadays represent an integrating part of the exam, with particular focus on the optimization of their use.

The last chapter of the introductive part is dedicated to image post processing; we present the techniques that are at present indispensable for obtaining a better interpretation of the native images and allow at the same time quantitative-qualitative evaluations facilitating the correlation with data obtained by other techniques of cardiovascular imaging.

The most extensive part of this book is dedicated to clinical diagnostic applications.

In reference to cardiology, we present the contribution of MRI in the most consolidated clinical sectors, providing an updated reference of positive practical value. At the same time we have wanted to analyze, in a prospective way, the most interesting applicative evolutions of what we foresee will find wide diffusion throughout cardiological diagnostics in the near future.

The second clinical diagnostic topic is represented by the study of the vessels: the subject has been approached to the full, spanning from the intracranial vasculature to the peripheral vessels of the limbs, in consideration of the *panexplorative* characteristics of MRI.

Wide space has also been dedicated to images, in order to allow the reader an immediate correlation of the description of the methods and disease on one hand, and the iconographic representation on the other.

This result has been achieved thanks to the Editor, who has permitted a full range of action as to the number of images reproduced and has assured us the best of quality. We are confident this aspect will be appreciated by those wishing to use this book as a reference text for the use of MRI in the cardio-vascular setting.

Pisa, December 2004

Carlo Bartolozzi
Director
Diagnostic and Interventional Radiology
University, AOUP, Pisa

Acknowledgements

A special message of acknowledgments to my colleagues involved in such a cumbersome task as the one we have just accomplished, an address that is more a letter of apology. Acknowledgements, which are even more due, as they have not been requested and perhaps arrive even unexpected.

In reality, along with the exciting scientific experience implicit to the preparation of a book of this type, there are surprising human aspects. During the argumentations born from different experiences, sometimes passionate, which dragged beyond dawn, the most sincere and spontaneous character traits were unveiled. The surprising aspect lies in the very enthusiasm and the constant tension my colleagues have shown throughout this journey from the planning to the printing of this book. This engagement added to the already many clinical, diagnostic, and professional duties, that seemingly would have left no spare time to any further workloads. What was unveiled to my eyes during these months can be summarized in two main aspects. The first is the enthusiasm towards a live, fulfilling – but also demanding – technique. The second aspect, which is quite flattering, is the friendship and availability shown by all the Authors to the Editors and especially to myself.

A special thanks goes to the technical, nursing, engineering and secretarial staff of the MRI laboratory of the IFC-CNR of Pisa, and in the same degree to the Diagnostic and Interventional Radiology Department of the University of Pisa that have allowed me to add further turbulence to the already chaotic daily activity without showing the slightest sign of restlessness or surrender, rather inspiring me to a even greater effort.

A special acknowledgment also to prof Alessandro Distante for his constant support, and to prof Antonio L'Abbate for his elegant and indulgent patience.

It must be remembered that this book would have lost, in terms of clarity, if I had not been assisted by the editorial staff of Springer-Verlag Italia, whose members have succeeded in interpreting many illogic statements and incongruities, which are overwhelming in a publication of this kind, notwithstanding the cryptic technical jargon. The attitude of the publishing, highly competent and collaborative staff was actually pleasant and made the technical decisions arising from the many technicalities in the transition from the manuscript to the definitive print easy.

A very special acknowledgment has to be reserved to Manuella Walker who has shown during these months the right mixture of patience, scientific curiosity, and friendly availability, which was necessary to translate the text into English according to the Authors' requests.

Lastly, I owe an apology to my family who watched over me with love and understanding in virtue of purely humanistic motivations, leaving me to my guilty absence.

I hope that the reader – if there will ever be one – will recall while judging this book, at least for a moment the hard work of all those who have made the publishing possible.

Pisa, December 2004   **Massimo Lombardi**
                                                         Director MRI Laboratory
                                     CNR, Institute of Clinical Physiology, Pisa

Contents

5   **Intracranial vascular district**.................................... **89**
       Raffaello Canapicchi, Francesco Lombardo, Fabio Scazzeri,
       Domenico Montanaro

6   **Vessels of the neck**.. **121**
       Mirco Cosottini, Maria Chiara Michelassi,
       Guido Lazzarotti

7   **Heart** **145**

List of Contributors

GIOVANNI AQUARO
MRI Laboratory
CNR, Institute of Clinical Physiology,
Pisa, Italy

IRENE BARGELLINI
Diagnostic and Interventional
Radiology
University, AOUP, Pisa, Italy

RAFFAELLO CANAPICCHI
MRI Laboratory
CNR, Institute of Clinical Physiology,
Pisa, Italy

MIRCO COSOTTINI
Department of Neuroscience
University of Pisa
and Diagnostic and Interventional
Radiology
University, AOUP, Pisa, Italy

MARIOLINA DEIANA
MRI Laboratory
CNR, Institute of Clinical Physiology,
Pisa, Italy

DANIELE DE MARCHI
MRI Laboratory
CNR, Institute of Clinical Physiology,
Pisa, Italy

BRUNELLA FAVILLI
MRI Laboratory
CNR, Institute of Clinical Physiology,
Pisa, Italy

PIERLUIGI FESTA
MRI Laboratory
CNR, Institute of Clinical Physiology,
Pisa, Italy

PIERO GHEDIN
GE Healthcare
Milan, Italy

GIULIA GRANAI
Diagnostic and Interventional
Radiology
University, AOUP, Pisa, Italy

PETRA KEILBERG
MRI Laboratory
CNR, Institute of Clinical Physiology,
Pisa, Italy

GUIDO LAZZAROTTI
Diagnostic and Interventional
Radiology
University, AOUP, Pisa, Italy

MASSIMO LOMBARDI
MRI Laboratory
CNR, Institute of Clinical Physiology,
Pisa, Italy

Francesco Lombardo
MRI Laboratory
CNR, Institute of Clinical Physiology,
Pisa, Italy

Paolo Marcheschi
MRI Laboratory
CNR, Institute of Clinical Physiology,
Pisa, Italy

Maria Chiara Michelassi
Diagnostic and Interventional
Radiology
University, AOUP, Pisa, Italy

Domenico Montanaro
MRI Laboratory
CNR, Institute of Clinical Physiology,
Pisa, Italy

Lorenzo Monti
MRI Laboratory
CNR, Institute of Clinical Physiology,
Pisa, Italy

Simona Ortori
Diagnostic and Interventional
Radiology
University, AOUP, Pisa, Italy

Alessia Pepe
MRI Laboratory
CNR, Institute of Clinical Physiology,
Pisa, Italy

Marzio Perri
Diagnostic and Interventional
Radiology
University, AOUP, Pisa, Italy

Alessandro Pingitore
MRI Laboratory
CNR, Institute of Clinical Physiology,
Pisa, Italy

Vincenzo Positano
MRI Laboratory
CNR, Institute of Clinical Physiology,
Pisa, Italy

Claudia Raineri
MRI Laboratory
CNR, Institute of Clinical Physiology,
Pisa, Italy

Maria Filomena Santarelli
MRI Laboratory
CNR, Institute of Clinical Physiology,
Pisa, Italy

Fabio Scazzeri
UO Neuroradiology Ospedale Civile
Livorno, Italy

Anna Maria Sironi
MRI Laboratory
CNR, Institute of Clinical Physiology,
Pisa, Italy

Elisabetta Strata
MRI Laboratory
CNR, Institute of Clinical Physiology,
Pisa, Italy

Paola Vagli
Diagnostic and Interventional
Radiology
University, AOUP, Pisa, Italy

Virna Zampa
Diagnostic and Interventional
Radiology
University, AOUP, Pisa, Italy

List of Acronyms

ACR	American College of Radiology
AFP	Alfa Feto Protein
AHA	American Heart Association
AO	Aorta
AoCo	Aortic Coarctation
APVR	Anomalous Pulmonary Venous Return
ARVC	Arrhythmogenic Right Ventricle Cardiomyopathy
ASD	Atrial Septal Defect
AVC	Atrio Ventricular Connection
AVM	Artero-Venous Malformations
A_1	Anterior cerebral a.
β-HCG	Beta-Human Chorionic Gonadotropin
BSA	Body Surface Area
CA	Cavernous Angiomas
CCD	Charging coupling device
CDP	Complex Difference Processing
CDROM	Compact Disk Read Only Memory
CEMRA	Contrast Enhanced Magnetic Resonance Angiography
CHESS	Chemical shift selective
c.m.	Contrast Medium
CNR	Contrast-to-Noise Ratio
CP-MRA	Contrast Phase Magnetic Resonance Angiography
CT	Capillary Telangiectasias
CT	Circulation Time
CT	Computed Tomography
CVT	Cerebral Venous Thrombosis
CX	Circumflex Coronary a.
DAF	Dural Artero-venous Fistula
DAT	Digital Audio Tape
DCCF	Direct Carotid-Cavernous Fistula
DE	Delayed-contrast Enhancement
DFT	Discrete Fourier Transform
DICOM	Digital Imaging and Communication in Medicine
DSA	Digital Subtraction Angiography
DVD	Digital Video Disk

DVDROM	Digital Video Disk Read Only Memory
DY-DTPA-BMA	Dysprosium diethylenetriamine pentaacetic acid-bismethylamide
EBT	Electron Beam Tomography
ECD	Echo Color Doppler
ECD	Endocardial Cushions Defect
ECG	Electrocardiography
EDV	End Diastolic Volume
EF	Ejection Fraction
EPI	Echo Planar Imaging
ESV	End Systolic Volume
FA	Flip Angle
FDG	18-Fluorodeoxyglucose
FFE	Fast Field Echo
FFT	Fast Fourier Transform
FGRE	Fast GRadient Echo
FID	Free Induction Decay
FIESTA	Fast Imaging Employing STeady –State Acquisition
FIS	Free Induction Signal
FISP	Fast Imaging with Steady-state free Precession
FLAIR	Fluid Attenuated Inversion Recovery
FLASH	Fast Low Angle Shot
FOV	Field Of View
FS	Fat Suppression
FSE	Fast Spin Echo
FSE-IR	Fast Spin Echo – Inversion Recovery
FT	Fallot's Tetralogy
Gd	Gadolinium
Gd-DTPA	Gadolinium-diethylenetriamine pentaacetic acid
Gd-DTPA-BMA	Gadolinium-diethylenetriamine pentaacetic acid-bismethylamide
Gd-HP-DO3A	Gadolinium 1,4,7- tris(carboxymethyl)-10-(2'-hydroxypropyl)-1,4,7,10-tetraazacycl ododecane
GRASS	Gradient Recalled Acquisition in Steady State
GRE	Gradient Echo
G-SPECT	Gated-Single Photon Emission Computed Tomography
HARP	HARmonic Analysis of Phase
HCM	Hypertrophic Cardiomyopathy
HU	Hounsfield Unit
IAD	Interatrial Defect
IP	Internet Protocol
IR	Inversion Recovery
IR-GRE	Inversion-Recovery Gradient Echo
IR-GRE DE	Inversion-Recovery Gradient Echo Delayed Enhancement
IT	Inversion delay Time
IV	Innominate Vein

IVC	Inferior Vena Cava
JIRA	Japan Industries Association Radiological systems
LA	Left Atrium
LAD	Left Anterior Descending a.
LAN	Local Area Network
LM	Left Main a.
LPA	Left Pulmonary Artery
LPV	Left Pulmonary Vein
LCD	Liquid Crystal Display
LV	Left Ventricle
MEDICOM	Medical Products Electronic Commerce
MEDICOM	MEdia Interchange COMunication
MIP	Maximum Intensity Projection
Mn-DPDP	Manganese-dipyridoxal diphosphate
MOTSA	Multiple Overlapping Thin-Slab Acquisition
MPR	Multiplanar Reconstruction
MPA	Main Pulmonary Artery
MPVR	Multiplanar Volume Reconstruction
MR	Magnetic Resonance
MRA	Magnetic Resonance Angiography
MRI	Magnetic Resonance Imaging
MT	Magnetization Transfer
MTT	Mean Transit Time
NASCET	North American Symptomatic Carotid Endoarterectomy Trial
NEMA	National Electrical Manufacturers Association
NEX	Number of Excitations
NVC	Neuro Vascular Conflict
PA	Pulmonary Artery
PAPVR	Partial Anomalous Pulmonary Venous Return
PC	Phase Contrast
PD	Proton Density
PDP	Phase Difference Processing
PDW	Proton Density Weight
PET	Positron Emission Tomography
PFR	Peak Filling Rate
PCr/ATP	Phospho Creatine/Adenosine Triphosphate
PICA	Postero Inferior Cerebellar Artery
PTA	Percutaneous Transluminal Angioplasty
PVC-MRI	Phase Velocity Cine Magnetic Resonance Imaging
QP/QS	Pulmonary Flow/ Systemic Flow
RA	Right Atrium
RC	Right Coronary
RF	Radio Frequency
RES	Reticuloendothelial system
REV	Réparation à l'Etage Ventriculaire
RIPV	Right Inferior Pulmonary Vein

ROI	Region Of Interest
RPA	Right Pulmonary Artery
RV	Right Ventricle
SA	Saccular Aneurysms
SVC	Superior Vena Cava
SE	Spin Echo
SENSE	SENSitivity Encoding techniques
SMASH	Simultaneous Acquisition of Spatial Harmonics
SNR	Signal-to-Noise Ratio
SPECT	Single Photon Emission Computed Tomography
SPGR	SPoiled Gradient Echo
SPGR-ET	SPoiled Gradient Echo Train
SSFP	Steady State Free Precession (Fiesta, True FISP, Balanced Echo)
STIR	Short Time Inversion Recovery
SV	Stroke Volume
T_1	Longitudinal relaxation time
T_2	Transverse relaxation time
TA	Time of Acquisition
TAPVR	Total Anomalous Pulmonary Venous Return
TCP	Transmission Control Protocol
TE	Time to Echo
TEA	Thromboendoarterectomy
TEE	Transesophageal Echography
TF	Tetralogy of Fallot
TGA	Transposition of Great Arteries
TIMI	Thrombolysis In Myocardial Infarction
TI	Time of Inversion
TOF	Time Of Flight
TOS	Thoracic Outlet Syndrome
TR	Time of Repetition
TRICKS	Time Resolved Imaging of Contrast Kinetics
TTE	Trans Thoracic Echocardiography
USPIO	Ultrasmall Superparamagnetic Iron Oxide
VENC	Velocity Encoding
VA	Venous Angiomas
VD	Venous Dysplasia
VSD	Ventricular Septal Defect
WMSI	Wall Motion Score Index
WHO	World Health Organization
2D	Bi-dimensional
3D	Three-dimensional

1 Physical principles of imaging with magnetic resonance

MARIA FILOMENA SANTARELLI

1.1 Introduction

Magnetic Resonance (MR) is a phenomenon involving magnetic fields and electromagnetic waves on the Radio Frequency (RF) domain. The discovery of this phenomenon is quite recent and was simultaneously made in 1946 by two independent groups of investigators at Stanford (directed by Bloch) and at Harvard (headed by Purcell) [1, 2]. Since its discovery, MR has become very popular, being an extremely useful tool, especially in the fields of analytical chemistry and biochemistry [3, 4].

The intuition of using MR on humans came from experiments by Jackson, who in 1967 acquired the first MR signals from a live animal. In 1972, Lauterbur [5] obtained the first MR image from a sample containing water and two years later generated the very first image from a live animal [6]. Later, many other groups, more or less independently, contributed to improving the technique toward those technologies that would allow the generation and reconstruction of MR images [7-12]. Magnetic Resonance Imaging (MRI) allows to generate images that yield excellent contrast between soft tissues, with high spatial resolution in each direction. Like other imaging techniques, MRI also employs electromagnetic radiation to examine the districts inside the human body; however, because it employs low energy radiation, it may be considered non-hazardous when used within tested limits.

In this chapter we will introduce the basic principles underlying the phenomenon of MR and the formation of MR images. The description of the single processes is not meant to be exhaustive. Because many of the principles we will deal with here are quite complex, we have put particular effort in keeping explanations simple avoiding details that would take the reader away from the main train of thought. For more exhaustive explanations on single processes or phenomena we suggest a list of specialist readings [13-16], while the principles of MR and their application to the cardiovascular system can be found on specific text books [17, 18].

1.2 The phenomenon of magnetic resonance

The phenomenon of Magnetic Resonance may be approached using different types of nuclei (^{1}H, ^{13}C, ^{19}F, ^{23}Na, ^{31}P), however the atom ^{1}H is generally uti-

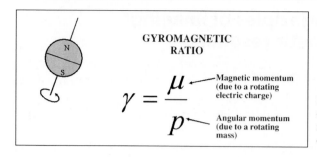

Fig. 1.1. Scheme of an electrically charged mass in rotational motion (spin) on its axis, producing a magnetic moment (μ)

lized for creating MR images. To get an idea of what nuclear magnetism is, we can imagine a similarity with an electrically charged mass rotating on its own axis that generates a tiny magnetic field with its own direction and orientation. This phenomenon is the so-called "spin" and is what attributes the magnetic momentum μ to the nucleus (Fig. 1.1).

In the case of ^1H, the nucleus is composed of a single proton (positive electric charge).

1.2.1 The nucleus

The property that allows each nucleus to interact with a magnetic field is the so-called intrinsic spin. It is a quantum phenomenon according to which the nucleus rotates on its axis, as illustrated in Figure 1.1. The values taken by the spin, I, depend on the number of protons and neutrons inside the nucleus.

If $I = 0$, there is no interaction between the nucleus and the external magnetic field. The atom of hydrogen ^1H has a single proton and its spin is $I = 1/2$.

The angular momentum, p, given by the spin I is given by:

$$\mathbf{p} = \hbar\ \mathbf{I} \tag{1}$$

where $\hbar$ is Planck's constant; $\mathbf{p}$ and $\mathbf{I}$ are vectors.

The so-called gyromagnetic ratio links the magnetic momentum μ to the angular momentum $\mathbf{p}$:

$$\gamma = \frac{\mu}{\mathbf{p}} \tag{2}$$

The value is a constant characteristic of the type of nucleus; for example, γ for ^1H, is 42.57 MHz/T (MHz: MegaHertz; T: Tesla).

1.3 Interaction with an external magnetic field

We can imagine the nucleus of hydrogen ^{1}H as a magnetic bar with a north and south pole (bipolar). According to the laws of quantum mechanics, the momentum of the dipole can take on the values of 2I+1 orientations in an external magnetic field, corresponding to the 2I+1 energy levels allowed. The "magnetic bar", the proton, can thus align with the external field in parallel or anti-parallel position, as represented in Figure 1.2.

In fact, the quantum model should be used to explain all the phenomena of nuclear magnetic resonance. However, from an intuitive point of view, the classical model in which the spin can assume any position in the external magnetic field shows to be the best for visualizing most of the experiments.

For I = 1/2, as in the nucleus of hydrogen, all the predictions of the classical model are in exact agreement with the quantum theory applied to a macroscopic system.

In the classical model, an electrically charged mass rotating on its axis will tend to align itself with B_0 when immersed in the magnetic field B_0. Thus the proton is affected by a rotating force that induces the proton to start precessing on B_0.

This could be compared to the spinning top that rotates on itself, moving with precessional motion about an axis perpendicular to the floor (force of gravity).

The precession rate (the number of rotations around the direction of B_0 over the unit of time) depends on the type of nucleus and the intensity of B_0.

The precession frequency can be calculated by means of Larmor's law:

$$\omega = \gamma B_0 \qquad\qquad (3)$$

where ω is the so-called "Larmor frequency" (measured in MHz); γ is the gyro-magnetic ratio (measured in MHz/Tesla, that describes the relationship of mechanical and magnetic properties of the nucleus considered and depends on the type of nucleus); B_0 is the intensity of the magnetic field in which the nucleus is immersed [(measured in Tesla T, where 1.0T = 10 kG = 10.000 G (Gauss)].

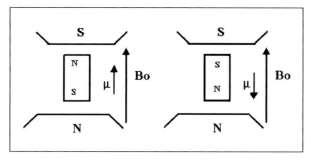

Fig. 1.2. Spin energy levels in a magnetic field; left: low energetic level, right: high energetic level

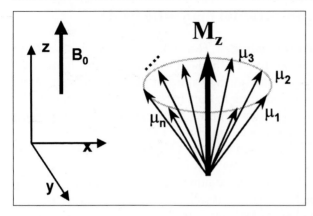

Fig. 1.3. Graphical representation of the total magnetization vector, **M**

Formula (3) indicates that by increasing the intensity of the magnetic field B_0, the frequency ω increases and thus also the nucleus rotation rate around B_0.

In reality, a single nucleus or a single magnetic momentum cannot be observed, but the combined effect of all the nuclei within a sample can be.

What can be observed is thus the total magnetization **M**, given by the vectorial summation of the single magnetic moments: $M = \sum \mu$, as shown in Figure 1.3.

Because magnetic moments tend to align each other to the magnetic field, there is only one component along B_0 at equilibrium.

1.3.1 Radio Frequency (RF) pulses

To evaluate the total magnetization, we must find a way of perturbing the system in its equilibrium state and force **M** to move away from B_0. Hence an excitation pulse is given by applying a second magnetic field B_1, which is perpendicular to B_0 and rotates around B_0 at a rate ω, exactly the same as the precession frequency of the nuclei.

The field B_1 causes **M** to move from its resting position, parallel to B_0, forcing **M** to take a spiral trajectory, Figure 1.4.

When B_1 is switched off, **M** continues precessing, describing a cone with an angle α to B_0.

The amplitude of this angle, the flip angle, depends on the amplitude of B_1 and on the duration of its application.

In fact:

$$\alpha = \gamma B_1 t \tag{4}$$

where t is the time during which the field B_1 is left on.

If B_1 is applied for sufficient time, it can cause **M** to position at 90° with respect to B_0. In such a case, the application of B_1 is called a 90° pulse. **M** may

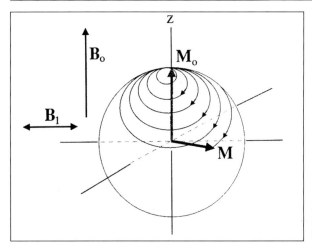

Fig. 1.4. Magnetization vector **M** during the activation of an additional field B_1

be also positioned in direction $-B_0$, which is called 180° pulse or inversion pulse.

Because $\omega/2\pi$ normally ranges between 1 MHz and 500 MHz (frequencies that fall within the radio frequency domain), B_1 pulses are also known as radio frequency pulses and B_1 as radio frequency magnetic field.

1.3.2 Free Induction Decay (FID)

After a 90° pulse has been applied, the magnetization vector **M** itself generates an oscillating RF magnetic field, which can be detected in virtue of the alternated current it produces in a coil – in this case the same coil used to apply the B_1 field. The signal induced by the magnetization vector increases during the 90° pulse and decays to zero after the pulse is switched off because of the relaxation that makes **M** return to its original equilibrium position M_0, parallel to B_0.

This type of decay signal obtained in absence of B_1, is called Free Induction Decay (FID), or Free Induction Signal (FIS), Figure 1.5. In this text we will refer to it as the FID MR signal.

1.3.2.1 The rotating reference system

What we are interested in here, is the behavior of the magnetization vector during the pulse sequences. The movement of the aforementioned vector **M** is quite complicated and difficult to visualize when considering all the involved phenomena together, especially when one or two pulses are applied. In order to facilitate the mathematical and visual description of the phenom-

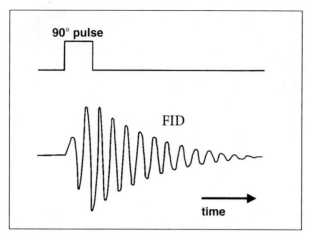

Fig. 1.5. Free decay signal following the 90° pulse

enon, it is best to describe it from the view of an observer who is rotating on an axis parallel to **B₀**, in synchrony with nuclear magnetic moments. This is the so-called "rotating reference system".

It is like observing moving objects from a rotating merry-go-round: if we are exclusively interested in the movement of the objects and not in the rotating merry-go-round, it is easier for us to observe it by being on the ride rotating with those object, than being in a fixed point on the ground.

Observing the objects being on the ground is the so called "static reference system", while observing the objects being on the merry-go-round is the "rotating reference system".

In the case of the rotating system, the protons precessing with **ω** frequency are still, while those protons that for some additional phenomenon (as we shall see later) precess at a minor speed are seen as rotating counterclockwise; likewise, the protons precessing at a speed higher than **ω** are seen as rotating clockwise (Fig. 1.6).

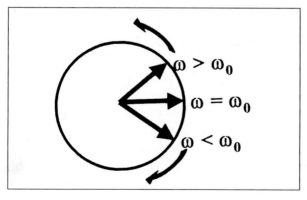

Fig. 1.6. Graphical representation, on a system of rotating axes, of protons precessing at different frequencies

1.4 Magnetic Resonance interaction with tissues

The contrast in the images of nuclear magnetic resonance depends on the different magnetic properties of the tissues. Although many parameters influence the signal coming from a sample under observation, the most commonly used are: proton density, T1 and T2, which are derived from the MR signal released from the material. These parameters may have different values for different tissues, but also have different values within the same tissue according to whether it is in a normal or diseased state.

1.4.1 Proton density

Most of the hydrogen molecules in the human body are bound in the molecules of water and fat, which is what we search for in the experiments of MR.

The term proton density simply refers to the number of protons per volume unit. Therefore, accordingly with the water contents, proton density in bones is low, high in liver, and very high in blood.

The proton density for a tissue examined is basically proportional to the initial amplitude of the MR signal immediately following the end of 90° excitation pulse (Fig. 1.7): the higher the proton density, the higher the amplitude of the signal.

1.4.2 Relaxation

The relaxation of the spin is caused by the exchange of energy between spins and between spins and the surrounding environment. These interactions generate two kinds of decay of the **M** vector, which are called spin-spin relaxation and spin-lattice relaxation. The result of relaxation is the return of **M** to its equilibrium state parallel to B_0.

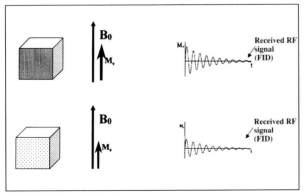

Fig. 1.7. Effect of the different proton density on the M_0 vector and on signal intensity

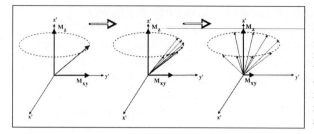

Fig. 1.8. Spin-spin relaxation causes the precession of nuclear magnetic moments at different velocities. The loss in phase coherence provokes the exponential decay of the transverse magnetization with time constant T_2

Spin-spin relaxation

The spin-spin relaxation, also said transversal relaxation, or T_2, is caused by the interaction between nuclear magnetic moments.

The magnetic field experimented in each instant by each nucleus is certainly dominated by the external field applied, however there is an additional contribution to the local field on behalf of the closer neighboring nuclei. These spin-spin interactions cause a weak change in the precessing frequencies of each nucleus. The result is a loss in phase coherence among the nuclei, with a reduction in the transverse component of the magnetization vector **M** (M_{xy}) – that is the component perpendicular to the field **B$_0$** (Fig. 1.8). The constant of the transverse relaxation time M_{xy} is given by T_2, that is the time necessary to reduce spin-lattice relaxation of the transverse component M_{xy} by 63%.

Spin-lattice relaxation

The spin-lattice relaxation, also called longitudinal relaxation time or T_1, causes a gradual realignment of the magnetic moments with **B$_0$**, as shown in Figure 1.9. This phenomenon depends on the intrinsic properties of the nucleus but also on the microenvironment in which the nucleus is immersed (surrounding nuclei, temperature, presence of large-sized molecules, paramagnetic molecules as those of contrast media, and so on) – from here the reference to spin-lattice interaction. Hence, the longitudinal component of **M** returns to the equilibrium value M_0 within a characteristic time, T_1. T_1 is the time needed for 63% of **M** to return to equilibrium M_0 after a 90° RF pulse.

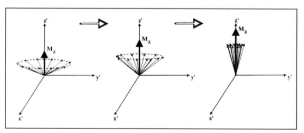

Fig. 1.9. Spin-lattice relaxation causes the longitudinal component of the magnetization vector to return to its **M$_0$** value at equilibrium

Generally, T1 for tissues is in the order of 1 second. Once the magnetization vector has returned to its equilibrium value Mo parallel to B_0, there are no chances of having a transverse magnetization different from zero. For this reason T2 is always minor than, or at the most, equal to T1.

Pseudo relaxation

The lack of homogeneity in the magnetic field within a sample inevitably causes a further relative dephasing among the protons, so that a relaxation time T2* is defined. The speed of transversal decay observed, 1/T2*, is then the sum of two contributions:

- contribution of spin-spin relaxation
- contribution of the relaxation given by the lack of homogeneity in the magnetic field.

Thus:

$$1/\ T_2^{\ *} = 1/\ T_2 + 1/\ T_2^{dishom} \tag{5}$$

Where:

$$1/\ T_2^{dishom} = \gamma\ \Delta B_0$$

in which ΔB_0 is the amplitude of the variation of the magnetic field in the volume where the sample is located.

1.4.3 RF pulse sequences

1.4.3.1 Inversion Recovery (IR)

Inversion Recovery (IR) is a 180° pulse, which is followed by a 90° pulse after a time of inversion (TI) (Fig. 1.10). This sequence is used in spectrometry to measure spin-lattice relaxation time in small samples and in MRI to create contrast regions with different T1 value.

In this latter case we must apply various pairs of 180° and 90° pulses.

The signal intensity S, immediately preceding the 90° pulse in an Inversion-Recovery experiment is proportional to the Mz amplitude at time TI, so that:

$$S \infty\ M_z\ (TI) = M_0\ (1 - 2\ exp\ (-\ TI\ /\ T_1)) \tag{6}$$

where M_0 is the equilibrium magnetization (equivalent to the proton density) and T1 is the sample's spin-lattice relaxation time.

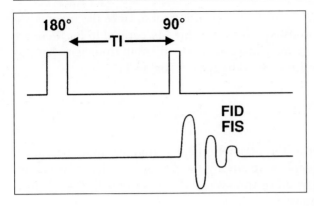

Fig. 1.10. Inversion recovery pulse sequence

The graph in Figure 1.11 shows the behavior of Mz in function of time, after a 180° pulse. The figure evidences how Mz depends on the value of T1.

The time t = 0 corresponds to the end of the 180° pulse, while the time t = TI is the instant in which the 90° pulse is applied. The three curves in Figure 1.11 refer to three samples with different T1 times.

1.4.3.2 Spin Echo (SE)

The base sequence consists in a 90° pulse followed by one of 180°. The time between the two pulses is TE/2 (Fig. 1.12), where TE is the Time of Echo (which will be described later in detail in Paragraph 1.4.4.2).

The Spin Echo sequence corrects the lack of homogeneity in the magnetic field, leaving only the decay signal due to the spin-spin relaxation. This correction is brought about with a 180° pulse, called refocusing pulse. The amplitude of the echo at TE is given by:

$$S_2 = S_1 \exp(-TE / T_2) \tag{7}$$

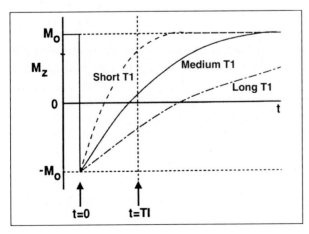

Fig. 1.11. M_z in function of time in an IR sequence

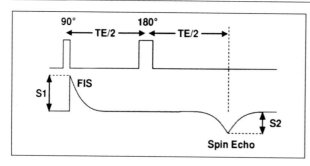

Fig. 1.12. Spin Echo base sequence

As illustrated in reference to Figure 1.13 the Spin Echo sequence consists in the following:

1. A 90° pulse is applied (Fig. 1.13a).
2. Because the lack of homogeneity in the magnetic field inevitably occurs inside the sample, the magnetization vectors that compose **M** start to lose phase concordance with each other (see Fig. 1.13b). For example, if part of the sample is in a region where the magnetic field is weaker than B_0, the nuclei in this region will precess at a speed lower than $\omega_0 = \gamma B_0$ in the static reference system; while according to the rotating reference system the magnetization vector will precess counterclockwise (because the relative system rotates exactly at speed ω_0 clockwise). On the contrary, the magnetization vectors relative to areas of the sample where the local magnetic field is higher than B_0 will precess clockwise in the rotating reference system.
   As final result, the transverse component of **M** (M_{xy}) decreases exponentially in time, while the resulting MR signal is proportional to $exp\ (-t/T_2^*)$.
3. A 180° pulse is applied after a time TE/2 following the first 90° pulse. The consequence is that all the magnetization vectors will rotate on the x' axis (Fig. 1.13c). At the end of the 180° pulse, the span of the magnetization vectors that previously opened away from the y' axis is now flipped onto the –y' axis.
4. The magnetization vectors that precess more quickly (in regions with higher magnetic fields) still precess clockwise in the relative reference system, but now move toward the –y' axis. Conversely, the vectors of the areas with lower magnetic fields precess counterclockwise in the relative system – they move toward the –y' axis too (Fig. 1.13d).
5. At the time TE after the first pulse, all vectors are aligned on the –y' axis; that is, they have been refocused by the 180° pulse. Because **M** is the net sum of these nuclear magnetic vectors, the transverse component M_{xy} reaches its maximum amplitude at this TE time (Fig. 1.13e).
6. The magnetic vectors dephase once again causing a decrease of the MR signal (Fig. 1.13f).

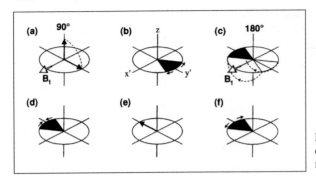

Fig. 1.13 a-f. A Spin Echo experiment seen from a rotating reference system

1.4.3.3 Gradient Echo (GRE)

The problems involved in measuring the free induction decay of the transverse magnetization (MR signal) immediately following the 90° excitation pulse in an experiment can be solved with the Gradient Echo sequence

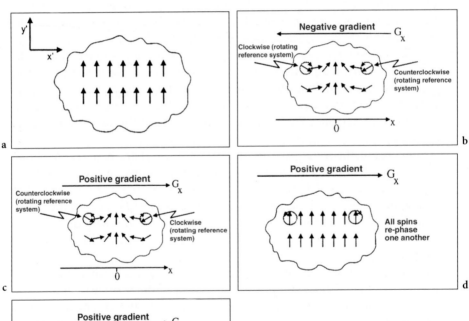

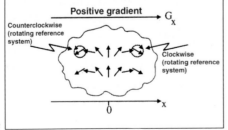

Fig. 1.14 a-e. (a) Instant following the 90° pulse; (b) Situation of the spins during application of the negative gradient; (c) Situation of the spins during application of the positive gradient; (d) Re-phasing of spins and formation of echo (e) dephasing of spins after the moment/instant of echo

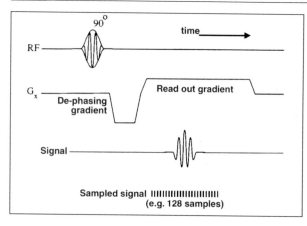

Fig. 1.15. Gradient Echo sequence

(GRE). Indeed this sequence exploits an inverse read-out gradient that re-phases spins, generating an echo signal. (For a detailed explanation please go to Paragraph 1.5.1 "Magnetic field gradients").

– The sample in the magnetic field B_0 is subjected to a 90° pulse, which puts the spins into phase to one another, so that the magnetization, thus the magnetic resonance signal, is highest (Fig. 1.14a)
– immediately after the 90° pulse, a negative magnetic field gradient is applied; the spins start precessing at a position-dependant speed, dephasing in an "ordinate" manner with one another (Fig. 1.14b)
– the following application of a gradient – this time a positive one – (Fig. 1.14c) causes a change in the direction of the spins' rotation and their re-phasing, which generates the echo known as echo of the gradient (Fig. 1.14d); the amplitude of the echo signal is the same as the FID immediately following the 90° pulse
– during the instants following TE, the spins start dephasing with one another and the magnetization (and the signal amplitude) decays (Fig. 1.14e).

The MR signal is sampled before and after the echo instant, as shown in Figure 1.15. Generally the GRE sequence uses α degree pulses, where α is ≤ 90°.

1.4.4 MR signal parameters

1.4.4.1 Time of Repetition (TR)

In a sequence of pulses the Time of Repetition (TR) is the time lapsing between two RF pulses. In the GRE sequences the TR parameter represents the time between 90° pulses (notice that the Spin Echo sequence includes two

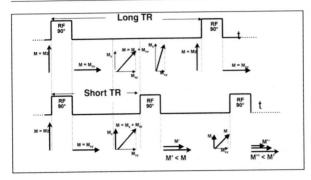

Fig. 1.16. Effects of TR values on magnetization M (and thus on the intensity of MR signal)

kinds of pulse: a 90° pulse first, followed by a 180° pulse); during Inversion Recovery (which includes a 180° pulse first, followed by a 90° pulse), TR equals the time between the 180° pulses.

Figure 1.16 shows how the parameter TR affects the intensity of the signal acquired. Indeed, taking for example a series of GRE pulses, if TR is sufficiently long to allow the total magnetization **M** to return completely parallel to **B$_0$** (Fig. 1.16, top) the amplitude of the signal acquired after the second pulse will be the same as that of the previous pulse. If instead TR is short (Fig. 1.16, bottom) the magnetization **M** has not yet returned completely to the position **M$_0$**, but part of the component remains on the xy plane; because only the z component is affected by the following RF pulse, the resulting signal will have a lower intensity than that acquired in the previous pulse.

This phenomenon is called signal saturation and usually should be avoided, as it slowly reduces the amplitude of the signal. On the other hand, in some cases saturation is purposely created for example to eliminate a specific tissue (such as fat) from the image and put into better evidence other neighboring tissues.

Figure 1.17 shows an example of how the TR parameter can be properly fixed to emphasize the contrast between different tissues with three different T1 values.

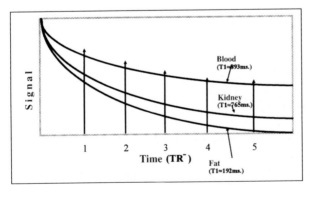

Fig. 1.17. Contrast between tissues with different T1 in function of different TR values

1.4.4.2 Time of Echo (TE)

The Time of Echo or echo time (TE) is the time between the RF excitation pulse and the center of the echo, that is where the signal has acquired its maximum intensity. The amplitude of the transverse magnetization Mxy (and thus of the echo signal acquired) at the peak of the echo signal depends on the TE and T2 of the tissue. For example, in a GRE sequence this amplitude is typically proportional to $exp^{-TE/T2}$; in particular if TE is equal to T2, the transverse magnetization (and thus the amplitude of the echo signal acquired) will be decayed by 37% compared to its amplitude immediately after the RF pulse.

For longer TEs (as seen in Figs. 1.18b with respect to 1.18a where TE is short) Mxy is reduced, as is the intensity of the signal acquired. This occurs because the spins have the possibility of dephasing progressively (see Fig. 1.18b) because of the T2 effect of the material and the time elapsed after the RF pulse.

The operator of the MR scanner can properly define the TE and search for the value that will generate the images with the greatest contrast among tissues. Figure 1.19 shows an example of three different curves relative to three different tissues; it can easily be seen that some TE values allow a better distinction between tissues than other TEs.

1.4.4.3 Flip Angle (FA)

The Flip Angle (FA) is the angle $\alpha = \gamma B_1 t$ between the direction of the field B_0 and the magnetization vector **M** (see paragraph 1.3.1 "Radio Frequency pulses"). As we can see from the formula, a high value of α is obtained with a longer RF activation pulse or with a greater amplitude of the B_1 field. So a FA = 90°

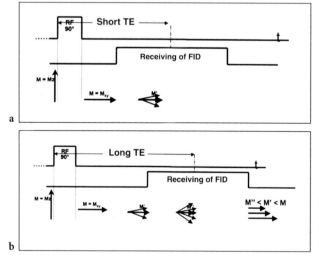

Fig. 1.18 a, b. Effects of TE values on magnetization M (and thus on the intensity of the echo signal). (a) short TE, (b) long TE

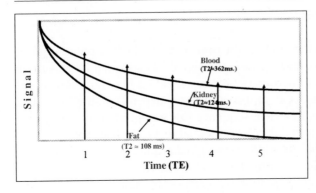

Fig. 1.19. Contrast between tissues with different T2 in function of different TE values

corresponds to a RF activation time twofold that of a FA = 45°; this explains the need for small FA values when the operator is monitoring extremely transient phenomena (as often happens for cardiovascular images) and images must be acquired very quickly. The inconvenience in these cases is that after the RF pulse, the magnetization component on the xy plane, M_{xy}, is lower than in the case with FA = 90° (see Fig. 1.20a, b) so that the amplitude of the signal acquired is lower. However, as it can be seen in the figure, using small FA values makes the magnetization **M** return to its initial position (parallel to B_0) in a shorter time compared to a FA of 90° (compare Figures 1.20a and b); this allows us to use shorter TRs without risking to saturate the signal.

1.5 MR imaging

Almost all images undergo a Fourier transformation analysis, a very efficient and versatile technique for identifying the spatial location of the MR signals released by the various sources of the body being examined.

Images can be 2D or 3D with several spatial characteristics and sizes.

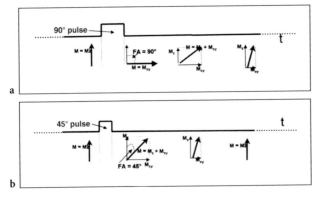

Fig. 1.20 a, b. Effect of FA values on total magnetization **M.** and consequently on the echo signal. (a) High FA (90°) and (b) low FA (45°)

MR images are shown as 2D planes divided into a grid of dots (pixels). The intensity of a pixel represents the amplitude of MR signal released from the corresponding region.

The following paragrahs will explain how the spatial information is encoded into MR signals and then decoded during the calculation of an MR image in a process called image reconstruction.

1.5.1 Magnetic field gradients

A field gradient is a magnetic field added to B_0, with an intensity that varies linearly with the position along the chosen axis. The MR measuring system has three gradients, one along each axis (x, y, and z). These axes are fixed in the scanner with the origin at the center of the magnet, while the field B_0 is conventionally set along z.

Whatever the gradient's direction, its magnetic field is always directed toward B_0 as shown in Figure 1.21. It can also be noticed how the intensity of B_0 varies along the x axis because of the gradient:

$$G_x = \frac{dB_z}{dx} \tag{8}$$

then the total magnetic field is given by:

$$B_z(x) = B_0 + xG_x \tag{9}$$

where B_z varies according to its position along the x axis.

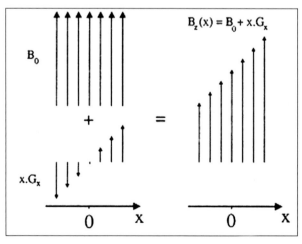

Fig. 1.21. Addition of a variable magnetic field along the x axis

According to the formula $\omega = \gamma B$ also the precession frequency of the protons, ω, changes with the variation of the field B_z to which the protons are subjected.

Figure 1.22 shows how the signal frequency released from different water containers changes in function of their spatial disposition along the x axis: container number 1 influenced by a field $B < B_0$ releases a signal with frequency $\omega < \omega_0$. Likewise, the contents of container 3 releases a signal with frequency $\omega > \omega_0$, while the signal from container 2 has frequency ω_0. The final signal is given by the sum of the three signals.

It is interesting to notice that the intensity of the three signals differs according to the quantity of water in the containers (which in fact depends on the number of hydrogen nuclei – hence on proton density). The spatial discrimination is performed by properly activating the three gradients (along x, y, z), in order to obtain three different encodings (one for each of the three spatial coordinates): 1) selective excitation, 2) frequency encoding, 3) phase encoding.

1. Selective excitation is a technique that limits the MR excitation, and thus the signal, to a specific region of a sample (or of a patient); hence the name of slice selection. This technique is performed applying a RF pulse together with a "slice selection gradient" perpendicular to the slice selected.

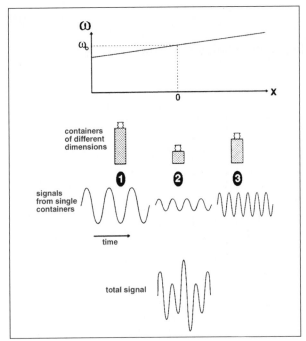

Fig. 1.22. Acquired MR signal, with active gradient in function of the spatial position of the hydrogen molecules

The effect of applying the gradient and the RF pulse simultaneously is that only those protons that are precessing exactly at the frequency $\omega = \gamma B_0$ within the slice are excited.

In fact the RF pulse has such an amplitude and temporal behavior to keep to a narrow interval of frequencies close to the fundamental frequency: only those spins whose resonance frequency fall within this interval will be excited. The slice thickness is given by:

$$\Delta Z = \frac{\Delta \omega}{\gamma G_z} \tag{10}$$

where $\Delta \omega$ is the interval of frequencies included in the selective RF pulse, and G_z is the intensity of the gradient applied for the selection of the single slice (Fig. 1.23).

2. Frequency encoding takes advantage of the property that resonance frequency in MR is directly proportional to the intensity of the magnetic field. When we apply a gradient (for example along x) we have a resonance frequency that is a function of the position along the gradient direction, according to the formula:

$$\omega(x) = \gamma(B_0 + xG_x) \tag{11}$$

The encoding gradient is activated during the MR signal acquisition. Knowing the intensity of the G_x gradient, the position of the object along direction can be derived from the information available on the frequency of the acquired signal. This is done by analyzing the frequencies of the signal.

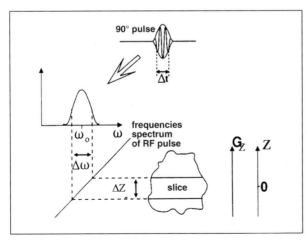

Fig. 1.23. Selective slice excitation

3. Phase encoding evaluates the phase variations of proton precessing during the activation of the gradient. The direction of the phase encoding is perpendicular to the direction of frequency encoding. If, for example, we apply a 90° pulse to a column of spins and then apply a phase encoding gradient, the spins will precess at different speeds (frequencies ω_i) dephasing from one another. When the gradient is switched off, the spins will experience the same magnetic field B_0 and thus begin once again to precess at the same frequency, maintaining however a dephasing (due to the previous activation of the phase gradient), the entity of which depends on the position along the direction of the phase encoding. Apart from the position, such dephasing also depends on the amplitude of the encoding gradient applied and on the total time during which it is switched on, as in the formula:

$$\Phi(y) = \int_0^T \omega\ (y)dt = \gamma y \int_0^T G_y dt \qquad (12)$$

where the phase encoding is applied along y; T is the time during which the phase encoding gradient is switched on, and G_y is the amplitude of this gradient. To create a MR image, the phase encoding gradient is alternatively switched on and off a number of times, varying amplitude of the gradient each time.

In summary, the alternating switching on and off of the gradients for spatial encoding that allows the creation of the images involves the following basic steps:

1. slice selection and spin excitation (interval 1, Fig. 1.24). The slice-selection gradient makes various protons precess at a specific frequency so that only those protons laying inside a slice and precessing at a specific frequency (ω_0) are affected by the RF pulse with frequency ω_0.
2. a phase-encoding gradient applied between the excitation and the read-out time (interval 2, Fig. 1.24). Immediately after the deactivation of the RF pulse and of the slice selection gradient, a phase gradient is applied for an extremely limited period so that the proton precession frequencies (and thus the phase) along the gradient direction differ from one another; then the phase gradient is deactivated so that the protons go back to precess at the initial frequency ω_0, yet dephased in relation to each other along the direction of the phase gradient.
    The spatial information in the direction of phase encoding may be solved by acquiring a great number of MR signals (from values of maximum amplitude, step by step down to minimum values until reaching negative values and negative minimums).

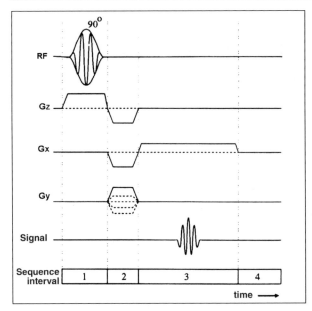

Fig. 1.24. Diagram of a basic sequence for generating a MR image

3. a readout gradient during which the MR signal is collected (interval 3, Fig. 1.24). As described in paragraph 1.4.3, the signals acquired are in the form of echoes; each echo is acquired during the activation of the frequency gradient in such a way to produce a distribution of different frequencies along the direction of the frequency gradient.

In order to obtain the image, this sequence is repeated a number of times, varying the amplitude of the gradient phase each time (interval 2, Fig. 1.24).

The series of signals obtained with such acquisition is then properly digitized and memorized into a matrix called K-space.

1.5.2 K-space

The evolution of a spin system after excitation can be studied more easily in K-space. K-space is important in forming MR images for the very reason that it is in K-space that MR signals are acquired: the samples of the signals acquired are exactly the samples of the K-space matrix! In reality such space is the dominium of the Fourier transformation of the MR image we want to obtain. K represents the wave number $k = 2\pi/\lambda$, where λ is the wavelenght with components K_x, K_y, K_z.

As a matter of fact the images can be broken down into the sum of the sine and cosine waves with different frequencies and orientation. K-space consists

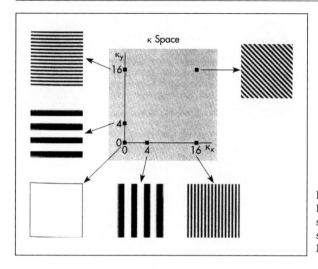

Fig. 1.25. Each single dot in the K-space corresponds to the sinusoidal coursing of a specific sequence and orientation in the MR image

in the set of coefficients that make up the weight factor of these sine and cosine waves. The coordinates of K-space are called spatial frequencies and their unit of measure is cycles per length unit. Hence, the spatial frequencies K_x, K_y, K_z correspond to a 2D image with x and y coordinates.

The K-space contains information on the intensity of the various points of the final image. The images are obtained from K-space by an inverse Fourier transformation, as we shall describe later on. Each point in K-space encloses information on the entire MR image (Fig. 1.25).

Figure 1.25 shows the contributions of 6 dots in the K-space in the final image. The distance of the dots from the center of the K-space determines the frequency of the repeated lines: the greater the distance from the center, the closer the lines (higher frequencies). The orientation of the sinusoidal wave is perpendicular to the direction of K.

Figure 1.25 shows only the positive panel (i.e. the values of K_x and $K_y>0$) of the K-space. In reality K-space also includes the negative values of K_x and K_y, thus at the center of K-space $K_x = K_y = 0$ are fixed (no spatial frequency).

The central region of K-space encloses information on the gross image while the areas farther from the center encode the details. Hence high frequencies (that is high values for K_x and K_y) provide information on the details of the image's elements, while low frequencies provide more approximate information.

The transition from approximate information to details is gradual from the center of the K-space towards its extremities. At times it can be useful not to acquire the entire K-space, especially when the aim is to reduce the acquisition time of MR imaging (as for cardiovascular images). Indeed, by applying the half-Fourier method, only the signals occupying the positive half of the K-space and the most central lines of the negative half are acquired.

1.6 From K-space to the MR image: the Fourier Transform

The Fourier transformation breaks up signals or curves in a sum of sine and cosine waves each having different frequencies [19].

To reconstruct MR images, the Discrete Fourier Transform (DFT) is used rather than the continuous transform. The data memorized in the K-space are in fact numerical, thus discrete. The DFT and its inverse are defined as a mathematical series (a sum of terms) in which the terms correspond to the number of samples of the curve to be transformed. The terms of the series are summed to calculate a pixel (that is a dot) in the final MR image. Fast Fourier Transform (FFT) is now recognized as the most efficient method for calculating the DFT and is implemented in all MR machines.

A bidimensional DFT (DFT-2D) recreates the 2D image from the K space. The DFT-2D is implemented as many separate FFTs, one for each line in the K-space, on which then we calculate the FFT along the columns. So if the K–space holds 256 lines and 256 columns, the recreation of the MR image will require 512 FFTs. The Volumetric Fourier Transform (3D) used to create volumetric images is an extension of the FFT-2D.

1.7 MRI hardware

A system for clinical MR generally is made up by the following parts:

- a coil that generates a static magnetic field (B_0) to align the protons to the axis of the field
- a RF pulse transmitter consisting in a coil that generates RF pulses for disturbing proton alignment along B_0
- a RF signal receiver consisting in a coil that receives the energy emitted by the protons
- three coils for generating magnetic field gradients for modifying the spatial homogeneity of the field B_0 so that each dot can be made spatially recognizable
- a computerized system for the amplification, digitization, and processing of the MR signals to reconstuct for composing the final MR image.

The diagram in Figure 1.26 shows the structure of MR hardware.

The next paragraph will briefly describe the various components, while the reader is invited to consult other specific references for a more detailed description [21, 22].

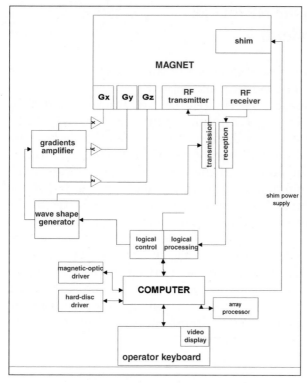

Fig. 1.26. Diagram of a MRI machine

1.7.1 The magnet

At present there are different kinds of magnets with different technical characteristics and also different purchase and management costs. The most used are:

- permanent magnet
- resistive magnet
- superconductive magnet.

1.7.1.1 Permanent magnet

It is made up of blocks of material with a strong magnetic memory that maintains the magnetic field created inside their assembly once they have been magnetized. These kinds of magnets only reach fields up to 0.3 T. Another inconvenience is that they are very heavy (which requires them to be installed in premises that can bear the excessive weight); moreover, the homogeneity of the field depends a lot on the block assembly and the variations of environmental temperature. On the other hand these magnets are relatively cheap and have low maintenance costs. In addition they have a vertical alignment of the main magnetic field, that added to its open configuration, greatly reduces claustrophobia in patients.

1.7.1.2 Resistive magnet

This magnet can be considered a huge electromagnet, made of coils of electric conductive material where high intensity current continuously flows. Because of phenomena of electrical resistance, the flow of current in the conductor creates a great amount of heat which poses a significant problem in terms of having adequate cooling systems; moreover, this system has a high energetic cost, while only yielding magnetic fields of medium-low intensity (0.2-0.3T). Other problems arise from the magnetic field homogeneity due to current fluctuations in time and sudden temperature changes. The main advantages of this type of magnet are in its open configuration, the easiness with which the field is generated and nulled (just by switching off the electricity) and the relatively limited maintenance costs.

1.7.1.3 Superconductive magnets

At present, it is the most used, thanks to its excellent level of intensity, homogeneity and temporal stability of the static magnetic field. The main advantages of these magnets are the possibility of reaching high magnetic fields (up to 3.0 T and above), the field's elevated temporal stability, and the possibility of having a homogeneous field also over big volumes; this permits the acquisition with large fields of view.

The superconductive magnet is based on the principle according to which electricity flows with practically no resistance at all through certain materials, the superconductors, at specific temperature conditions (close to the absolute zero). This way the current passing through the superconductor coil generates a magnetic field of great intensity, indefinitely as long as temperature conditions are kept close to zero.

The main problems concerning these magnets are their closed tunnel-like configuration and high maintenance costs; in fact the creation of the cold environment in which the superconductor is immersed requires costly cryogens such as helium. In order to assure a constant temperature (about 4K, that is −269 °C) these liquids must be periodically integrated into the circuit.

1.7.1.4 Magnetic field homogeneity

One of the fundamental requirements of the magnetic field generated by a magnet consists in the homogeneity of the field. A low field homogeneity will lead to poor quality images owing to the fact that the protons of the sample being examined do not experience the same magnetic field intensity and thus will not all be affected by the RF pulse that will instead selectively act on the protons that precess at the resonance frequency established. The homogeneity of the magnetic field is measured in parts per million (ppm); the quality of the magnet is characterized by its having a limited lack of homogeneity-within few ppm.

The MR machine is equipped with "shim" systems that control the homogeneity of the static magnetic field, these systems are distinguished as passive and active. Passive shimming is created during the creation stage of of the magnet and corrects the lack of homogeneity in the field due to the metal structures used to build the magnet. On the other hand active shimming is a system for correcting the lack of homogeneity in the field by exploiting the coils inside the machine (shimming coils, see diagram in Fig. 1.26) aimed at correcting the lack of homogeneity inside the central volume of the magnet with maximum accuracy.

1.7.2 Radio frequency coils

RF coils are antennas used to emit the radio frequency signals required to disturb the alignment of the protons with the magnetic field B_0 (transmission coils) and to receive the signals emitted by the tissue during the proton relaxation phase (receiving coils). This latter type of coil (receiving coils) is variable in size and morphology according to the body part to be analyzed.

1.7.2.1 Transmission coils

Potentially each coil or antenna can both transmit and receive RF signals, and this was the case with the first tomographic scans; nowadays, the modern MR systems are equipped with a single coil fixed in the inner part of the magnet, which transmits RF signals. This antenna is called a body coil and is usually used in transmission, while it is used both for transmission and reception when large body volumes need to be studied.

1.7.2.2 Receiver coils

On the market there are now many types of receiver coils differing in shape, building strategy, and receiving quality in function of the body part to be analyzed. For what concerns acquisition of signals from the cardiovascular system, receiver coils can be distinguished into three families: volume coils, surface coils, and phased array coils.

1.7.2.2.1 Volume coils

Usually they have the shape of a carved cylinder, which hosts the structure that needs to be examined. They have an excellent receiving homogeneity and greatly enhance the Signal-to-Noise-Ratio (SNR) when they are "filled" (but not touched) by the object under examination. Because the body parts vary in size (skull, neck, abdomen, knee, and so on), there are also different sizes of coils. Nowadays, the most used volume coils are the so-called birdcages that are formed by a set of bars in which each cage bar receives the signal originating from the sample part closest to its structure.

1.7.2.2.2 Surface coils

Their particular configuration allows them to receive the signal from the structure contiguous to the coil; in fact increasing the distance between the sample and the coil, the signal is reduced quadratically. This kind of coil allows the acquisition of images with small fields of view, yet maintaining the SNR (for example in the carotid district). Another distinguishing characteristic of surface coils is their morphology that can vary in relation to the body part for which they were specifically built (flat, circular, or wrapping coils).

1.7.2.2.3 Phased array

These are antennas made up of various units, arranged in an appropriate manner; each unit independently receives the signals from the regions of the sample of their pertinence, examined with a preestablished delay. Later, the signals received by each coil are elaborated to form a global image given by the appropriate processing of the single images received by each coil. This way images with a high SNR and with a large field of view can be obtained: in fact the spatial resolution is determined by the single units, while the image's total field of view is given by the sum of the fields of view of the single units of the coil.

1.7.3 Field gradient

Field gradients are coils that are switched on and off with the purpose of creating magnetic fields variable in time and space. The coils of the gradient are positioned externally to the magnet.

The appropriate switching on and off of the gradients generates three spatial encodings (slice selection, phase encoding, and frequency encoding) that make the position of each point of the sample recognizable. There are three gradients inside a scanner, each of which is oriented along one of the three spatial directions (x, y, z, with z generally defined as parallel to B_0), in a way that allows the selection of axial, sagittal, and coronal sections. Moreover, the combination of the gradients allows to perform scanning along any other plane.

Important parameters for evaluating the efficiency of a gradient are the maximum amplitude (measured in T/m, Tesla on meter), the time required to reach the peak amplitude (measured in milliseconds, msec), the speed at which the gradient reaches the maximum amplitude ("slew rate" measured in T/m/sec). The MR equipment used today in cardiology with B_0 1.5 T, have typical field gradients with an amplitude between 20 a 50 mT/m, time to peak 150-250 msec, and a slew rate between 70-150 T/m/sec.

1.7.4 Computer

The computer in a MR system is the core unit for the instructions and control of all the components of the scanner. It manages all the functions required to generate MR images: from the management of the RF wave shapes and the switching on and off of RF pulses, to the management of the gradients and data acquisition, processing, memorization, and the search and presentation of the final data. Figure 1.26 illustrates the central role of the computer within the system.

In addition to the computer, there is also an array processor for performing high-speed calculations such as the Fast Fourier Transform.

The drivers allow the memorization of the images acquired on mass memory devices such as magnetic-optic discs or DVDs.

References

1. Bloch F, Hanson WW, Packard M (1946) Nuclear induction. Phys Rev 69:127
2. Purcell EM, Torrey HC, Pound RV (1946) Resonance absorption by nuclear magnetic moments in a solid. Phys Rev 69:37-38
3. Abragam A (1961) The principles of nuclear magnetism. London, Oxford University Press
4. Allen PS. Some fundamental principles of nuclear magnetic resonance. In: Medical Physics monograph No. 21: The Physics of MRI (1992) AAPM Summer School Proceedings, American Institute of Physics 21:15
5. Lauterbur PC (1973) Image formation by induced local interactions: examples employing nuclear magnetic resonance. Nature 242:190
6. Lauterbur PC (1974) Image formation by induced local interactions: examples employing nuclear magnetic resonance. Pure Appl Chem 40:149
7. Hinshaw WS, Bottomley PA, Holland GN et al (1977) Radiographic thin-section of the human wrist by nuclear magnetic resonance imaging. Nature 270:722-723

8. Mansfield P, Pykett IL (1978) Biological and medical imaging by NMR. Journal of Magn Reson 29:355

9. Hedelstein WA, Hutchinson JMS, Johnson G et al (1980) Spin-Warp NMR imaging and applications to human whole body imaging. Phys Med Biol 25:751

10. Pykett IL, Mansfield P (1978) A line scan image study of a tumorous rat leg by NMR. Phys Med Biol 23:961-967

11. Maudsley A (1980) Multiple line-scanning spin-density imaging. Journal of Magn Reson 41:112

12. Makovski A (1985) Volumetric NMR imaging with time-varying gradients. Magn Reson Med 2:29

13. Mansfield P (1976) Proton spin imaging by nuclear magnetic resonance. Contemp Physics 17:553

14. Magnetic resonance in medicine. The basic textbook of the European Magnetic Resonance Forum (1993). P. Rinck Ed. 3rd ed. Oxford, UK, Blackwell Scientific Pubblications

15. Stark DD, Bradley WG (1999) Magnetic resonance imaging. Mosby Edts.

16. University of Aberdeen (1988) Physical Basis of Magnetic Resonance Imaging-Summer School Material

17. Underwood R, Firmin D (eds) (1991) Magnetic resonance of the cardiovascular system. London, Oxford, Edinburgh, Blackwell Scientific Publications

18. Higgins CB, De Roos A (2003) Cardiovascular MRI and MRA. Lippincott Williams & Wilkins. Philadelphia, PA, U.S.A.

19. Lombardi M, Santarelli F (2000) Risonanza Magnetica Cardiovascolare. Da: Trattato di cardiologia. ANMCO (Associazione Nazionale Medici Cardiologi Ospedalieri). Excerpta Medica Ed.

20. Verrazzani L (1990) Teoria dei segnali determinati. ETS Università Editore

21. Del Pozzi G (2001) Compendio di risonanza magnetica – cranio e rachide. UTET Diagnostica per immagini

22. Stetter Eckart Instrumentation (1996) In: Edelmann RR, Esselink SR, Zlakin MB (eds) MRI clinical imaging. WB Saunders Co., vol. 1, pp 435-455

2 Techniques of fast MR imaging for studying the cardiovascular system

Maria Filomena Santarelli

2.1 Introduction

The use of Magnetic Resonance Imaging (MRI) in cardiovascular applications has developed with the introduction of new techniques for the control of artifacts caused by movement and flow. Indeed, until the last decade, the acquisition of cardiac MR images was suboptimal because of problems of compensation in respiratory movement; nowadays, instead, excellent images can be acquired by simply having the patient hold its breath. Alternatively, excellent cardiac images can be acquired even with free breathing by relying on the so-called navigator technique. There are a number of techniques available, the choice spanning from Gradient Echo (GRE) synchronized with ECG, or the more sophisticated segmented breath-hold and navigator techniques that produce excellent quality images in a short time (seconds) and practically void of artifacts if the patient is collaborative.

The advanced MRI machines in use today also reflect great developments in hardware: very quick gradient activation and disactivation times (slew-rates), high sensitivity radiofrequency coils, and very high gradient amplitude allow numerous clinical evaluations in the cardiovascular setting. An MR exam today makes it possible to evaluate the morphology of the heart, perfusion, myocardial viability, flows and coronary anatomy.

This chapter will briefly illustrate the basic concepts of fast MR image formation [1, 2], which are those that can be applied to the acquisition of cardiovascular images.

2.2 Methods for optimizing K-space covering

2.2.1 Scanning time

The total acquisition time T_{tot} is determined by the Time of Repetition (TR) (that is, the time between radiofrequency pulses), by the number of phase encodings N_y, by the number of sections N_z, and by the number of excitations (NEX):

$$T_{tot} = NEX \cdot N_z N_y \cdot TR \tag{1}$$

So reducing the total scanning time translates into reducing the value of at least one of the parameters above.

2.2.1.1 TR reduction

In one of the following paragraphs we shall see more in detail which methodologies allow the reduction of TR, and of values $\ll T_1$. However, we must underline that when $TR \rightarrow \lambda TR$ with $\lambda < 1$, also the Signal-to-Noise Ratio (SNR) decreases by at least $\sqrt{\lambda}$ and hence, at the best: $SNR \rightarrow \sqrt{\lambda} \, SNR$. Moreover, when TR is modified, there is a consequent change also in tissue contrast. It is thus necessary to evaluate properly whether it is best to reduce TR and by how much, which is why the scanning time should be reduced by trying to find a compromise between signal quality and time acquisition.

2.2.1.2 Reduction of the phase encoding number N_y, and/or the slice number N_z

Another way of reducing the total scanning time is to cut the number of phase encodings or sections. As this method does not affect the contrast, this could represent a valid solution, although it could induce artifacts due to partial volume effect. There are two ways for reducing N_y or N_z. The first way is to keep the Field Of View (FOV) constant along the directions y ($L_y = \Delta_y \cdot N_y$) and/or z ($L_z = \Delta_z \cdot N_z$), so that for $N_y \rightarrow \lambda N_y$, with $\lambda < 1$, the acquisition time is reduced by a factor l; although spatial resolution worsens by a factor λ (that is: $\Delta_y \rightarrow \Delta_y / \lambda$), on the other hand SNR increases by a factor $1/\sqrt{\lambda}$. If we do not want to reduce spatial resolution, then the reduction of N_y is not a good solution for shortening the total acquisition time.

The second way to reduce the total scanning time is to maintain the spatial resolution, reducing N_y and L_y by a same factor λ so to keep the value Δ_y fixed. In this case $T_{tot} \rightarrow \lambda T_{tot}$, but the SNR is reduced to $\sqrt{\lambda} \, SNR$. This reduction of the SNR is unavoidable when choosing to reduce the FOV.

2.2.1.3 Reduction of the Number of Excitations (NEX)

A third way to reduce the total acquisition time is to fix the Number of Excitations (NEX) at 1 – a possible solution only in the case a high SNR is present. As we have already seen, when we use a small FOV, SNR decreases by a factor $\sqrt{\lambda}$, therefore we should need to use a value NEX>1. However, we can increase the SNR by using purposely-designed RF coils, similar to small surface coils or array coils.

A better SNR also allows to reduce TR; therefore, also the design of the RF coil can be considered as an important factor for reducing the total acquisition time T_{tot}.

On the other hand, we could also use a value NEX< 1 to reduce the acquisition time. This is usually referred to as partial data acquisition on the Fourier plane; this method, which is extensively used in the acquisition of cardiovascular images, will be described in detail below.

2.2.2 Cardiac Gating

Acquisition of cardiac images not only requires the use of sequences with short acquisition time but also that the organ being examined stay as still as possible, in order to avoid causing the so-called motion artifacts in the image. A movement in the direction of the readout gradient will create a blurry final image (blurring), while a longer movement in the direction of the phase gradient will create rippled borders (ghosting). One way to reduce these artifacts is to make sure every RF pulse in the sequence occurs at the same instant of the cardiac cycle. This can be obtained by the electrocardiogram synchronization (also called ECG-gating). Such ECG-gating is created between the R wave and the RF pulse for resonance signal acquisition, as shown in Figure 2.1.

As we see from the figure, an image with a matrix of 128×128 dots can be rebuilt after 128 pulses and thus after 128 cardiac cycles. However, it is also possible to perform more than one RF pulse per cardiac cycle, activating each pulse at a different phase of the cycle. This way, during a single cardiac cycle, more lines of the K-space that belong simultaneously to more images can be covered. Each line acquired is relevant to different times after the wave R peak (see Fig. 2.2). Figure 2.2 shows how to acquire 4 images relevant to 4 different phases of the cardiac cycle. Yet, many more images could be acquired by applying the methods already described above (TR reduction, and so on) or

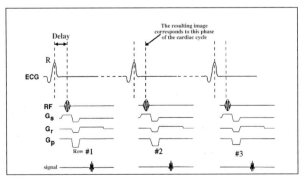

Fig. 2.1. MRI sequence synchronized with ECG, with one image per cardiac cycle. Each RF pulse is activated at a set time established by the peak of the R wave; the image so obtained shows the heart in that particular phase of the cardiac cycle

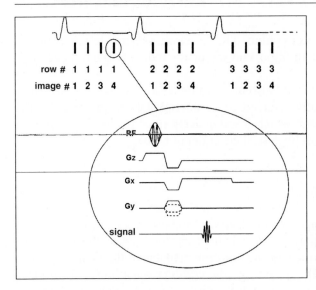

row # 1 1 1 1   2 2 2 2   3 3 3 3

image # 1 2 3 4   1 2 3 4   1 2 3 4

RF

Gz

Gx

Gy

signal

Fig. 2.2. ECG synchronized sequence for the acquisition of 4 different images relevant to 4 phases of the cardiac cycle

the methods of partial covering of K-space, single pulse acquisition, and segmenting that will be explained in the following paragraphs. By employing the various methods for the optimization of acquisition times, we can now acquire up to 10 sections of the heart with 16-50 frames (temporal images) per second.

2.2.2.1 Breath-hold

Breathing is another cause for motion artifacts. Synchrony with breathing could help reduce these artifacts but does not actually contribute to feasibility since single breathing cycles last over a couple of seconds, and the image acquisition would require too much time.

An alternative solution is to ask the patient to hold his breath for at least half of the scan time, which covers the time necessary for acquiring the central lines of the K-space. The central lines in fact correspond to the lowest space frequencies; because the main information of the image is mostly in low frequencies, it is best to reduce motion artifacts during this phase of acquisition as much as possible. However, the quality of the image increases if the image is acquired in synchrony to ECG and with a complete breath-hold on behalf of the patient. Sometimes, depending on the images required and the sequences used, the procedure might require repeated apneas – each of which should present a number of phases in which the data acquisition can be segmented. This method will work efficiently if each breath-hold maintains the chest in the same position at each cycle, a condition which is achieved by using the navigator echo technique as shown in Figure 2.3.

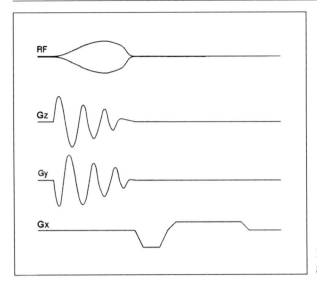

Fig. 2.3. Diagram of the "navigator echo" sequence

An appropriate RF pulse is applied during the activation of the slice gradient and phase selections (G_z and G_y in the figure). This involves a filling of the spiral K-space. Such sequence selectively excites a narrow column of spins along the readout gradient (x in figure). The readout gradient allows the acquisition of an echo from the column of spins, and the Fourier Transform of this echo signal is a mono-dimensional projection along the column. The column to be acquired is located in an adequate way so that it intersects the diaphragm in proximity of the border between the lung and the liver. An edge detection algorithm allows to detect the position of this border over time; hence the position of the diaphragm can be detected at each breath-hold, before acquiring a set of images.

Another empirical method for keeping the chest always in the same position is to have patients hold their breath for their data-acquisition time in the expiration phase rather than during inspiration.

2.2.3 Partial filling of K-space

The partial filling of K-space consists in reducing the number of phase encodings, causing a reduction in SNR, which is compensated by keeping spatial resolution constant. Partial data acquisition in the Fourier plane can be obtained in virtue of the symmetry properties of the Fourier Transform to be applied on the raw data, as are the signals acquired in MR. In this case, the use of adequate algorithms would allow to reconstruct the entire set of data by acquiring only half of the data.

Initially, this method was utilized acquiring half K-space, thus including either the positive or the negative lines; in such cases the final images had a loss in SNR by a factor of √2 with no loss in spatial resolution. However, by trying to reduce phase distortions, also additional lines beyond the exact half were acquired.

One of the most recent methods consists in making acquisitions with a rectangular FOV, in place of a square one. This method is applicable to all the MRI sequences and preserves the conventional image sizes. This solution consists in reducing the size of the data acquired along the direction of phase encoding to the exact dimensions of the object that should be in the image.

In other words we avoid measuring the data in K-space outside the object, obtaining a rectangular K-space rather than the conventional square one. As shown in Figure 2.4c, the data acquired and memorized in the K-space are more distant but the bandwidth in the phase encoding is left the same, so that the spatial resolution remains unchanged. This result can be obtained by increasing the amplitude of the gradient as it is increased for the phase encoding, so that the reduced number of steps (lines of K-space) leads to the original dimensions of the K-space. After the reconstruction, the final image contains information in the central area of the matrix, with no signal in the relative extreme areas (upper and lower, if this was the phase encoding direction).

Obviously the method of rectangular FOV and that of partial acquisition can be combined (see Fig. 2.4d) in order to have a greater reduction in acquisition time, without a great loss in SNR, since the original acquisition is of a sufficiently satisfying quality.

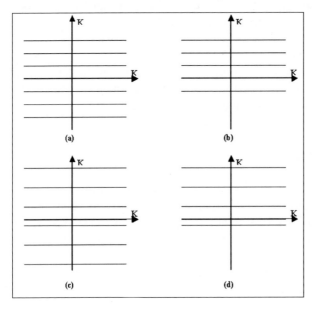

Fig. 2.4 a-d. Simplified representation of the K-space coverage: (a) with complete line filling; (b) with partial filling (half Fourier); (c) with rectangular FOV; (d) with a combination of Half Fourier and rectangular FOV

2.2.4 Segmentation

In all the methods discussed so far for reducing image acquisition time for each RF excitation (that is, within the repetition interval) the procedure analyzes and memorizes only one single line of the K-space. Moreover, before a new RF pulse can be activated some sequences require a waiting period (as the longitudinal relaxation or the transverse dephasing of spins); for this reason, in many conventional sequences, excitations are performed simultaneously on different slices properly distanced one from the other. This solution is known as "interleaved multislice excitation" and will be approached later on in more detail.

Alternatively, a greater number of lines of the K-space can be acquired within a TR interval; this is performed by activating the phase and readout gradients over again within a single TR. Hence, the result will be a series of signals (echoes) acquired with a single RF pulse; for this reason, the method is also called *echo train*. The corresponding image can therefore be seen as fractioned in more segments, where each segment consists in the acquisition of a certain number of lines with a single RF pulse. For example, if the image includes N = 256 lines and is segmented into 4 (S = 4), that means that the phase and readout gradients are switched on and off during each TR for N/S = 64 times and that each segment includes 64 lines of K-space. Figure 2.5 presents a sketch of the segmented K-space.

With the segmented K-space the total acquisition time is reduced S-fold, also if the total number of signals acquired (that is of the K-space) remains unchanged. The SNR of the resulting image is affected in this case by the attenuation between one phase encoding and another, caused by the spin-lattice (longitudinal, T1), spin-spin (transverse, T2), or effective (T2*) relaxations. Segmentation can be applied by both Gradient Echo and Spin Echo acquisitions.

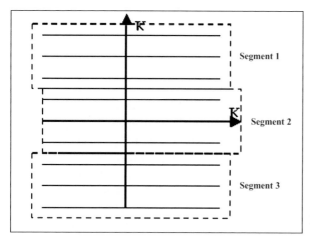

Fig. 2.5. Simplified diagram of the segmenting technique

2.2.5 Single pulse

The limit case for acquiring a higher number of lines during a TR interval occurs with the "single shot" method, or single pulse, where the entire K-space is filled by adequately activating and dis-activating phase and readout gradients in a single TR interval. In such a case the number of echoes in the echo train corresponds exactly to the number of lines of the K-space, and thus of the final image. The Echo Planar Imaging (EPI) was the first sequence to implement such methodology; actually, EPI today – and the sequences derived from it – also includes the possibility of acquiring images in multiple shots (multiple RF pulses), covering the K-space in a segmented and/or interleaved way. It is the user's task to establish whether it is best to acquire images very quickly but with a reduced SNR and more or less significant artifacts or to acquire images by more repetitions of RF pulses.

In the EPI single shot sequences, all the data needed to reconstruct the image are obtained using a set or train of echoes after a single RF pulse, followed by a *blipped* activation and disactivation time of the phase gradient between the activation and disactivation of the readout gradient, with simultaneous acquisition and memorization of the echo. Figure 2.6 represents a diagram of the single shot EPI sequence, and the consequent K-space filling.

With this technique the total acquisition time of the images does not depend on TR; what matters is the duration of the switch-on and switch-off times for the gradients and the how many times the switch is performed (the number of echoes, that is the number of lines of the K-space):

$$\text{Ttot} = N_x N_y \Delta t + N_y \Delta T \tag{2}$$

where ΔT is the time interval between the beginning of disactivation of the readout gradient and the beginning of the reactivation of the that same gradient for the reading of the following echo (see Figure 2.6); Δt instead is the time interval between one piece of data and another in a single line of the K-space.

2.2.6 Echo Planar Imaging (EPI)

There is a limit to the number of K-space lines that can actually be memorized after a single RF pulse; such a limit basically implies the signal decay caused by the effect of T_2 and the amplitude and speed of activation/disactivation of the readout gradient. This is particularly relevant when it is desirable to obtain images with high spatial resolution; in such cases it is best to repeat the sequence over and over again to fill in the K-space with intermediate lines. This filling is achieved by using the same sequence (EPI) with the same shape of gradients – except for Gy, the phase gradient that is initialized

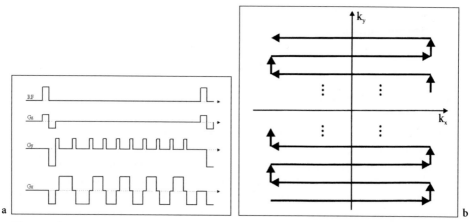

Fig. 2.6 a, b. Representation of single-pulse EPI sequence (a), and the consequent K-space filling (b)

with a slightly different value to allow the filling of the K-space starting from a line intermediate to the previous pulses. In Figure 2.7 the continuous lines show the K-space filling with the first RF pulse, while the dashed lines show the filling with the second RF pulse (second sequence).

The EPI sequences may also include a preparation phase (prepared EPI). For example, for a T2 contrast, we can address the event as a Spin Echo pulse. Alternatively, we can include an inversion-recovery pulse to obtain a T1 contrast. To obtain cardiac images with sequences from the EPI family, there is no need to acquire the entire image in a single-shot, in a single cardiac cycle.

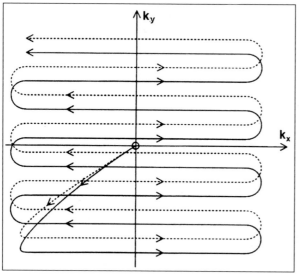

Fig. 2.7. Example of K-space filling with a number of repeated EPI sequences

Indeed, because heart activity is repetitive and quite regular, the sequence can be synchronized with the heart cycle, acquiring an image with more RF pulses each synchronized with the ECG.

2.2.7 Interleaved image acquisition

The interleaved acquisition of MR images (interleaved imaging) is used to obtain more slices in the shortest acquisition time. This method allows taking advantage of the "lag times" between RF pulses that cause the saturation of the echo signal to be acquired. In particular, at the end of the readout gradient the spins in the selected slice have little longitudinal magnetization and a pause will be necessary, in the order of T1 or even longer, before the spins can be used again. However, the spins in the slice's neighboring regions have not been subjected to the previous pulses and may be used immediately, while the original spins are returning to their longitudinal position. This method can be extended to a set of equally spaced slices, to which we alternatively apply the sequences so that the spins of the interlaced slices are activated, while the spins of the previously activated slices are returning to their longitudinal position.

Figure 2.8 schematically shows how the interlaced slices are acquired, with ECG synchrony.

Let us suppose that each RF pulse takes 50 msec, with a 1 sec recovery time for the spins to return to their longitudinal position; in this case there would be enough time to fill 20 slices with 20 separate sequences. The best temporal order for slice acquisition is not spatial order as the slices do not have a perfectly rectangular edge and the neighboring slices overlap. The best order consists in first acquiring all the odd numbered slices and then all the even ones then again odd ones and so on. For example, if we have 10 slices numbered in spatial order, the temporal order for acquisition will be: ...1,3,5,7,9,2,4,6,8,10,1,3,...

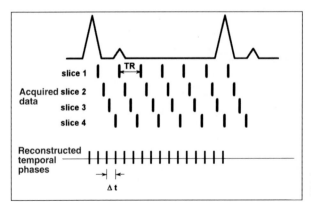

Fig. 2.8. Representation of interleaved image acquisition

2.2.8 Spiral

As we have already mentioned, the EPI sequence was the first example of single shot pulse sequence, many others have followed in diverse forms thanks to advances in gradient technology and the improved rapidity of processing and memory capacity of computers. Among these sequences, the spiral has recently met interest for its use also in cardiac applications. The sequence traced in the Figure 2.9 consists of a Gradient Echo pulse with the successive activation of gradients of phase and frequency in a sinusoidal fashion (Fig. 2.9a). This method allows the memorization of the K-space signal in the form of an expanding spiral as shown in Figure 2.9b.

The acquisition of the data that are memorized and acquired filling K-space with a spiral trajectory, involve a very short acquisition time. The data are acquired during the gradient amplitude, both in increasing and decreasing phases. Furthermore, there are no quick increases or decreases in gradient amplitude. However, this method implies a rather high processing time. As a matter of fact, data are not acquired in a form to which we can directly apply the Fourier Transform; the spiral data must be transferred to a rectangular grid through appropriate interpolation algorithms that request additional calculation time.

A positive aspect in using the spiral sequence is its potential in increasing spatial resolution; indeed, the spiral allows acquisition at gradually increasing resolutions: by increasing the activation time, the K-space coverage increases, thus providing a better spatial resolution.

Obviously, just as for the EPI sequences, so can the spiral sequences be utilized as multiple RF pulses: the spiral is repeated with a small motion of the phase gradient so as to fill intermediate spirals.

Preparation prepulses (as Spin Echo or Inversion Recovery) can be also performed for the spiral sequence.

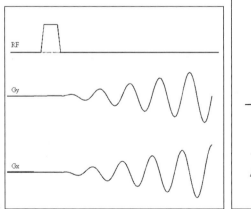
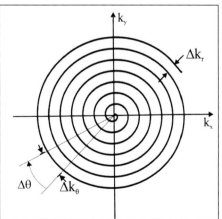

Fig. 2.9 a, b. (a) Diagram of a spiral sequence; (b) Filling of the K-space with the spiral sequence

2.3 Fast sequences in GRE

In this paragraph we shall briefly show the main strategies presently used for reducing the time for forming and acquiring images in GRE. Notice that the use of different strategies leads to different sequence nomenclatures, but it may well happen that sequences employing the same strategies may have different names because of the trademarks assigned by different producing companies. For example the sequence called FLASH in the Siemens machine exploits the same strategy of the sequence named GRASS in the machine by General Electric. However, it must be said that the physical principles governing such strategies are similar. For this purpose in this and the following paragraph we will illustrate the different principles using sequence names only when citing examples.

2.3.1 Low Angle GRE

As seen in the previous paragraph, one of the strategies for getting GRE images quickly is to utilize very short repetition times. However, such a solution may lead to signal saturation and thus to the reduction of the amplitude of the signal acquired. To avoid this, GRE acquisitions are performed setting very narrow Flip Angles (FAs). This strategy was first exploited in 1986 with FLASH by Siemens (Fast Low Angle SHot) [3].

The acquisition of signals with narrow FAs allows very low TRs—even below the T_1 of the tissue that is being acquired. In fact, we can use 1 msec $\leq$ TR$\leq$ 200 msec for tissues like the heart muscle with $T_1 \approx 800$ msec; therefore if we set TR = 1 msec, the scanning time for an image will be about 128 msec. In this case if the RF pulse were 90°, the spin system would saturate after very few TRs and thus a very low signal would be acquired; conversely, if we use a FA much narrower than 90°, no saturation occurs, if not after many TRs. Let us suppose we set FA=30°; if M_0 is the total magnetization available immediately before the first RF pulse, the component of **M** laying on the plane transverse to z after the 30° pulse is $M_0\sin30° = M_0/2$, which means that a 30° pulse generates a signal with half the amplitude of that of a 90° pulse; moreover it means that about 87% of the magnetization stays along z and is thus ready to undergo another 30° pulse – differently from the 90° pulse that makes the **M** component along z null, excluding the possibility of applying another RF pulse. Figure 2.10 shows the orientation of M_0 after the 30° pulse.

Therefore, we can avoid saturating the signals by utilizing a succession of TR (TR<<T_1) with small FAs; which is paid with a reduced amplitude of the signals. Mathematically, the amplitude of the signal acquired with small FAs can be so described:

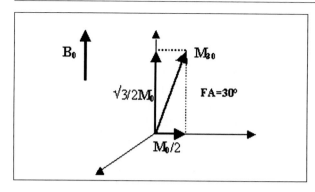

Fig. 2.10. Graphical representation of **M** after a 30° RF pulse

$$S = S_0 \frac{\left(1 - e^{-TR/T_1}\right) \sin(\alpha) \cdot e^{-TE/T_2^*}}{1 - \cos(\alpha) \cdot e^{-TR/T_1}} \tag{3}$$

with S_0 the maximum signal amplitude (obtainable with TR>>T₁, TE = 0 msec and FA = α = 90°). From this formula we can calculate, after a series of mathematical steps, the optimal FA – also called the Ernst angle α_E [4] – by fixing TR and TE for given values of T₁, we have the maximum signal at:

$$\alpha_E = \cos^{-1}\left(e^{-TR/T_1}\right) \tag{4}$$

Let us consider, for example a typical value of TR = 20 msec and the T₁ of the heart muscle ≈ 800 msec; from the formula, we will have that the Ernst angle is α_E ≈ 13° with the magnetization available for the next RF pulse of 0.9M₀, that is 90% of the maximum amplitude **M₀**.

In practice, different tissues have different T₁ values, so that it is impossible to optimize the contrast for all, as each have their own Ernst angle. In medical imaging, the most important factor is the Contrast-to-Noise Ratio (CNR) between tissues, while the Ernst angle is basically a useful guide for identifying which is the most suitable FA.

With the sequences in GRE, image contrast can be manipulated simply by changing the FA: higher FA values yield a T₁-weighed contrast (T₁W); lower angles yield Proton Density weighted images (PDW) when using brief echo times and T2* weighted images (T2*W) when using longer TEs.

2.3.2 Spoiled Gradient Echo (SPGR)

In order to obtain images in Gradient Echo without artifacts, the transverse magnetization M_{xy} along the plane perpendicular to $\mathbf{B}_0$ needs to be completely null at the end of the TR interval so that only the longitudinal component M_z is left when the next RF pulse occurs. This way the amplitude of the signal that we obtain depends uniquely on the longitudinal relaxation during TR, void of any possible effects caused by transverse magnetization remaining at the end of the TR interval. Such an assumption is true if $T_1 << TR$, but in many cases (when the image includes areas with a high T_1, such as in blood for example) this is not true and the remaining magnetization creates artifacts in the final image. At present, one of the methods used to avoid the problems above consists in the so called "spoiling" operation – from which the name of Spoiled Gradient Echo. This method spoils the phase coherence in transverse magnetization between successive TR intervals [5].

This disturbance, called "gradient spoiling" is usually performed after data acquisition. An alternative method consists in the casual variation of the RF pulse phase (RF spoiling) at each pulse. This method is, at the moment, the most used in the machines for cardiovascular images as it guarantees a homogeneous spoiling effect over the entire FOV.

2.3.3 Steady State Free Precession (SSFP)

An alternative way of treating the remaining transverse component before the following RF pulse – that is, at the end of the TR interval – is to utilize this very same component to improve the SNR and increase the phase coherence between successive TR intervals [1]. In other words, this technique recycles the remaining transverse component by exploiting the physical phenomenon known as Steady State Free Precession. This technique enables the operator to make acquisitions, even in conditions of wide FAs and very brief TRs, without risking saturation. Hence the sequences that exploit such a method (FIESTA, True FISP, Balanced Echo) include a first phase involving an appropriate succession of RF pulses until the steady state is reached, and then a real sequence of data acquisition for generating the image.

In the acquisition of cardiovascular images, such an approach is extensively used, especially for anatomo-functional images in which it is absolutely necessary to have images very rapidly, and with high SNR and CNR.

2.4 Fast sequences in SE

Images acquired using the standard Spin Echo sequence (SE) require long acquisition times (minutes) and are therefore inadequate in cardiovascular settings. The long acquisition times are due to the fact that at least two RF pulses must be generated (the first at 90°, the second at 180°) and a TE/2 time lapse must run between the two pulses. However, from the SE images we can extrapolate some extremely useful information for the diagnosis in cardio-vascular settings. Therefore, diverse strategies have been studied in the attempt of obtaining SE images having acquisition times compatible with those that may be proposed for acquiring cardiovascular images.

Such new technologies belong to the large family of Fast Spin Echo sequences.

2.4.1 Fast Spin Echo (FSE)

One of the strategies implemented in the FSE sequences involves the use of echo-trains. With this technique, each Spin Echo is subjected to a different phase encoding gradient; therefore, if we collect P spin echoes at each TR interval, we will have P lines of the K-space acquired in a single TR, with the result that the image acquisition time is P-fold faster than a conventional SE sequence. Therefore, in general, if the image matrix has N_y pixels in the direction of the phase encoding and P echoes (hence P lines in K-space) are memorized at each TR, the sequence must be repeated N_y/P times to memorize all the data (i.e., to fill all the K-space). The total acquisition time will then be:

$$T_{acq} = TR^*N_y/P \qquad\qquad\qquad (5)$$

With this methodology each echo is memorized at a particular segment of the K-space at each TR; the most simple strategy is to memorize the first echoes after having activated the phase gradient with negative maximum value, memorize the central echoes after having activated phase gradient with amplitude close to 0; and finally the last echoes after having activated the gradient with the positive maximum amplitude. Figure 2.11a shows the diagram of a typical FSE sequence, while Figure 2.11b schematically shows the memorization process according to this strategy.

From the graph we can notice the way such a gradient is activated with negative amplitude ("rewind" of phase gradient) just briefly before the RF 180° pulse. This operation is performed in the FSE sequence for the purpose of eliminating any dephasing owed to the phase gradient; in fact the 180° pulse must have the role of rephasing uniquely those spins that have been dephased by the T2 effect alone, and not those dephased by the phase gradient effect also. In the case in which an echo train is acquired, as happens for the FSE sequences, the TE time (also called effective TE) corresponds to the echo memorized when the amplitude of phase encoding gradient is null. Therefore, the segment of the K-space containing the low spatial frequencies

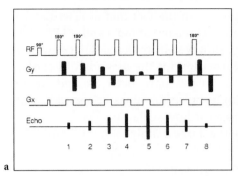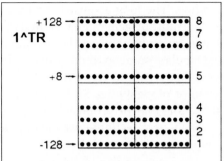

Fig. 2.11 a, b. Diagram of one of the most used data memorization methods in FSE echo trains. The figure shows 8 echo trains: (**a**) the diagram of the sequence; (**b**) the consequent filling of the K-space

determines the TE. It must be remembered that in MRI the contrast is determined especially by low spatial frequencies, while the details are enclosed in the higher frequencies.

2.5 Rapid images with parallel imaging techniques

The term parallel imaging is used in MR to describe the strategies by which a number of signals are acquired simultaneously, contrarily to what conventionally happens with one signal acquired at a time. Parallel imaging requires the simultaneous use of several receiving coils, from each of which spatial information of the image is acquired separately. In optics, an analogy is represented by the CCD charging coupling device monitor that is a parallel image device, unlike the fax that is a line-by-line scanning device.

The techniques of parallel imaging in MR are very recent, indeed the first publications on the theoretical aspects of this methodology with the first in-vivo results only date back to the late nineties [6, 7]. Such techniques are based on the appropriate use of several RF receiving coils (array coils) and on software algorithms enabling image reconstruction; these procedures drastically reduce image-formation and reconstruction times and are thus suitable in cardiovascular setting. Historically, parallel imaging was first implemented in the Philips machines, although today many companies are implementing the same methodologies in different machine models, assigning – as always – different names to the corresponding sequences!

Literature reports on two categories of parallel imaging: massively parallel strategies and partially parallel strategies. The category of massively parallel strategies includes those techniques in which the number of the coils receiving the RF signal corresponds to the number of signals to be acquired (that is the number of lines of the K-space). This solution would substitute completely the use of gradients for phase encoding with a remarkable increase in velocity in image acquisition. Yet at present, this technique has not been implemented although there are several proposals from a theoretical point of view, along with the projects for the relative coils. The number of receiving coils in the partially parallel methods is instead much less than the number of the lines of data. With this last solution space encoding is obtained by the combination of encoding through the gradients and the RF coils. To date, these are the solutions that are implemented in the MR scanners. Therefore, when speaking of parallel imaging we refer to the latter.

The different parallel imaging methods mentioned above share the common characteristic of using multiple RF-signal receiving coils, but differ in the way they elaborate the signals received and the way they form the final image. The SMASH (Simultaneous Acquisition of Spatial Harmonics) technique for example uses a linear combination of the various signals acquired by the different coils (refer to [6] for details); such an operation depends by the positioning of the coils and the geometry of the section. The more recent SENSE (SENSitivity Encoding) technique depends instead on coil sensitivity and not on the geometry of the coils or of the section [7]. Figure 2.12 schematically shows the different stages of signal acquisition in the parallel imaging technique (in particular an example of the SMASH technique) and how the final image is obtained after appropriate algorithmic steps. Figure 2.12.a illustrates (left) how the signals are acquired by 3 different coils and memorized in the K- space, while the right side of the figure shows the respective images of each coil as they would appear if they were actually acquired separately by the single coils; as we can see from the figure, the images contain data belonging to distanced points overlapping one another, as a consequence of data undersampling. Figure 2.12b evidences how the SMASH technique "exploits" the different signals acquired by the different coils: the algorithm performs a specific linear combination of the spatial harmonics (2 in the case of the example represented in the Figure). Finally, Figure 2.12c shows, on the left, how the lines of the K-space have been properly defined and, on the right, the reconstruction of the final image.

2.6 Vascular imaging sequences

This section will briefly describe the three major families of sequences utilized to acquire vascular images (also called angio-MR, or Magnetic Resonance Angiography, MRA). For more detailed information we invite the reader to consult other scientific publications [8-12]. These sequences exploit the physical principles that link the behavior of moving tissue (like blood) to the phenomenon of resonance and to the proper succession of switching on and off of RF pulses and gradients.

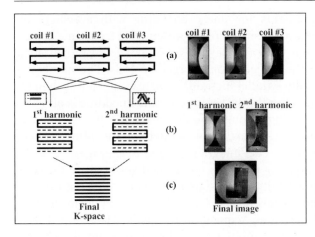

Fig. 2.12 a-c. Simplified representation of a parallel-imaging strategy

2.6.1 Time Of Flight (TOF)

The Time Of Flight sequence is a GRE sequence having a TR shorter than the T1 of stationary tissues, to an extent that it determines saturation of stationary spins. Let us imagine submitting to MR a volume of stationary tissue, not too thick, and which is orthogonally crossed by vessels of flowing blood. After a first radio frequency pulse all the tissue volume has been excited. If a second RF pulse is given after a short TR, the stationary tissue has yet to recover the longitudinal magnetization and is thus saturated ,while the blood that has flown by is substituted by fresh blood, obviously different from the blood flowing during the first RF pulse, and may be excited again to re-generate an MR signal.

This produces a high contrast between the blood flowing inside the excited layer and the absence of a signal in the stationary tissue. The entity of such contrast depends on the flow rate and on the thickness of the layer: the higher the flow rate and the thinner the layer, the higher the signal of the circulating blood.

T1 GRE sequences, are used with the shortest TR and TE possible and an intermediate FA (approximately 40°) in 2D or 3D acquisition modality.

2.6.1.1 Angio-MR 2D TOF

Sequential acquisition is made on two dimension images, with a thickness of 1.5-4 mm so that a sufficient spatial resolution is obtained. Figure 2.13a schematically shows how the single slices are acquired perpendicularly to the flow.

The sequential acquisition of each layer minimizes the saturation phenomena as each layer acts as an "entry slice" in which the accentuation of the signal linked to the flow has its highest expression.

2.6.1.2 Angio-MR 3D TOF

A 3D volumetric GRE T1 sequence is used (spoiled to null the T2 residual component of the signal). The sequence allows the simultaneous acquisition of a tissue volume (slab) composed of very thin (submillimetric) partitions with a high acquisition matrix that are formed by small voxels as shown in Figure 2.13b.

Volumes thicker than 6 cm can not be examined because of progressive saturation phenomena within the slab; however these phenomena can also occur in cases of slowed flow because the path covered by the spins across the slab can be long enough to cause a loss in signal.

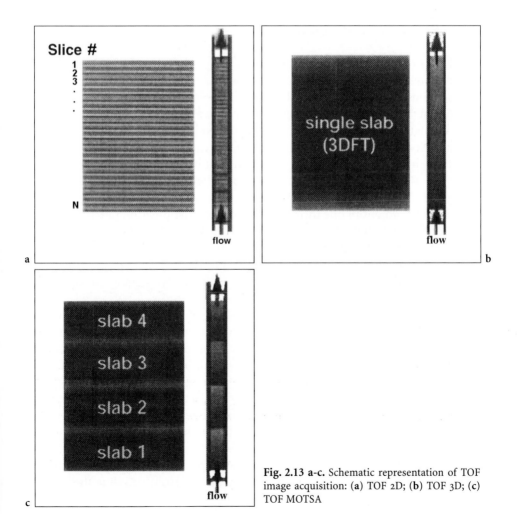

Fig. 2.13 a-c. Schematic representation of TOF image acquisition: (a) TOF 2D; (b) TOF 3D; (c) TOF MOTSA

2.6.1.3 Angio-MR 3D TOF MOTSA (Multiple Overlapping Thin Slab)

An angio-MR TOF-MOTSA method puts together the advantages of the 2D and 3D sequences. Actually, this method utilizes multiple, partially overlapped slabs of reduced thickness (Figure 2.13c). Each slab is acquired separately and in theory can be assimilated to an entry slice, then all the slabs are rebuilt together. On one hand this allows to minimize the phenomenon of intra-voxel phase dispersion and to have images with high spatial and contrast resolution, on the other to reduce saturation effects inside each slab with a better evaluation of slow flows. The method is particularly suited for covering a wide FOV but requires a longer acquisition time than the 3D TOF single slab and the reconstruction is burdened by the "Venetian blind" artifact that can be seen on the interface between the two slabs.

2.6.2 Phase Contrast Images

The Phase Contrast (PC) methods exploit the phenomenon of phase shift as a signal source. The angio-MR PC enables to evaluate the blood flow in the arterial and venous districts qualitatively and quantitatively providing information on volume, speed and direction of blood flow.

Both stationary spins and spins moving inside an excited sample along the direction of field gradient undergo phase variations. These variations in the spins that make up stationary tissue depends exclusively on their spatial position and always maintains the same intensity (linear function). Conversely, the mobile spins behave differently, as the phase variation induced by the field gradient in one direction depends on the position but also on the speed and direction of flow and varies in function of time (square function, that is proportional to the square of the time).

Let us suppose to firstly apply a positive gradient, then a negative one to a GRE sequence. This gradient will have to be bipolar with equal but opposite amplitude.

During the application of the positive lobe of the gradient both mobile and stationary spins build up a phase shift that the stationary spins give off during the application of the negative lobe. The mobile spins instead return to their phase of origin only partially, maintaining a shift proportional to their speed of motion and to the time the gradient is applied. This very difference between stationary and mobile spins is the underlying concept of Phase Contrast MRA. The bipolar gradient must be applied separately in each direction of the magnetic field (x, y, z) and must have an amplitude proportional to the blood flow the operator wishes to acquire (VENC, Velocity Encoding Value). Figure 2.14 shows an example of a PC acquired image (Figure 2.14a illustrates the anatomic image, while Figure 2.14b is the corre-

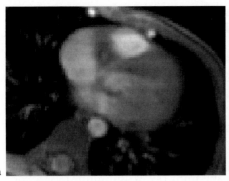

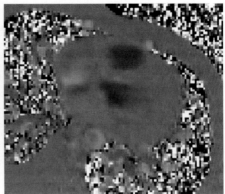

a

b

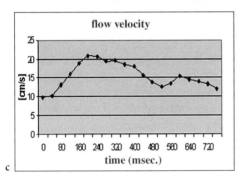

c

Fig. 2.14 a-c. Example of PC image: (a) conventional image; (b) corresponding image in PC; (c) graph plotting flow-velocity vs time for a specific ROI in the PC image

sponding image in PC) and a diagram of flow velocity evaluated by PC in a Region Of Interest (ROI) of the area pictured above.

Although stationary spins do not accumulate phase dispersion, a minimum amount of the signal comes from field inhomogeneities because of phenomena of magnetic susceptibility. This is avoided by acquiring two identical sequences that differ only in the activation of the bipolar gradient; then the two sets of data are subtracted, completely eliminating the signal of the stationary tissue. The subtraction of the signal of the stationary spins from that of the mobile spins therefore yields the signal exclusively emitted by the flow.

This passage is fundamental as it allows to eliminate an eventual signal coming from tissues with brief T1 or with high magnetic susceptibility while maintaining only the signal relating to the blood flow.

The data so obtained can be processed in three ways:

a) by obtaining anatomical details or relating to the flow velocity according to the VENC chosen (Complex Difference Processing, CDP)
b) by obtaining information on the direction of flow (Phase Difference Processing, PDP) by encoding the blood flow along the x, y, z axes separately, so as to obtain images with different signs according to whether the flow is in the same or opposite direction to the gradient

c) by obtaining dynamic images and volume and blood flow measurements acquiring a single section repeated at the same level during the cardiac sample and synchronized to it.

The PC MRA, as the TOF can be performed in 2D or 3D.

2.6.3 Contrast Enhanced Magnetic Resonance Angiography (CEMRA)

CEMRA foresees the use of a contrast medium (ex. gadolinium-based contrast agent). Intravenously infused gadolinium determines a reduction in T1 of blood that in turn translates in a hyperintensity of flow signal over other surrounding tissue.

The contrast medium routinely used is a chelate of gadolinium, with low molecular weight that crosses the capillary membrane and has a distribution outside the capillary bed into the extra-cellular space, thus behaving as an interstitial contrast medium. For its use in MRA it is therefore necessary that the acquisition occurs during the phase of arterial distribution of the contrast medium. Figure 2.15 illustrates an example of CEMRA.

The success of an MRA with contrast bolus depends on the synchronysm between acquisition of data and concentration of the contrast medium in the vascular district of interest. To assure a high quality of images, data from the central portion of the K-space of the sequence, which are responsible for the image's contrast resolution, have to be obtained when the contrast media concentration is the highest. It is therefore fundamental to know both the acquisition time for the sequence and the circulation time. A scanning time

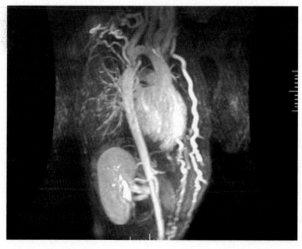

Fig. 2.15. Example of a CEMRA image

of 18 seconds will fill the central portion of the K-space between the sixth and the twelfth second from the beginning of the scanning. If the circulating time is 15 seconds, we will have a scanning delay of 9 seconds; the scanning delay, that is the time elapsing between the beginning of the injection with contrast medium and the beginning of acquisition, is given by the formula:

$$RS = TC - 1/3 \ TS \tag{6}$$

where RS is the scanning delay, TS is the sequence scanning, and TC is the time of circulation. The unknown circulating time can be calculated with the bolus test. The test consists in injecting 1-2 ml of paramagnetic contrast solution and acquiring a scan perpendicular to the vascular axis under examination with high temporal resolution (1 scanning with acquisition time of 1-2 seconds), repeated a number of times so to be able to appreciate the arrival of the contrast medium in the vessel lumen. A ROI positioned inside the vessel examined allows one to trace a graph for signal intensity in function of time, where the peak corresponds to the maximum concentration of the contrast medium in the vessel, at that specific time, that is at the circulating time. Nowadays there are automatic bolus detection systems (bolus tracking) with automatic synchronization of the CEMRA scanning that disengage the operator from calculating the circulating time. For example, with the "smart prep" technique we can register the variations in signal intensity upon arrival of the bolus by positioning an echo navigator over the aortic arc. Once the signal reaches the preestablished threshold indicating the arrival of the bolus, the CEMRA scanning is automatically synchronized. An analogous method is the fluoroscopic triggering, which consists in the serial acquisition of ultra rapid bidimensional T1-weighted images that are obtained each second, visualizing the arrival of the contrast medium. The operator is required to start the acquisition of the 3D data set upon arrival of the bolus in the artery.

Venous opacification can be reduced by using sequences with elliptic filling of the K-space. This method allows the acquisition of data in a time frame over 30 seconds, avoiding venous overlay since the portion of the K-space deputed to the difference of image contrast is rapidly filled at the beginning and the remaining portion of the K-space is used to increment the spatial resolution, thus the image's resolution. Given the narrowness of the window used to create the contrast, it is necessary to use automatic detection methods for the arrival of the bolus, like the smart prep or the fluoroscopic triggering.

Another method that enables to obtain MR angiograms independent from circulating time is 3D Time-Resolved Imaging of Contrast Kinetics sequence (TRICKS).

The imaging techniques available today are not fast enough to acquire all of the necessary data of the K-space data with the desired temporal resolution in angiography. In fact, to resolve arterial and venous phases, good temporal resolution is required (e.g., ~5 sec, depending on the anatomical region). Unfortunately, acquiring a time frame with the needed spatial resolution and coverage may require significantly more than just a few seconds (i.e., 15-20 sec might be considered typical).

Accordingly, in a time interval comparable to the temporal resolution required, one may be able to acquire only 1/4 to 1/2 of the necessary K-space data.

TRICKS [13-14] is a method capable of converting an acquired partial dataset into a full frame. To do this, TRICKS assumes that the high spatial frequency content of the image does not require as high a temporal resolution as the low spatial frequency content.

Basically, TRICKS sequence includes K-space acquisition into sub-regions (usually 3 or 4) along the phase-encoding direction; each region is acquired in separated times (or frames). During each TRICKS time frame, a segment of K-space, corresponding to a single region, is acquired. The first region contains the lowest part of the spatial frequencies in the phase-encoding direction, and the successive regions correspond to higher spatial frequencies in this direction. Complete K-space volumes are formed from these segments by retrospectively combining the acquired regions.

This temporal interpolation scheme ensures that region acquired near the peak arterial signal intensity enhancement (i.e., the lowest spatial frequencies) is combined with the regions that are acquired after the contrast agent filled the targeted blood vessels.

This method allows one to obtain a single set of 3D data in short time (2-10 sec) with the aim of solving temporarily the arterial, parenchomigraphic, and venous phases of the angiogram. The method however, allows a gain in temporal resolution at the expenses of spatial resolution.

2.7 Conclusions

In this chapter we have seen a rapid overview of different strategies applied for obtaining cardiovascular MR images. Obviously, the aim of using such methods is to obtain images in the least time possible, but also that they be of the best quality. The parameters most often used to determine whether the images are of good quality are the SNR and the CNR. Therefore the primary objective of the techniques mentioned above is to obtain images rapidly with high SNR and CNR; this objective is pursued thanks to the use of methods that allow to best exploit the physical principles on which they are based , and the hardware and software tools available today. It is obvious that the study and development of new techniques for fast imaging are evolving in parallel to the new instruments designed and developed in the field of electronics, informatics, and material science.

References

1. Haacke EM, Brown RW, Thompson MR, Venkatesan R (1999) Magnetic resonance imaging – Physical principles and sequence design. J. Wiley & Sons, Inc., Publication
2. University of Aberdeen – Department of Bio-medical Physics and Bio-Engineering (1998) Physical basis of MRI. Summer School Notes
3. Haase A, Frahm J, Matthaei D, Haenicke W, Merboldt KD (1986) FLASH imaging – Rapid NMR imaging using low flip-angle pulses. Journal of Magn Reson 67:258-266
4. Ernst RR, Anderson WA (1966) Application of Fourier Transform spectroscopy to magnetic Resonance. Rev Sci Instrum 37:93-102
5. Frahm J, Haenicke W, Merboldt KD (1987) Transverse coherence in rapid FLASH NMR imaging. Journal of Magn Reson 72:307-314
6. Sodickson DK, Manning WJ (1997) Simultaneous acquisition of spatial harmonics (SMASH): fast imaging with radiofrequency coil arrays. Magn Reson Med 38:591-603
7. Pruessmann KP, Weiger M, Scheidegger MB, Boesiger P (1999) SENSE: Sensitivity encoding for fast MRI. Magn Reson Med 42:952-962
8. Debatin JF, Spritzer CE, Grist TM et al (1991) Imaging of the renal arteries. Value of MR angiography. AJR 157:981-990
9. Keller PJ (1992) Time of flight magnetic resonance angiography. Neuroim Clin NA 2:639-656
10. Dumoulin CL (1992) Phase-contrast magnetic resonance angiography. Neuroim Clin NA 2:657-676
11. Turski P, Korosec F (1993) Phase contrast angiography. In: Anderson CM, Edelman R, Turski P (eds). Clinical Magnetic Resonance angiography. New York, Raven Press
12. Snidow JJ, Matthew SJ, Harris VJ et al (1996) Three-dimensional gadolinium-enhanced MR angiography for aortoiliac inflow assessment plus renal artery screening in a single breath-hold. Radiology 198:725-732
13. Korosec FR, Frayne R, Grist TM, Mistretta CA (1996) Time-resolved contrast-enhanced 3D MR angiography. Magn Reson Med 36:345–351
14. Carroll TJ, Korosec FR, Petermann GM, Grist TM, Turski PA (2001) Carotid bifurcation: evaluation of time-resolved three-dimensional contrast-enhanced MR angiography. Radiology 220:525–532

3 Post-processing

VINCENZO POSITANO

3.1 Introduction

In the past years the computerized analysis of digital images in Magnetic Resonance (MR), and particularly in cardiovascular magnetic resonance, has gained an increasing relevance and has become as important as the traditional procedures of direct printing on radiographic film. In fact the use of digital images allows to produce, store and interchange great quantities of data in a simple and inexpensive way, while preserving the possibility of examining and distributing some of the images produced as traditional radiographic films. Moreover, the use of digital images has allowed the development of advanced postprocessing techniques, with the possibility of obtaining 3D images of the organs under examination and making quantitative measurements of physiological parameters useful at the diagnostic phase.

Typically, the Magnetic Resonance Imaging (MRI) scanner is connected to a console – generally a calculator equipped with a UNIX operating system – where the images are produced directly in digital format. The images obtained can be stored through a proper memorizing device that can utilize magneto-optical disks, DAT, CDROM, DVD, and others. A Local Area Network (LAN) connects the console to a digital printer, which is usually adapted for printing on radiographic film. In addition there can be a second workstation to which the images can be sent for examination and storage via LAN, also when the main console is engaged in acquisitions. Further extensions dedicated to reporting or image processing can be connected either directly through the LAN or indirectly through a remote connection via internet.

3.2 Digital images

In digital imaging the basic element of an image is the pixel – a geometrical element, generally square, of the same size of the image's spatial resolution, which can take on a certain number of levels of gray. If, for example, the res-

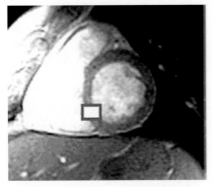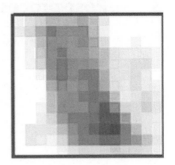

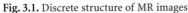

Fig. 3.1. Discrete structure of MR images

olution of a MR image is 1.2×1.2 mm, then each pixel of the image will be a square with a side of 1.2 mm. The overall image is formed by a matrix of pixels. Figure 3.1 shows a typical image of MR and the enlargement of a detail that evidences the discrete structure of the very image. The number of gray levels that the pixel can take on is called image depth and is usually expressed as a number of bits. Without going into detail on binary codes, it can be stated that the depth of an image can be considered as 2 raised to the power of number of bits available, as can be seen in Table 3.1. Images only 1 pixel deep are binary images and therefore in black and white. The typical depth of most electronic devices such as monitors and video cameras is 8 bits. MRI utilizes a maximum image depth of 16 bits, often reduced to 12.

Generally, each digital image is memorized in a particular format in which the information relating to an image is encoded according to a particular algorithm in a digital file. Clearly, in order to read an image encoded in such a way, it is necessary to run a program that can interpret the format used to produce that image.

For what concerns MRI machines, the digital image must enclose, apart from the image itself, also all the information pertaining to the examination

Table 3.1. Depth of digital images

Number of bits	Depth of image	Notes
1	2	Black and white image
8	256	Image displayed on monitor
12	4096	Typical MR image
16	65536	Max depth of MR image

which the image is part of. The data required are the patient's personal data (name, date of birth, etc.) which are inserted by the operator, and then the data referring to the sequence adopted, the characteristics of the MRI machine being used, the spatial and temporal information of the images acquired, and in general any information that can be useful for interpreting the image correctly.

Speaking in terms of computer jargon, the part of the image containing such information is called *header*, and the unprocessed numerical data relative to the image itself are called *raw data*.

Therefore, it appears evident that MR images can be used only with a program that can correctly interpret the encoding of the header and the raw data the manufacturer made use of to build the scanner. Otherwise, the MR images are absolutely unusable.

3.2.1 Proprietary formats and DICOM formats

The moment the companies manufacturing MR machines began to use digital images, each company produced images employing its own encodings. Therefore, encodings differ from one manufacturer to another but also from one model to another. These formats are called *proprietary*, as they are company property, developed by the manufacturer for their exclusive use, and are usually not made public. Normally the manufacturer does not provide any guarantee on the possibility of exchanging the data contained in such formats with the outside world. The reality is that the use of a proprietary format for digital images ties the user to the software and hardware provided by the manufacturer of that given MR machine and there is no guarantee of the possibility to access the stored data in the case of substitution of the MR equipment. Moreover, the exchange of data with other centers is extremely difficult, if not impossible.

In recent years, a common DICOM (Digital Imaging and Communications in Medicine) format has been developed to overcome the obstacles limiting the use of proprietary formats; this format allows the exchange of medical images and is compatible with almost all the cardiovascular MR equipment in use today [1].

The DICOM format is a standard set of rules for transmitting biomedical digital images and healthcare information to and from different pieces of equipment (acquisition machines, computers, printers, digital databases...), through the definition of a communication protocol and the use of standard web protocols and technologies (Ethernet, Transmission Control Protocol/ Internet Protocol, TCP/IP). The original project was developed by two American associations: *The American College of Radiology* (ACR), responsible for developing the technical and medical aspects, and the *National Electrical Manufacturers Association* (NEMA), a consortium of manufacturers responsible, among other things, for the legal aspects covering patent regulations. At international level, the European standardization committee has accepted DICOM in MEDICOM (MEDia Interchange COMmunication), and the JIRA (Japan Industries Association Radiological Systems) has approved its development. From 1985 to 2001 the DICOM 3 standard underwent many changes and integrations before reaching its actual state in the DICOM regulations set out in 15 volumes for a total of 15000 pages. It should be underlined that DICOM 3 is an industrial standard and not an ISO (International Standard Organization) universal one: this allows a certain tolerance in the implementation of its specifications to the point that, at present, there are no truly DICOM *compliant* machines, in the rigorous sense a standard would impose. Indeed, in the vast majority of cases a machine will conform to the standard in some parts (for example, the image storage modality), while it will adopt proprietary functions in others (as for managing patient lists).

The DICOM compatibility of MR equipment, and more in general any DICOM compatible device, must be certified by the manufacturer through the auto-certification document, called Conformance Statement, which lists properties and functions of the equipment. Certainly, DICOM is extremely practical as it allows us to efficiently store, elaborate, and exchange digital images. Moreover, DICOM frees the user from having to buy hardware or software extensions from the manufacturer of the MR scanner. Yet, before purchasing a DICOM compatible device it is advisable to make a compatibility enquiry and an on-the-field trial.

Many programs also allow the vision of DICOM images on a Personal Computer, and often can even be downloaded from the internet. Many of these programs also allow elementary postprocessing operations such as linear and surface measurements.

3.2.2 Memory devices

The first concern in a MR lab is storing the digital images acquired. The backup and the storage of images over long periods of time is required by the present regulations but also by issues of scientific/diagnostic relevance. The amount of data that needs to be preserved can be evaluated keeping in mind that a cardiac MR image is encoded on 16 bits (2 bytes), and that each pixel can take on $2^{16} = 65536$ values. The typical acquisition format is 256x256 pixel, and thus the size of raw data is $256 \times 256 \times 2 = 131,072$ bytes. To these, we must add the bytes of the titles and annotations (approximately 10.000 for the DICOM format) up to about 140,000 bytes (149 Kb) for a typical cardiac MR image. Other typical acquisition formats are 128×128, 512×512 and 1024×1024, which correspond respectively to image sizes of 42Kb, 522Kb and 2058 Kb. Considering that a cardiac MR exam usually includes from several hundreds to several thousands of images, the average size of one study can range between 50 and 200 Mbytes.

There are basically three memory devices used for saving images:

1) Magneto-optical disks
2) DAT (magnetic tapes)
3) CDROM and DVDROM

The storage on magneto-optical disks is the most popular technique and is implemented on most MR machines on the market. The disks are quite small sized (5.3"×0.25") and utilize a double-control data transcription system: the disk contents can only be modified when there is the simultaneous activation of the magnetic head and the laser ray that heats the disk. This system avoids accidental damages to the disk that may occur in the presence of contaminating magnetic fields (monitor, acoustic speakers, the MR equipment itself). Disk capacity ranges from 1.2 Mb to 5 Gb; moreover, the disks can be written over countless times and be reused. On the other hand, these magneto-optical disks present some disadvantages such as their elevated cost (50 Euro), as compared to other memory devices, and the difficulty of using the recorded disks outside the laboratory owing to problems in finding the drivers and often to problems of incompatibility. There are, however, devices (called Jukeboxes) that can manage several hundred magneto-optical disks automatically, allowing the user to easily handle reading and writing operations on a great number of disks. These apparatuses can remarkably simplify the management of a MR data storage system.

The Digital Audio Tape (DAT) are magnetic tapes similar to normal music cassettes but smaller in size. Data are memorized sequentially by magnetic heads. The main advantage of DAT is the elevated capacity (up to 10 Gb) and the limited cost of the memory media (about 10 Euro). The drawback is the sequential nature of the device which makes access to stored data quite lengthy: if we are interested in a study memorized at the end of the tape, we are forced to play the entire tape. Notwithstanding these inconveniences, the DAT can be useful as an emergency support when data on the main disk are accidentally deleted or destroyed. As DAT are sensitive to magnetic fields they must be stored away from the MR scanner or other electromagnetic devices.

Compact Disks Read-Only-Memory (CDROMs) are extremely popular optical storage devices on which data are memorized by a laser ray. CDROMs are totally insensitive to magnetic and electrical fields. Because the memory media is not enclosed in a container as for magneto-optical disks, it is vulnerable to chipping and scratching. The typical capacity of a CDROM is 700 MB. The main advantage is the inexpensive cost of both the memory support (less than one Euro) and the device (writer/burner) for writing on disk (100 Euro). In addition, CD readers are practically installed on almost every computer.

The Digital Video Disks Read-Only-Memory (DVDROMs) are optical disks similar to CDROMs but with a much higher memory capacity (approximately 10 Gb). The prices of the DVD support are already quite accessible (about 10 Euro) and are likely to decrease in the future in virtue to the wide diffusion of DVDs in the field of multimedia. Although CDROMs and DVDROMs have not reached the reliability of the magneto-optical supports, they will probably become the most widespread memorization platform also in the medical setting.

3.2.3 Data transfer via network

In modern laboratories of cardiac MR, the standard way of transferring data from and to different working stations is by LAN. The LAN can be installed at the same time the machine is installed, otherwise a preexisting LAN can be used instead, in which case the several workstations can also be set far apart from one another. The exchange of data between workstations may be done using proprietary formats, with the limits mentioned above, or with the DICOM format and its relative advantages.

The exchange of data according to the DICOM protocol foresees an authenticating system between the stations involved in the exchange. The model adopted is the classical client-server: one machine, generally the MR console, hosts the images and a DICOM program called DICOM server that waits to receive requests coming from programs (client) residing on other machines, such as the workstation where the images are processed. Each client must be authorized to the connection and configured through an appropriate code. This allows to protect the data located on the different stations from unwanted intrusions. It is important to notice, however, that the DICOM protocol foresees that data transmission occur uncripted; thus to assure the protection of confidential data it is advisable that the LAN connecting the different stations be isolated from the rest of the network and protected by security devices (firewall). An interesting aspect of the use of the DICOM protocol is the possibility of exchanging data via network not only among stations of the same lab but also between different labs, at the condition they are both connected by an internet connection. Because of the difficulty of rendering this type of connection secure, the transfer of data should occur only after the data have been encoded in an anonymous form to preserve the confidential part of data intact. In the case we wish to implement permanently a protocol for the exchange of data between two physically distant laboratories using the internet, data can be protected during the transfer with the use of specific cryptographic algorithms.

Another very important aspect is the possibility of exchanging data also outside the workstations provided by the manufacturer of the scanner, with the use of low cost computers. This is made possible through the use of appropriate software that allows access to DICOM data on the MR machine and the possibility to view and elaborate the images received.

3.2.4 Printing devices

Each MRI lab foresees the presence of a digital printer for radiographic films. The printer can be connected either directly to the MR console or to the other stations via LAN. A radiographic printer can also utilize the DICOM protocol for printing images; the main advantage in applying the protocol is that the same printer can be used from different stations and by different labs.

3.3 Image visualization

3.3.1 Windowing

Generally, MR images are encoded on 16 bits, that is each pixel of the image can take on $2^{16} = 65536$ values, which corresponds to a same number of gray levels. Actually, the number of levels employed is less – in cardiac magnetic imaging, usually a few thousand.

The viewing instruments used, traditional video screens or Liquid Cristal Display (LCD), can visualize up to 256 levels of grey. This does not constitute a limit as greater resolutions would be useless: the human eye can only distinguish a limited number of grey levels simultaneously [2]. But because the human eye can separate a much greater number of colors, medical images often characterize images representing false colors; in other words, they match each hue of grey to a specific color through a predetermined map. This application, however, is not widely used in cardiac MRI.

Hence, all the devices for displaying images must approach the problem of representing a number of grey levels higher than the ones they can manage. The images visualized or printed are, therefore, strongly characterized by the

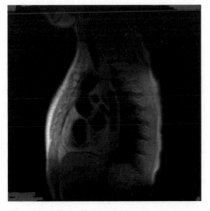 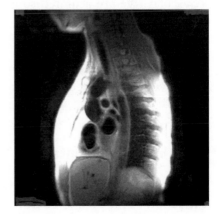

Fig. 3.2. Effect of the windowing operation

way in which this inconvenience is approached; because the solution is all but univocal one must consider that each image printed or viewed on the monitor may represent only in part the global information actually enclosed in the data acquired by the scanner.

The process by which the image's levels of gray are represented on screen or printed is generally called windowing. The pixels lying within a certain range of values (a window) – established by the user – are represented using all grey levels available (typically 256).

The values below the chosen window are all set to zero, and they are hence represented in black. All the values above are, instead, assigned the highest value of the scale (typically 255) and are thus represented in white. Figure 3.2 shows an example of the differences of visualization that can be obtained through different selections of the window to be used. In the picture on the left, gray levels are displayed in a proportional way. The picture on the right shows the same image after appropriate windowing to optimize the visualization of the heart. However, as it can be noticed, the area of the anterior chest loses some detail owing to a compression of the relative gray levels.

3.3.2 Visualizing in 3D

In many cases cardiac magnetic resonance images are acquired in 3D, covering an entire area of interest such as the heart or a cluster of vessels, through a series of parallel sections. These 3D acquisitions can then be repeated over time so to follow the evolution of a certain phenomenon like a cardiac cycle over an R-R interval, or the diffusion of a paramagnetic contrast medium.

Typical examples are the fast-cine sequences, in which 8-12 parallel sections on short axis are acquired 20-30 times in different instances of the R-R interval, and the sequences used in MRA, in which a set of parallel sections of a vascular tree are acquired so as to obtain a 3D view of the vascular tree itself.

The visual representation of a volume of tridimensional data naturally involves the use of algorithms for visualizing an image in 3D on a bidimensional support such as a monitor or photographic film [3, 4]. Ahead we will analyze some of the techniques for 3D viewing, underlining the characteristics with the respective advantages and disadvantages.

3.3.3 Image segmentation

All the 3D viewing procedures involve a segmenting operation – that is, the extraction of the area of interest from the global image. More in detail, the segmenting consists in partitioning the image in homogeneous regions, each corresponding to a real object (for example a cardiac vessel or a cardiac wall). Literature reports of many algorithms for segmenting MR images. An important group of methods is based on the identification of two threshold values, a minimum and maximum that define the anatomical item to be located. This technique allows to locate regions of a scene sharing the same properties and which thus belong to the same tissue. Typically, the user can define an interval of values to separate the object of interest from the surrounding scene and transform the latter into background. Usually, a preview of the segmented image is provided so that the segmentation parameters can be adjusted interactively. Often the threshold values are implicitly provided by the program used, based on the types of images that have to be elaborated. Therefore, the threshold method is very simple to apply and efficient in those images in which the regions of interest are well distinguishable, like in vascular images by MRA. Another option foreseen by visualization programs is the manual selection of an area and the limitation of the viewing procedure to that selected area. For other kinds of images, due to reduced Signal-to-Noise Ratio (SNR) and Contrast-to-Noise Ratio (CNR), more sophisticated methods are employed, an example of which (active contour/algorithm) will be described later.

3.3.4 MIP and RaySum algorithms

These are algorithms that mimic the principle underlying the production of radiographic images.

The starting images are made up of a series of equally distanced parallel slices (Fig. 3.3). Once the direction of projection has been established (see Fig. 3.3) the algorithm locates a series of rays parallel to the direction of projection that crosses the slices. In particular each projecting ray crosses all the slices in a specific number of dots (see Fig. 3.3). Therefore each ray will have a set of values corresponding to the signal intensity of the pixel crossed in

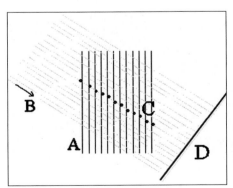

Fig. 3.3. Maximum Intensity projection (MIP) and RAYSUM algorithms for 3D visualization. A: Series of parallel slices; B: Direction of projection; C: Projecting rays crossing the slices; D: Angle of observation

each slice. In the MIP algorithm (Maximum Intensity Projection), the maximum value is chosen and is transferred onto the projected image that constitutes the visualization of the 3D image wanted (see Fig. 3.3). In the RaySum algorithm all the values obtained are summed and the resulting value is tracked on the projected image. Other algorithms employed are the projection at minimum intensity, in which the minimum value is adopted, and the projection at medium intensity in which the average of values is utilized.

Another further variant foresees the projection rays to be non-parallel, leaving from a source and spreading with a certain angle. While the first hypothesis of parallel rays means hypothesizing a far point of view for 3D visualization, this latter approach hypothesizes a close-up point of view. Usually the MRA visualization utilizes the MIP parallel ray technique. Figure 3.4 illustrates the steps of 3D reconstruction obtained with the technique explained above. In the upper part of the figure there are some of the 72 images that make up the starting acquisition (the sections indicated as A in Fig. 3.3) and hence of the parallel sections that cover the upper part of the trunk, neck and the inferior part of the head. In the lower part three different MIP reconstructions are visualized. The first is the global reconstruction with

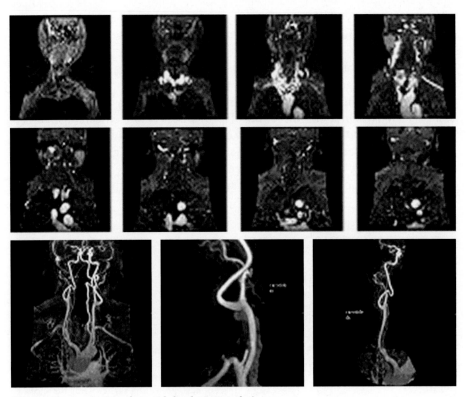

Fig. 3.4. Reconstruction of carotids by the MIP technique

a view direction perpendicular to the plane of the sections acquired; the other two are details of the left and right carotid obtained from the global image through an operation of manual segmentation.

3.3.5 Approach to surfaces

The approach to surfaces uses bidimensional primitives, generally triangles or polygons, to represent tridimensional objects. In practice, the surface of the object to be visualized is approximated with a certain number of adjacent polygons (often triangles). Algorithms that have been optimized for this purpose, and which often utilize particular video cards, visualize the polygons thus providing a three-dimensional representation of the object. Obviously, the higher the number of polygons, the better the accuracy of the representation. Figure 3.5 shows the triangle representation of the left and right ventricle, and the ensuing 3D image. The main advantage of surface representation is the reduction of the data to be elaborated down into a list of polygons and connections, with the consequential reduction in time lost in calculations. Since the surface approach is extensively employed in popular commercial items such as videogames, the market offers of wide selection of inexpensive highly advanced video boards that support this type of approach. The fundamental limit to this approach is the need to separate or segment the object of interest, in our case a vessel or the heart, from the surrounding objects. An error in the segmenting procedure inevitably leads to errors in the 3D representation [5].

Another important aspect in the 3D reconstruction by surface algorithms is the introduction of shading, an effect for conveying the three-dimensional information. Without going into detail of the various algorithms, the underlying concept is to define one or more light sources and mimic the illuminating effect of those sources on the rebuilt surfaces to create the illusion of 3D representation.

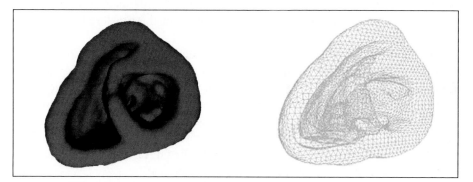

Fig. 3.5. 3D surface rendering of heart. The 3D representation of left and right ventricle (right); the underlying grid of triangles (left)

3.4 Quantitative measures of mass and volume

The importance of wall thickness, ventricular mass and volumes as fundamental diagnostic parameters is well known, as they allow us to estimate indices such as the ejection fraction, wall function, etc. Cardiovascular MRI allows the evaluation of these indices in an extremely precise way thanks to high image resolution and the possibility of acquiring images on a series of parallel planes, whichever way they may be oriented.

The software tools that allow the quantitative mass and volume evaluation typically use short axis images of the fast-cine type, i.e. a certain number of parallel slices (8-12) covering the whole ventricle. For each slice there are a high number of frames (16-30) that allow to rebuild the entire cardiac cycle. As we can imagine, the number of images to be examined is significant (200-540), and a manual measurement would not be proposable. Many programs have been developed for the automatic analysis of the images which could be adopted to reduce the time of postprocessing; this software is usually provided along with MR equipment intended for use in cardiology [6]. At present, the software available does not yet allow a totally automatic elaboration of the images but requires considerable interaction on behalf of the user. Generally, to reduce elaboration time, the operator chooses to examine only two temporal phases of the R-R interval, typically end-diastole and end-systole, thus reducing the number of images to be examined to about 16-24 and preserving at the same time the option of evaluating efficiently the diagnostic indices desired.

The key point of the procedure of automatic elaboration is a segmentation algorithm: this divides the image into a series of primitive portions topologically connected (in our case right ventricle, left ventricle, myocardial wall), and then catalogues every single region and reassembles those portions that belong to the same tissue.

The segmenting algorithms used are of various nature but a detailed dissertation of these would go beyond the scope of this paragraph. Speaking in general terms, the algorithms used are referred to as edge segmentation, where intensity discontinuity inside the image is evidenced as sharp variations in grey scales. Such discontinuities represent the borders between different tissues.

One of the most utilized techniques for detecting edges is that proposed by Canny, which consists in the use of the first derivative of the voxel intensity function: the points where the max values of the derivative make up the edge.

In general the user is asked to insert a *seed* for the automatic segmentation algorithm, which can either be an approximate border of the inside of the left ventricle or a marker at the center of the ventricle itself. At this point the algorithm goes on automatically, trying to locate the edges desired, typically the endocardium and the epicardium of the left ventricle.

Figure 3.6 shows the edges detected on six slices relative to the diastolic phase. The algorithm used in this example is called "active contours" and

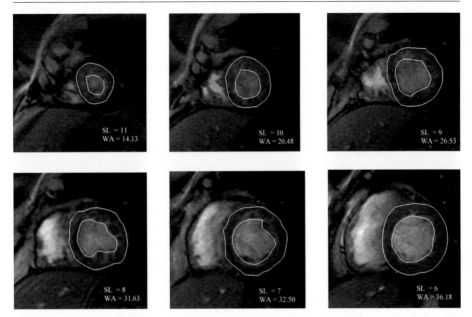

Fig. 3.6. Detection of endocardial and epicardial borders on MR cardiac images

defines a closed curve that simulates the physical behavior of an elastic band. The ring is deformed by external forces which are represented, as we described earlier, by the portions of maximum intensity of the first derivative of the image and by internal forces that oppose the deformation. When the equilibrium between the two forces is reached, the curve stabilizes and locates the contour desired [7]. Since the information enclosed in the DICOM format provides both the planar resolution of the single slice and the distance between two adjacent slices, the program can automatically calculate the ventricular mass and volume in the phase considered by evaluating the area of the curves that define the endocardium and epicardium. Because the ventricular volume is approximated with a series of parallel planes, there will obviously be an error proportional to the distance between the slices. This happens because the volume is approximated by an operation of interpolation, typically when using the Simpson method or its variants.

By repeating the calculation of the volume and mass for the systolic phase, we can evaluate the first diagnostic index, the Ejection Fraction (EF). If the software calculates the value of the ventricular volume for each phase of the cardiac cycle, then the diastolic and systolic phase are automatically calculated and consequentially also the value of EF.

Other parameters of interest from a diagnostic point of view are the wall thickness and wall thickening that measure respectively the absolute thickness of the ventricular wall (in mm) and the relative wall thickening during the cardiac cycle with respect to the diastolic phase.

Table 3.2. Number and type of contours to be drawn in order to obtain a quantitative analysis

Quantitative measurement	Contours to be detected	Frames to be processed
End-diastolic volume	Endocardium	All end-diastolic frames
End-systolic volume	Endocardium	All end-systolic frames
Ejection fraction	Endocardium	All end-diast. and end-syst. frames
Stroke volume	Endocardium	All end-diast. and end-syst. frames
Myocardial mass	Endocardium and Epicardium	All end-diastolic frames
Wall thickness	Endocardium and Epicardium	All frames in the selected cardiac phase
Wall thickening	Endocardium and Epicardium	All end-diast. and end-syst. frames
Wall function	Endocardium and Epicardium	All frames in the selected cardiac phase

Generally, the number of edges to detect and validate depends on the information desired. Table 3.2 shows the types and number of contours necessary for the most common types of analysis. The results of the quantitative analyses are made available in both numerical and graphical format, often using colored representations such as the bull's eye.

3.5 Flow analysis

By using appropriate acquisition sequences, it is possible to obtain images containing information on the velocity of the blood inside a vessel. Such images, known by the name of Phase Contrast (PC), can be elaborated through appropriate algorithms in order to acquire information on the speed of the haematic fluid in a vessel, and therefore on the volume transported.

An image sequence of PC type is made up of anatomical images, which serve as reference for the analysis, and by a series of PC images that enclose information on the velocity of flow in time, usually in an R-R interval. In Figure 3.7b we can see the anatomical image of reference, and on the left the first of the series of PC images (usually 20-40 images per cardiac cycle). To perform the analysis, the user must establish the edges of the vessel on all images. The procedure usually adopted foresees the definition of a starting contour on an anatomical image where the vessel is well defined. At this point the automatic procedure continues defining the edges on all the anatomical and the PC images. The user can eventually intervene to correct any errors manually.

Once the contours have all been defined, the program extracts the mean value of the signal from the Region Of Interest (ROI) thereby defined. The mean value will be proportional to the velocity of the blood in the vessel con-

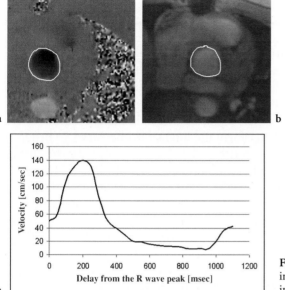

a

b

c

Fig. 3.7 a-c. Flow analysis with PC images (**a**) PC image; (**b**) anatomical image; (**c**) velocity vs time plot

sidered. In some cases it is advisable to define a reference area far away from the vessel in order to normalize the amplitude of the signal detected in relation to variations in background intensity. This operation is particularly important when making measurements on vessels close to the heart where the baseline signal may be subject to oscillations due to cardiac motion.

Once the value of the velocity has been extracted for each temporal instant, we can obtain graphs on the velocity itself, flow, and volume. Indeed, by knowing the area of the vessel through the contours defined earlier, and the blood velocity through the analysis of grey levels, it is possible to derive the volume that passes through the vessel over the unit of time, and thus, the actual flow. Figure 3.7 illustrates a typical graph of blood velocity over time, measured on PC images. Similar graphs can be obtained for volume also.

3.6 Measures of myocardial perfusion

The use of cardiac MR in evaluating myocardial perfusion is made possible by the use of paramagnetic contrast mediums and the relationship between their concentrations in the myocardium and signal intensity over time. To this purpose a set of parallel sections of the left ventricle are acquired over time (typically three every R-R interval) during the passage of the contrast medium – generally gadolinium based. The acquisition is synchronized with ECG to acquire all the images in the diastolic phase. Myocardial perfusion is measured by evaluating the dynamic changes of the magnetic properties of the wall caused by the presence of the contrast medium. In particular, after the injection of the contrast medium, an increase of signal intensity is detected in the cavity of the right ventricle first, then in the cavity of the left one, and finally in the wall. Apart from the visual analysis of eventual perfusion defects, it is possible to perform a quantitative analysis through the use of proper software. The method is based on the extraction of the intensity vs time curves (I/T) from a region of the myocardium and from the ventricular cavity, which is considered representative of the medium input function. Considering a certain section, the average value of the signal in a certain area is measured for each time frame, which all together form the intensity/time curve. In order to compensate any spatial variations in the signal's baseline intensity, the curves are normalized to the value measured before the arrival of the contrast medium. Various parameters can be extracted from the curve, such as slope, peak time, integrals, etc. Given the kinetic characteristics of the contrast medium in use in cardiovascular MR, the most representative parameter is the slope, which is usually normalized to the maximum slope of the input function [8-10]. Figure 3.8 illustrates from left to right, a typical I/T curve extracted from the left ventricle cavity and the I/T curve extracted from the myocardium of healthy heart. The slope of the line, which approximates the curve in the point of maximum inclination, represents the diagnostic index extracted.

One of the fundamental issues to address here is represented by the misalignment of the images in the time sequence. In fact, even if the acquisition is performed with the breath-hold technique, the patient's movements often cause a misaligning of the images, which produces artifacts on the I/T curve since the same geometrical location no longer corresponds to the same anatomical location. Indeed, the programs for quantitative analysis of myocardial perfusion images often include tools for automatic realignment. In gener-

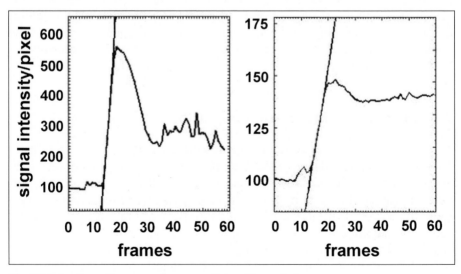

Fig. 3.8. Intensity vs. time curves for myocardial cardiac perfusion

al the steps in quantitative analysis of MR perfusion images may be summarized as follows:

1. The user performs the realignment of the images, a procedure known as registration. Usually, an area corresponding to the left ventricle is selected from the global image, and the automatic registration starts.
2. The user defines the limits of the ventricular wall on an image of the temporal sequence, usually the one in which the ventricle is best defined. The two edges (endocardium and epicardium) are copied and pasted over to all the temporal frames. If the registration was successful then the edges match on all the images of the time sequence, otherwise the edges must be corrected manually.
3. The myocardium is divided into ROIs. The user establishes a reference marker, for example the anterior intersection of the right and left ventricle walls, and establishes a number of radial and angular divisions. The subdivision of the myocardium is performed automatically and the I/T curves for each ROI are extracted. Figure 3.9 illustrates two example of automatic subdivision of the myocardium.

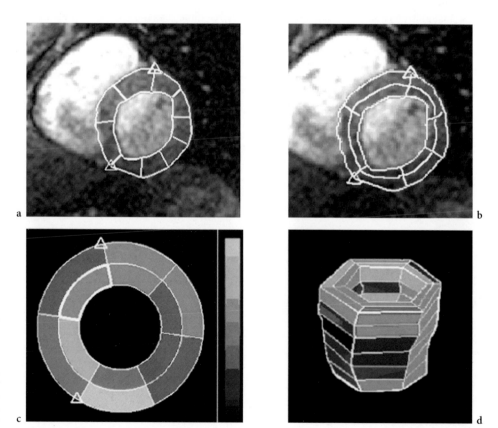

Fig. 3.9 a-d. Two examples of myocardial segmentation (**a, b**) and 2D (**c**) and 3D (**d**) perfusion maps

4. The parameters extracted from the curves are viewed through colored maps in which the color intensity corresponds to a value of the perfusion index chosen (see Fig. 3.9). The value of the indices can be saved for future analyses.
5. The same procedure may be repeated on a different slice.
6. If more than one slice is examined, we can obtain a 3D visualization of the perfusion indices (see Fig. 3.9).

References

1. Digital Imaging and Communication in Medicine (DICOM) Set. ACR-NEMA. Rosslyn, VA, USA
2. Russ John C. (ed) (1999) The Image Processing Handbook. 3rd ed. CRC Press
3. Barillot C (1993) Surface and volume rendering techniques to display 3D data. IEEE Eng Med and Biol 12:111-119
4. Pommert A, Pflesser B, Riemer M et al (1994) Advances in medical volume visualization state of art report Eurographics '94, Vol. E694STAR, 111-139
5. Foley JD, van Dam A, Feiner SK, Hughes JF, Phillips RL (1993) Introduction to computer graphics. Addison-Wesley
6. Frangi AF, Niessen WJ, Viergever MA (2001) Three-dimensional modeling for functional analysis of cardiac images: a review. IEEE Trans Med Imaging 20:2-25
7. Santarelli MF, Positano V, Michelassi C, Lombardi M, Landini L (2003) Automated cardiac MR image segmentation: theory and measurement evaluation. Med Eng Phys 25:149-159
8. Schwitter J, Nanz D, Kneifel S et al (2001) Assessment of myocardial perfusion in coronary artery disease by magnetic resonance: a comparison with positron emission tomography and coronary angiography. Circulation 103:2230-2235
9. Wilke N, Jerosch-Herold M (1998) Assessing myocardial perfusion in coronary artery disease with magnetic resonance first-pass imaging. Cardiol Clin 16:1227-1246
10. Positano V, Santarelli MF, Landini L (2003) Automatic characterization of myocardial perfusion in contrast enhanced MRI. EURASIP Journal on Applied Signal Processing 5:413-422

4 Contrast agents in cardiovascular magnetic resonance

Massimo Lombardi, Virna Zampa

4.1 General characteristics

The contrast agents used in Magnetic Resonance Imaging (MRI) feature some peculiarities that distinguish them from the agents used in other imaging techniques. Their most original characteristic is that they are indirect contrast agents, in the sense that the molecules of the contrast alter the magnetization state of the surrounding protons, which are the only atoms competing for the formation of the images. The interaction between the molecules of the contrast and the protons becomes visible with the alteration of the relaxation times T_1 and T_2 of the ^1H nuclei that are within a 100 nm distance from the molecule of the contrast medium (Fig. 4.1). The alteration of the relaxation times is exploited to increase the contrast both between tissues and between the regions with contrast medium and those without (or less enriched regions) within the same tissue. According to whether the longitudinal (T_1) or transverse (T_2) relaxation is more affected, we distinguish between relaxation agents and susceptibility agents. The first cause a shortening in relaxation time T_1 and induce a positive enhancement of the signal in T_1-weighted images and are therefore identified as positive contrast agents. The latter act by creating a local lack of homogeneity in the magnetic field at a macroscopic level which induces a marked fluctuation of the magnetic momentum between the blood and intracellular compartments, causing a shortening of T_2^* of the neighboring ^1H nuclei, thus determining a decrease in signal. Hence the term of negative contrast agents.

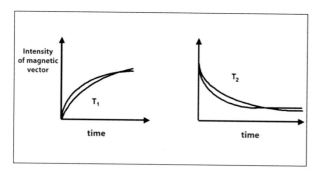

Fig. 4.1. The curve on the left shows the effect of the contrast agent on longitudinal relaxation time, on the right the effect on the transversal relaxation time. The presence of the contrast agent induces a much quicker recovery of base magnetization in both T_1 and T_2 (downward shift of the curve entity of magnetic vector/time)

It must however be said that, although this classification is still in use, it is now widely acknowledged that the phenomenon varies according to the dosage of the contrast medium and to the type of sequence used.

For example, let us consider the paramagnetic substances such as the Gd complexes, which are traditionally included in the group of positive agents; when these substances are present in low concentrations, they determine an increase in the signal of T1-weighted images; while when they are in high concentrations they determine a decrease in signal because of the prevailing effect of T2* over the signal detected (Fig. 4.2).

Among the susceptibility agents, there are microcrystals of ferrous oxide and dysprosium-based agents (such as DY-DTPA-BMA), which principally act on the relaxation time T2.

It must be underlined that with the acquisition techniques in use today, cardiovascular MRI exclusively employs the association between positive contrast agents and the sequences that generate T1-weighted images.

Another way by which contrasts are classified is linked to their behavior in the magnetic field; therefore, we distinguish diamagnetic, paramagnetic, ferromagnetic, and superparamagnetic contrast agents.

Diamagnetic substances do not have unpaired electrons in their outer orbital and, therefore, do not have a magnetic momentum (ratio of induced magnetization inside the material over the external magnetic field) and are not used in clinical settings.

Paramagnetic substances (gadolinium, manganese, dysprosium), the most used in MRI today [1-5], have one or more unpaired electrons in the outer orbitals. These electrons generate local fluctuating magnetic fields that determine a non-null magnetic momentum once they are immersed into a stationary magnetic field. This magnetic momentum is nulled when the paramagnetic substance is removed from the magnetic field. The most utilized paramagnetic substances are the lanthanides, among which the most used is

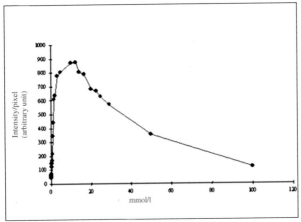

Fig. 4.2. The relation between concentration of the contrast agent and signal intensity in an *in vitro* experiment employing a T1 sequence with a short TR (10 msec). For relatively small changes in concentration, the relation remains linear until a plateau is reached a further increases of concentration above a threshold value there is a consequent fall in signal (susceptibility effect)

gadolinium – the first to be employed for this purpose thanks to the intuition of H. Weinman. Gadolinium (Gd) has 7 unpaired electrons in its last orbital and thus has a strong magnetic field. By its nature, it is extremely toxic and is, therefore, chelated with a molecule that binds it very tightly into a very low toxic product. The first chelating agent for Gd was DTPA (diethylene-tri-amine-pentaacetic acid). Gd-DTPA has long been the only agent on the market; however in recent years the number of contrast agents containing lanthanides, and in particular gadolinium, together with different chelating substances, has increased symmetrically with the growth of MRI. The chelating agent represents the main determinant of the pharmacokinetics, the ionization and the relaxivity of the molecule (Fig. 4.3a-c).

Ferromagnetic and superparamagnetic agents are composed of micro-crystals of ferrous oxide: the first by larger particles, the second by smaller ones.

Iron itself (Fe III) is a weak paramagnetic ion, and can form ferrous oxide crystals ($FeO\text{-}Fe_2O_3$), also called magnetite, when bonded to a bivalent ion (Fe II). A ferromagnetic substance has the characteristic of maintaining the magnetic momentum acquired during exposition to a strong stationary

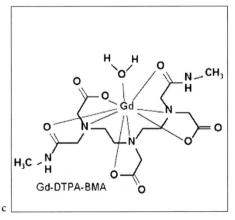

Fig. 4.3 a-c. Examples of molecules of three Gd-based contrast agents that differ for how Gd is chelated inside the molecule; the shell-like structure of the molecule avoids any contact between the Gd ion and the tissue components

magnetic field also after the removal from the field. Superparamagnetic substances (nanometric-sized microcrystals) acquire once more reversibility characteristics in consequence of the microscopic dimension itself. Ferromagnetic substances are non-soluble and are administered in an aqueous suspension. Their atoms have unpaired electrons but are not used in cardiovascular MRI.

Superparamagnetic substances share the common characteristic of having a strong electromagnetic momentum and of influencing the atoms of hydrogen within a radius that is 100 times larger than that influenced by other paramagnetic substances (10 micrometers). Compared to paramagnetic agents, these contrast agents can be used in much smaller concentrations (about 1/10th the usual gadolinium based contrast agents).

The strong effect produced on proton magnetization by these substances influences the relaxation of both T_1 and T_2^*. When these superparamagnetic molecules are circulating in the blood stream and suspended in the plasma they can manifest a strong contrast effect in T_1-weighed sequences. These substances are then eliminated in a few hours through the endothelial reticular system.

Superparamagnetic contrast agents have also been proposed for studies on the cardiovascular system with satisfying results both in animal and human studies [6-8]. Yet these preliminary experiences are still limited to the research labs.

Another important classification of contrast agents in MRI is linked to their pharmacokinetics, and particularly to their distribution throughout compartments. Hence, the division into: multi-compartmental or interstitial distribution agents, mono-compartmental or intravascular distribution agents, and intracellular or organ-specific agents.

Given that there are basically 4 compartments at the myocardial level (plasma, blood cells, interstitium, and tissue cells), the extracellular agents have low molecular weights, are hydro-soluble, have a rapid distribution from plasma to interstitial space and are rapidly eliminated (mainly through the kidney). Although these agents have a low molecular weight, they do not penetrate significantly into the cellular structures. At present they are the only agents used in clinical routine since they are the only ones available on the market for the cardiovascular apparatus [1-5]. However, they present the inconvenience of not keeping within a single compartment of a tissue. Indeed, the permeability of the spaces between endothelial cells (100-200 Å) allows their rapid transfer to the interstitial level with a high partitioning coefficient. Therefore, the enhancement of the signal depends on the contrast medium both distributed intravascularly and at an interstitial level (Fig. 4.4a).

Intravascular contrast agents (or blood pool agents) stay confined within the plasma without entering the extravascular compartment. The use of these agents provides information relative to haematic tissue volume, absolute blood flow, and endothelial permeability, which cannot be obtained using extra-cellular agents (Fig. 4.4b).

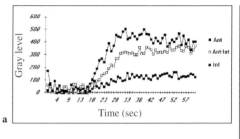
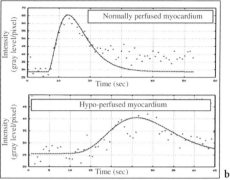

a

b

Fig. 4.4 a, b. (a) Time/intensity curves of the first passage of the contrast medium through the myocardium, in all cases either it be or normally perfused tissues (Ant = anterior myocardial wall, Ant-lat = anterior-lateral myocardial wall) of hypoperfused tissue (Inf = inferior myocardial wall), once the signal has reached a peak concentration the signal remains high, indicating the presence of the agent within the myocardium, as a result of the presence of the agent within the interstitium, which begins after a few heart beats and remains up to the equilibrium phase. (b) Time-intensity curves obtained in an animal model of myocardial perfusion, using ferrous oxide as a contrast agent with intravascular behavior. It can be noticed that there is a rapid washout of the agent prior to the equilibrium phase both in the case of normally perfused tissue and hypoperfused tissue

Blood-pool contrast agents have been obtained using macromolecules containing gadolinium, with molecular weights such that confine the molecule within the vessels, yet allowing them to be eliminated through the kidney glomerules. Molecules such as Gd-DTPA-albumine, Gd-DTPA-destrane, Gd-DTPA polylysine have been used. Yet the main drawback remains the long half-life (Gd-DTPA-destrane has an half-life of several hours) that causes a larger risk for toxicity and immunological reactions.

Finally, also microcrystals of ferrous oxide have been utilized: coated with polymeric structures of particular sizes, they stay confined to the vessels before they are eliminated by the endothelial reticular system of the liver, spleen, and bone marrow.

As for the blood-pool contrast agents, studies of phase II and III are being completed with favorable results (see Paragraph 7.3.2).

4.2 Behavior of extra-vascular contrast agents at myocardial level

The local concentration of extravascular contrast agents with low molecular weight at the cardiac level are remarkably affected by the changes in distribution volumes, which in turn are affected by the tissue's physiopathological status – as occurs for example in the case of the loss of compartmentalization following the destruction of the cell membrane. The pharmacogentic characteristics of Gd-DTPA have been studied in an animal model characterized by a precisely defined ischemic territory [9] where the kinetics of the contrast medium can be modelled according to Kety's modified model [9-12]:

$$[Gd\text{-}DTPA]_i(t) = FE\sum_{o}^{t}[Gd\text{-}DTPA]_a(\tau)\cdot e^{FE/\lambda(t-\tau)d\tau}$$

where F is the regional perfusion, E is the extraction fraction of the Gd-DTPA, [Gd-DTPA] is the concentration of the arterial (a) and tissue (i) contrast medium, and λ is the partition coefficient for Gd-DTPA. In agreement with this equation, if the input of the arterial function is kept constant so that the concentration of tissue and blood Gd-DTPA is in equilibrium, then λ will be the ratio between the tissue and arterial concentrations of Gd-DTPA. If these considerations are true, an increase in distribution volume – the effect of the loss of ischemic myocardial cell-membrane integrity – origins an increased mass of Gd-DPTA per tissue-mass unit, which results in a higher increase of the signal compared to normal tissue in T1-weighed images. It is apparent that whenever the regional perfusion (F) is altered or unbalanced, the local kinetics of the contrast medium are heavily affected. Figure 4.4a shows the intensity vs time curves (signal intensity that is in turn a function of the local concentration of the contrast medium). It is apparent that once the intensity plateau is reached, the washout is influenced by the presence of the contrast medium within the interstitial space, where during this first phase it is distributed according to the principles mentioned above.

Another application that derives from other pharmacokinetic considerations on low molecular weight contrast agents has recently become widespread. In presence of necrotic myocardium and during the phase of post-ischemic reparation, severe structural alterations occur (increase of collagen component, alterations of local perfusion, etc.) and determine an accumulation and delayed contrast medium washout. The result is a wide difference in the concentration of the contrast medium in the necrotic and non-necrotic tissue, which reaches the maximum differential after 10-15 minutes from the i.v. administration. By utilizing adequate acquisition techniques, the diverse concentration in necrotic and non-necrotic (hence viable) tissues is amplified (see Paragraph 7.3.3).

4.3 Distinctive behavior of intravascular contrast agents at myocardial level

In the study of myocardial perfusion based on the first pass technique, one of the implicit problems in the use of blood-pool contrast agents is the fact that the concentration (number of molecules per volume unit) is inevitably

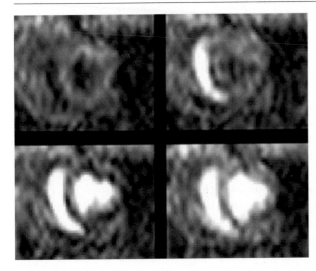

Fig. 4.5. Myocardial perfusion study performed with an intravascular contrast agent (iron dioxide) in an animal model

reduced as compared to the extra-cellular agents, which makes the signal weaker (Fig. 4.5) as compared to the enhancement effect obtained with a standard dosage of extra-cellular contrast agents (Fig. 4.6). Moreover, this problem seems to be overcome through the increased effectiveness in terms of relaxivity (that is, the capacity of modifying the T1 of the neighboring protons) of the more recent intravascular contrast agents. The first indications as to the use of intravascular contrast agents in the visualization of the vessels appear univocally positive [13].

In reality the concept of indirect contrast agents has much more complex implications. For example, we must consider that hydrogen atoms in water – notwithstanding their compartment of origin (red blood cells, plasma, inter-

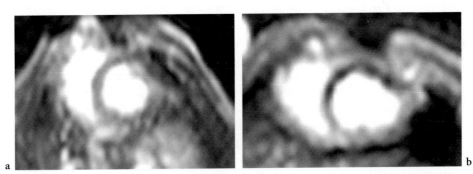

Fig. 4.6 a, b. Study of myocardial perfusion performed with an extravascular contrast agent (gadodiamide) in an animal model. The wide ischemic territory can be well appreciated in figure (**b**) as a region of reduced signal intensity, pertaining to the anterior descending coronary artery, if compared with the other myocardial regions

stitium or tissue cells) – change their compartment between the intracellular space and the interstitial space with a rate of 8-27 times per sec, and about 7 times per sec between the interstitium and the plasma. Therefore, there are about 40 water exchanges between the blood and the interstitium at each single passage through the capillaries. Such frequency of water exchanges presupposes movements within times shorter than those required for proton relaxation that the agents cause in the ^1H atoms. Thus the effect of the contrast agents largely depends on the concentration in the voxels but is, at least in part, independent from the distribution of the contrast medium in the voxel and thus independent from its compartmentalization. The above is especially true in the case of paramagnetic contrast agents. In the case of superparamagnetic contrasts agents that induce distortion of the magnetic field only in the point where they create a lack of homogeneity in the magnetic distribution, their action is not only markedly influenced by the concentration, but also by the compartmentalization inside the voxel. If, for example, as a consequence of a heart attack the compartmentalization between plasma, interstitium and the cells (being lysated) is lost, there will be a reduced contrast effect (in the perfusion images) caused by these agents, since the expanded volume of distribution will lessen the influence of these compounds on the magnetic susceptibility.

These movements of water protons between compartments significantly influence the signal variations induced by the contrast agents and thus must be considered, and perhaps corrected, from a modellistic point of view, when one passes to a semi-quantitative or quantitative evaluation of regional perfusion distribution [14].

All the first pass acquisition techniques must overcome the above problem of the water exchange between vasculature and interstitium. The contrast medium acts indirectly through its effect on the signal coming from the hydrogen nuclei, therefore the phenomenon of water exchange through different compartments can cause problems relative to the evaluation of the presence of the contrast medium in the vessels of the tissue under examination. Hence, even if the contrast medium is confined to the vascular compartment where it has a reducing effect on T1, because of the very exchange of water molecules between vessels and insterstitium, we can obtain magnetization outside the compartment where the proton had contact with the contrast medium, and thus a contamination of the signal coming from other compartments. The relaxation time T1 of a voxel in which there are several distinct compartments depends indeed, not only on the characteristic T1 of the given compartment, but also on the water exchange between the various compartments. This phenomenon can interfere with the quantification of the flow when using a no-exchange model that does not foresee exchanges. In such cases, the hematic volume can be overestimated, which can consequently lead to an erroneous assessment of regional perfusion.

The opposite situation would occur with models that take into account fast exchanges. However, by using a sequence prepared with a saturation recovery pulse performed setting a short TR (<4 ms) and a wide flip angle (>20°) a situation comparable to the non-exchange condition can be obtained.

4.4 Intracellular or organ-specific contrast agents

Noteworthy of mention are the intracellular or organ-specific contrast agents that can penetrate cells. Manganese (Mn), a paramagnetic contrast medium, can be towed inside cells through the calcium channels of myocardiocytes. However, free Mn is highly toxic and perhaps even teratogenic. The only Mn-based contrast medium on the market is Mn-DPDP (Mn-dipyridoxal diphosphate), the use of which is limited to studies on hepatic imaging. To date, the necessity of administering high dosages to increase the myocardial signal has limited its use in humans, at least for what concerns the cardiovascular district.

4.5 Guide to the use of contrast agents in cardiovascular magnetic resonance

In cardiologic studies, contrast agents are generally employed on a routine basis for three purposes: inducing or excluding the enhancement of pathologic structures (e.g. neoplastic masses, thrombotic formations), gaining diagnostic benefits in agreement with what might be defined as the semiotics of "classic" magnetic resonance; to study myocardial viability [15]; and assess myocardial perfusion [16]. For details on the use of the contrast agents we invite the reader to the pertaining chapters.

In the case of angiography with magnetic resonance (MRA) we can briefly say that the use of contrast agents is practically unavoidable in all districts – with the exception of intracranial vessels – also when, as in the case of the thoracic aorta, the images that can be obtained with static and dynamic images already offer a wealth of diagnostic information. In the case of Contrast Enhanced Magnetic Resonance Angiography (CEMRA) there are a few pragmatic principles (see pertaining chapters) that guide the choice on the dosage and velocity of administration, along with the presupposition that the shortening effect on T1 is a function of the local concentration (Fig. 4.7) that can be reached only with high dosages and rapid administration.

The use of contrast agents with intravascular distribution (blood-pool) seems quite promising for MRA in that these agents have a better Contrast-to-Noise Ratio (CNR) than the extravascular ones. However, the use of such contrast agents is not void of negative effects, among which their permanence

Effect on T_1 :
$$\frac{1}{T_1 post} = \frac{1}{T_1 pre} + r_1 \cdot c$$

Effect on T_2 :
$$\frac{1}{T_2 post} = \frac{1}{T_2 pre} + r_2 \cdot c$$

Fig. 4.7. The ratio linking the concentration of the contrast agent to the length of relaxation times T1 and T2 (post: after administration, pre: before administration of the contrast agent, r1: relaxility pertaining T1, r2: relaxility pertaining to T2, c: concentration of contrast agent)

within the venous system, which inevitably contaminates the images obtained at the equilibrium state. Yet it is early to understand what the impact of the use of blood-pool agents in MRA will be and whether such use will involve substantial changes in techniques and acquisition sequences.

4.6 Toxicity of contrast agents in magnetic resonance

This is an issue of particular interest especially for MRA. In fact, MRA employs higher volumes of contrast medium (the maximum limit that should not be exceeded is 4 mmol/kg corresponding to 8 ml of contrast medium 0.05 mmol every 10 kg of body weight) with the purpose of obtaining the shortest T1 possible and having the optimal contrast with the surrounding structures that are still almost void, of contrast medium. Generally, however, lower dosages of about 0.2-0.3 mmol/kg are used.

The toxicity of the contrast agents used in MRI (at least those in use today, employed in over a million of individuals) has been shown to be extremely low as to the major collateral effects (very few documented cases of severe idiosyncrasy or lethal effects) and minor effects (skin rashes, itching, etc.). For this reason the agents are administered without any particular patient preparation or preliminary check-ups. The low toxicity is explained, among other reasons, by the high molecular stability (dissociation constant) that remains practically unchanged all the way until the elimination of the molecules through the kidney and through the liver (the latter representing 5-10% of the whole ammount administered) (Fig. 4.8), without freeing Gd in ionic, and thus toxic form. This high stability remains unchanged for many hours after administration. As for the iodate contrast agents, also in this family of contrast agents for magnetic resonance, many non-ionic molecules for reducing toxicity have been developed. Low toxicity apart, the true advantage remains however in general quite modest, although useful when dealing with patients with a pluri-allergic status.

A completely different issue is the use of these agents in patients with kidney failure, since the kidney is the main path for elimination of the medium.

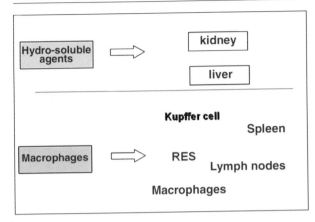

Fig. 4.8. Simplified diagram of the elimination/washout of the contrast agent from the body. Top of figure refers to elimination of hydro-soluble molecules (mainly through the kidney) bottom refers to particles that cannot filtrate through glomerular structures. RES = Reticulo Endothelial System

Yet, there are studies that document their usability in patients with creatinine plasmatic levels >5 mg/dl or, however, with a reduction of creatinine clearance below 30 ml/min [17-24]. Therefore, in clinical practice, these patients too, are administered high volumes of contrast medium (up to 0.4 mmol/kg) without particular precautions.

4.7 Way of administration

Intravenous administration of contrast agents can be performed manually in the case of tumor masses or in case of viability studies (delayed enhancement), but requires a pressure injector in all other cases. In the case of high volumes, as for the MRA exam (30-50 ml of contrast agents), there are no precise guidelines regulating the injection rate since every scanner is different with its own acquisition time procedure. Consequently, the velocity of infusion must be optimized in function of the equipment's rapidity of acquisition. Some studies however indicate an injection velocity of 2 and 4 ml/sec. In the case of the study of myocardial perfusion, the aim is to have the bolus arrive in the left sections of the heart as compact as possible, so as to obtain an input function characterized by a rapid rise and minimize the variability between injections. For perfusion studies, it is pragmatically advisable not to exceed the injection time of 3 seconds, whatever the volume administered. Elevated flows obviously require the positioning of a tube of adequate dimensions certified or tested for such flow levels. The suggestion is just as trivial as useful! For the dosage in single applications we invite the reader to the chapters on the specific organ.

References

1. Amparo EG, Higgins CB, Farmer D, Gasmu G, MacNamara M (1984) Gated MRI of cardiac

and paracardiac masses: initial experience. AJR 143:1151-1156

2. Barakos JA, Brown JJ, Higgins CB (1989) MR imaging of secondary cardiac and paracardiac lesions. AJR 153:47-50

3. Gomes AS, Lois JF, Child JS, Bown K, Batra P (1987) Cardiac tumors and thrombus: evaluation with MR imaging. AJR 149:895-899

4. Lund JT, Ehman RL, Julsrud PR, Sinak LJ, Tajik AJ (1989) Cardiac masses: assessment by MR imaging. AJR 152:469-473

5. Prince MR (1994) Gadolinium-enhanced MR aortography. Radiology 191:155-164

6. Canet E, Revel D, Forrat R et al (1993) Superparamagnetic iron oxide particles and positive enhancement for myocardial perfusion studies assessed by subsecond T1-weighted MRI. Magn Reson Med 11:1139-1145

7. Stillman AE et al (1996) Ultrasmall superparamagnetic iron oxide to enhance MRA of the renal and coronary arteries: studies in human patients. J Comput Assist Tomogr 20:51-55

8. Stillman AE (2001) New contrast agents for cardiovascular MRI and MRA. Int J Cardiovasc Imaging 17:471-472

9. De Roos A, Van Rossum AC, Van der Wall EE et al (1989) Reperfused and non reperfused myocardial infarction: potential of Gd-DTPA enhanced MR imaging. Radiology 172:717-720

10. Pereira RS, Prato FS, Wisenberg G, Sykes J (1996) The determination of myocardial viability using Gd-DTPA in a canine model of acute myocardial ischemia and reperfusion. Magn Reson Med 36:684-693

11. Diesbourg LD, Proat FS, Wisemberg G et al (1992) Quantification of myocardial blood flow and extracellular volumes using a bolus injection of Gd-DTPA: kinetic modelling in canine ischemic disease. Magn Reson Med 23:239-253

12. Larsson HBW, Stubgaard M, Søndergaard L, Henriksen O (1994) In vivo quantification of the unidirectional influx constant for Gd-DTPA diffusion across the myocardial capillaries with MR imaging. J Magn Reson Imaging 4:433-440

13. Kroft LJ, De Roos A (1999) Blood pool contrast agents for cardiovascular MR imaging. J Magn Reson Imaging 10:395-403

14. Lombardi M, Jones RA, Westby J et al (1997) MRI for the evaluation of regional myocardial perfusion in an experimental animal model. J Magn Reson Imaging 7:987-995

15. Kim RJ, Fieno DS, Parrish TB et al (1999) Relationship of MRI delayed contrast enhancement to irreversible injury, infarct age, and contractile function. Circulation 100:1992-2002

16. Wilke N, Simm C, Zhang J et al (1993) Contrast-enhanced first pass myocardial perfusion imaging: correlation between myocardial blood flow in dogs at rest and during hyperemia. Magn Reson Med 29:485-497

17. Tombach B, Bremer C, Reimer P et al (2002) Using highly concentrated gadobutrol as an MR contrast agent in patients also requiring hemodialysis: safety and dialysability. Am J Roentgenol 178:105-109

18. Rai AT, Hogg JP (2001) Persistence of gadolinium in CSF: a diagnostic pitfall in patients with end-stage renal disease. Am J Neuroradiol 22:1357-1361

19. Tombach B, Bremer C, Reimer P et al (2001) Renal tolerance of a neutral gadolinium chelate (gadobutrol) in patients with chronic renal failure: results of a randomized study. Radiology 218:651-657

20. Townsend RR, Cohen DL, Katholi R et al (2000) Safety of intravenous gadolinium (Gd-BOPTA) infusion in patients with renal insufficiency. Am J Kidney Dis 36:1207-1212

21. Swan SK, Lambrecht LJ, Townsend R et al (1999) Safety and pharmacokinetic profile of gadobenate dimeglumine in subjects with renal impairment. Invest Radiol 34:443-448

22. Joffe P, Thomsen HS, Meusel M (1998) Pharmacokinetics of gadodiamide injection in patients with severe renal insufficiency and patients undergoing hemodialysis or continu-

ous ambulatory peritoneal dialysis. Acad Radiol 5:491-502

23. Arsenault TM, King BF, Marsh JW Jr et al (1996) Systemic gadolinium toxicity in patients with renal insufficiency and renal failure: retrospective analysis of an initial experience. Mayo Clin Proc 71:1150-1154

24. Haustein J, Niendorf HP, Krestin G et al (1992) Renal tolerance of gadolinium-DTPA/dimeglumine in patients with chronic renal failure. Invest Radiol 27:153-156

5   Intracranial vascular district

Raffaello Canapicchi, Francesco Lombardo, Fabio Scazzeri, Domenico Montanaro

5.1 Introduction

The diagnosis of cerebral pathology currently employs Computed Tomography (CT), Digital Subtraction Angiography (DSA) and Magnetic Resonance Imaging (MRI). The latter plays an important role as it provides structural information through the study of the encephalic parenchyma, and functional information through the analysis of molecular motion (diffusion), cell metabolism (spectroscopy), and blood flow (perfusion and MR Angiography – MRA).

Although DSA is an invasive and expensive technique, it is still considered irreplaceable in image diagnostics of many cerebro-vascular pathologies. However, the implementation of fast sequences and of sophisticated application software on high-field MR equipment today allows, to obtain vascular images iconographically similar to those of DSA and with a sufficient spatial resolution in a non-invasive and relatively inexpensive way.

Hence, MRA has gained its place among the neuroradiologist's diagnostic tools and is successfully gaining ground in clinical practice.

This chapter will deal with the potential and the limits of MRA methodologies in the neuroradiological assessment of major intra-cranial vascular lesions; for didactic purposes MRA types will be treated based on the distinction between arterial and venous abnormalities. For many of these abnormalities, DSA is still the method of choice, although MRA is increasingly being considered, as new sequences are being provided by technological progress.

Here, the technical aspects of MRA will not be treated as they have already been approached in the previous chapters.

5.2 Arterial compartment

5.2.1 Anatomical variants and persistence of fetal anastomoses

The circle of Willis connects the arterial vessels of the base of the skull and forms the main way for collateral flow in the case of obstructive pathology of the large cerebro-ascending arterial trunks. Unfortunately, the circle is complete only in 21% of cases, which explains the variability of clinical presentation (which can go from a simple transient ischemic attack to a definitive hemi-plegia), for example, in the case of a carotid occlusion [1].

Therefore, in the occurence of an ischemic event, knowing the morphology of the circle can be useful. In approximately 10% of cases, the supra-optic tract of the anterior cerebral a. (A1) is missing or hypoplasic with supply of the pericallosal a. from the anterior communicating a. (Fig. 5.1a).

In 20% of individuals the communicating posterior a. arises from the carotid siphon (fetal origin) and continues directly in the posterior cerebral a. with absence or hypoplasia of its premesencephalic tract [2] (Fig 5.1b). Asymmetry between the two vertebral aa, with one side dominating over the other, is frequent.

The most common form of persistent fetal anastomosis (0.55% of cases) is the primitive trigeminal artery, and derives from the missed involution of the embryonic circulation system. Less frequent are the hypoglossal a., the ophthalmic a., and the proatlantal a. [3]. The primitive trigeminal a. connects the intracavernous tract of the carotid siphon to the intermediate tract of the basilar a. at the point of origin of the trigeminal nerve (Fig. 5.1c). Often the proximal segment of the basilar a. is hypoplastic.

Less frequent anatomical variants are the duplication of the superior cerebellar a. (Fig. 5.1d), the fenestration of the basilar a., the azygos pericallosal a. (Fig 5.1a) [4].

The presence of such anatomic abnormalities can be detected in a simple way by adding a 3D Time of Flight (TOF) sequence to the MR structural study.

5.2.2 Arterial lumen abnormalities: steno-occlusion and ectasia

This group gathers luminal abnormalities of the intra-cranial portions of the cerebro-afferent arterial vessels and the consequences of the obstructive pathology of the extra-cranial arterial cerebro-afferent compartment on the intra-cranial circulation.

Atherosclerotic disease is the most frequent cause of arterial canalization damage, followed by dissections, vasculitis, dysplasia (fibro muscular dysplasia, moya-moya, carotid aplasia-hypoplasia), coagulopathies and extrinsic compressions (tumors).

Atheromas mostly affect arterial cerebro-afferent vessels in the extra-cranial district but also in the intra-cranial compartment, both directly and as a consequence of a number of pathologic situations (embolization, reduction in blood supply, and thereby O_2, in the designated territories). Atherosclerotic disease causes artery wall alterations that can lead to stenosis, ulceration, thrombosis or ectasia [5].

Stenosis of the main arterial trunks appears in MRA as a focal narrowing

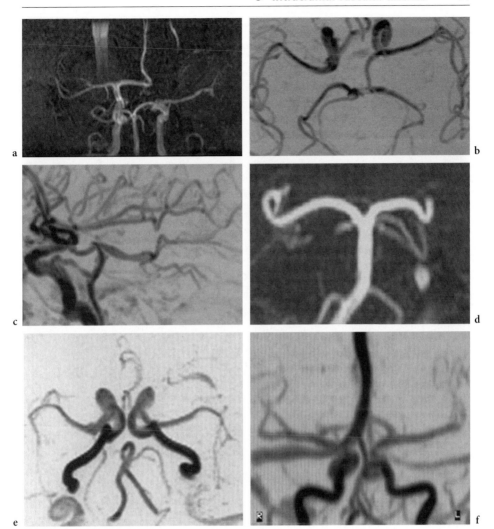

Fig. 5.1 a-f. (a) MRA, 3D TOF, MIP reconstruction, coronal view: unique pericallosal (Azygos) artery associated to hypoplasia of the left A1 tract; (b) MRA, 3D TOF, MIP reconstruction, axial view: fetal origin of the left posterior cerebral a. from the carotid siphon with hypoplasia of the pre-mesencefalic portion; (c) MRA, 3D TOF, MIP reconstruction, sagittal view: primitive trigeminal a. connecting the intrapetrosus segment of the left carotid siphon with the intermediate tract of the basilar a. (d) MPR of the partitions on the coronal plane: Fenestration of left superior cerebellar a.: double origin of the artery with fusion of the two branches in an unique peri-pontine branch. (e, f) Axial and coronal views, MRA, 3D PC: kissing carotids

of the flow signal delimited by smooth or irregular edges, with poststenotic apparent normalization. In the presurgical assessment of the extra-cranial carotid artery stenoses, the study of the intra-cranial circulation aims to exclude coexisting stenoses of the carotid siphon (tandem lesions) [6] which would contraindicate endarterectomy (Fig. 5.2a,b).

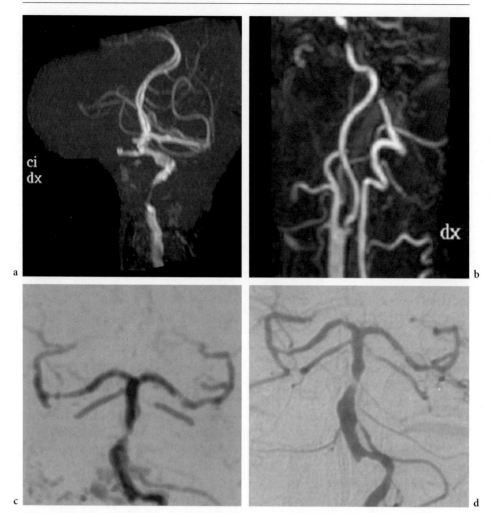

Fig. 5.2 a-d. (a) MRA, 3D TOF, Target MIP reconstruction: high degree stenosis of the intrapetrosus tract of the right internal carotid a. **(b)** Same case, 3D TOF + contrast agent, Target MIP reconstruction of the carotid a. and vertebral a.: stenosating ulcered plaque at the origin of the extra-cranial internal carotid a. Evidence of concomitant stenosis at the intrapetrosus tract (tandem lesion) **(c)** MRA, 3D TOF, Target MIP reconstruction: hemodynamic stenosis of the intermediate tract of the basilar a. with focal absence of flow signal **(d)** Same case: confirmation and better definition with DSA

Usually, the TOF sequence is employed, even if it overestimates the degree of stenosis due to saturation phenomena linked to turbulent flow appearing near the luminal stenosis, and to intravoxel phase dispersion. As these are more marked in the 2D TOF sequences, 3D is preferable as it has the further advantage of a better spatial resolution [7].

Stenoses over 70% of the lumen can appear as a focal absence of flow signal (Fig. 5.2c,d).

Lumen abnormalities are not easy to locate at the level of the petrous, cavernous and supraclinoid segments of the carotid siphon, as the course of the vessels is irregular and not perfectly orthogonal to the acquisition plane. This fact give rise to saturation phenomena artifacts that, simulating arterial lumen narrowing, may lead to diagnostic error. Generally, the signal loss of artifactual origin concerns both carotid siphons and is perfectly symmetrical; however, if there is any doubt concerning the morphology, it is recommended to rely on complementary sequences, such as the 2D Phase Contrast (PC) with the appropriate Velocity ENCoding (VENC) [8], or on the injection of a contrast agent (such as in the 3D TOF CEMRA sequence) that minimizes the inflow effect and exploits the T1 shortening caused by the Gd in the circulating blood [9] (Fig. 5.2a,b).

About 50% of severe ischemic events are due to thrombo-embolic occlusion of the internal carotid a. in its supraclinoid tract, of sylvian a. (main branch or first degree branching), or of posterior cerebral a. [10].

MRA, performed in the acute phase, has a diagnostic sensitivity close to 100% [11], therefore, in the case of stroke, it is recomended to complete the traditional MRI exam and the diffusion and perfusion sequences with a 3D TOF sequence.

Occlusion causes absence of signal inside the artery lumen being examined, generally with sharp edges, with the disappearance or reduction of flow in the territory of dependant supply, according to whether there are collateral circles or not, and to their extent. Much more difficult is the diagnosis in case of occlusion of the peripheral intra-cranial arterial branches. In fact, the ischemic oedema can slow down the flow in small vessels, causing a saturation phenomenon that obstacles their identification also in case of maintained lumen patency (Fig. 5.3a-c).

Also hemodynamically-significant stenoses of the carotids and basilar first-degree arterial branches appear as absence or marked focal decrease of flow signal [12] (Fig. 5.3d).

If the diagnosis of steno-occlusion is confirmed, the following step consists in the search for signs of any compensation by collateral vascular branches. This can be achieved by using either TOF sequences with selective positioning of presaturation bands, or – more simply and rapidly – 2D PC Phase Difference Processing (PDP) after choosing an appropriate VENC [13]. The circle of Willis and the ophtalmic aa. can be evaluated by juxtaposing two 1 cm-thick slabs at the cranial base.

This allows us to identify separately the direction of the flow according to the orientation of the single gradients. Indeed, in the image processed for evidencing the PDP, the flow oriented toward the versus of the gradient is codified with a high signal, while the opposite flow is codified with a low signal thus suggesting which arterial afferents are involved in the revascularizing the ischemic territory (Fig 5.4a-e).

Because MRA is a non-invasive procedure, it is suitable in follow-up for

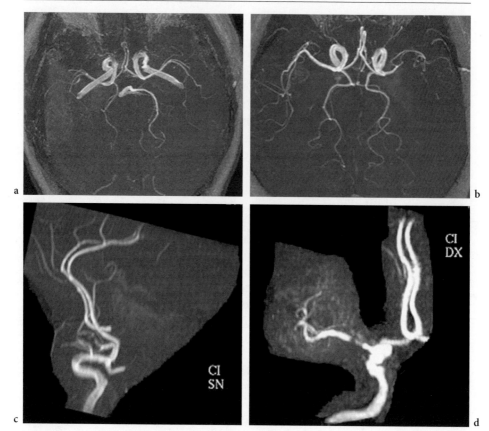

Fig. 5.3 a-d. (a) MRA, 3D TOF, MIP reconstruction, axial view. Right Temporal hemorrhagic infarction: the periferal sylvian branches are much less evident for saturation phenomena due to the
delayed flow. (b) MRA, 3D TOF, MIP reconstruction, axial view. Bare left sylvian tree for partial
occlusion. (c) Same case: MRA, 3D TOF, Target MIP sagittal view. Subtotal occlusion of the left sylvian a. (d) MRA, 3D TOF, Target MIP, coronal view : stenosis of the horizontal tract of the right sylvian a.

documenting the re-canalization after fibrinolytic therapy of an obstructed
arterial lumen.

In cases of vasculitis structural MRI has an important role in the diagnostic work-up demonstrating brain injury, but the same cannot be said for
MRA. In fact, the disease affects small vessels, causing multiple focal narrowing and ectasia which are hard to detect with the MRA techniques available
today [14]. Therefore, although the DSA does not reach 100% diagnostic sensitivity, it still remains the current standard of reference.

In vasculitis that involve also larger vessels (Takayasu syndrome) MRA
can result useful, but the findings are similar to those of atheromasic disease.

Atherosclerosis of the intra-cranial arterial district causes degeneration in
the tunica media, which may determine in elder patients ectasia and tortuosity of the vessels. The event may involve the whole main artery (dolico-ectasia)

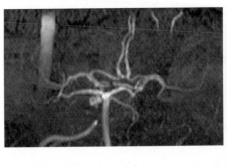

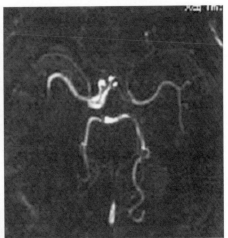

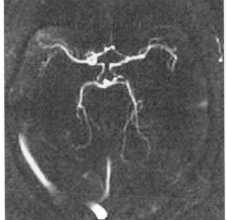

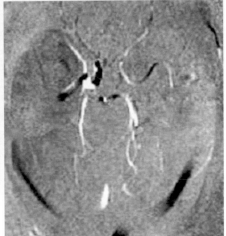

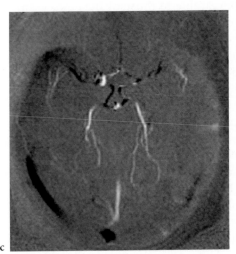

Fig. 5.4 a-e. (a) MRA, 3D TOF, MIP reconstruction, coronal view. Occlusion of the left extra-cranial internal carotid a. and preocclusive stenosis of the right carotid siphon. (b) Same case, MRA, 2D PC CDP VENC 80, axial view. Absence of flow signal of the left carotid siphon. Good representation of the intra-cranial vasculature. (c) Same case, MRA, 2D PC, PDP VENC 80, flow direction anterior/posterior. Inversion of flow direction in the Ophthalmic aa. and in the Posterior Communicants that contribute to the rehabitation of the intra-cranic carotidal circulation. (d) Occlusion of left Internal Carotid a., MRA, 2D PC, CDP VENC 80. Absence of flow signal of the left carotid siphon. Good representation of the intra-cranial vasculature. (e) Same case, MRA, 2D PC, PDP VENC 80 direction of flow gradient anterior/posterior. Inversion of flow direction in the left ophthalmic a. which appears hyperintense. Notice the contro-lateral a. appears hypointense the flow being regularly directed

or a portion of it (fusiform aneurysm). Dolico-ectasia more frequently involves the vertebro-basilar district and less often the carotid siphons [15].

The most informative MRA sequence is the 3D TOF. The affected artery becomes ectatic and elongated, with irregular walls due both to the presence of atheromasic plaques and to intramural hemorrhage and wall thrombi. This determines turbulence and slowing of the flow, with a focal signal loss which is difficult to differentiate from a lumen narrowing. Therefore, for diagnostic purposes, the use of PC sequences or contrast agents may be required to complete the study [16].

The ectatic carotid siphons can run medially within the sella turcica, instead of coursing laterally along the carotid sulcus, approaching the median line and assuming the so called aspect of "kissing carotids" (Fig. 5.1e,f).

Fusiform aneurysms most often have an atheromasic origin. Less frequent origins are collagenopathies and viral infections (chicken pox, HIV). They involve the basilar a., where MRA detects a focal elongated arterial ectasia with variable extension that does not usually involve the main branches. Inside the lumen there are haematic clots that slow down the flow and cause turbulences that originate signal loss due to spin saturation and intravoxel phase dispersion when 3D TOF sequences are used (Fig. 5.5a,b). The use of contrast agents does not always solve the problem because the signal emitted by the meta-hemoglobin in the clot overlaps the signal emitted by blood flow and can be responsible for false negatives. More reliable information can be obtained with PC sequences but the exam of choice for the most accurate balance is still the DSA.

Arterial dissection causes 10-15% of ischemic strokes occurring among young adults.

Intra-cranial dissection of arteries is often traumatic in origin and is mostly localized at the supra-clinoid carotid siphons, distal segments of vertebral aa, and basilar a.

The MRI and MRA findings are comparable to those of the extra-cranial cerebro-afferent arteries but are more difficult to recognize because of the small size and tortuosity of the vessels.

The moya-moya syndrome is a vascular dysplasia characterized by a progressive occlusion of the intra-cranial arteries, with unusual collateral compensative circulation coming from lepto-meningeal, trans-dural, lenticulostriate and thalamus-perforating anastomoses. The latter take on the aspect of a cigarette smoke puff (in Japanese moya-moya). The syndrome can affect both children and adults and may be associated with various pathologies such as neurofibromatosis, sickle cell disease, atherosclerosis, and radiotherapy.

The most informative MRA sequence is the 3D TOF, which evidences the narrowing of the arterial tracts involved (generally the supra-clinoid segments of carotid siphons) and the collateral circulation that have a typical aspect when they involve the lenticulostriate a. and appear as high-signal contorted tubular structures. The analysis of single sections and of the structur-

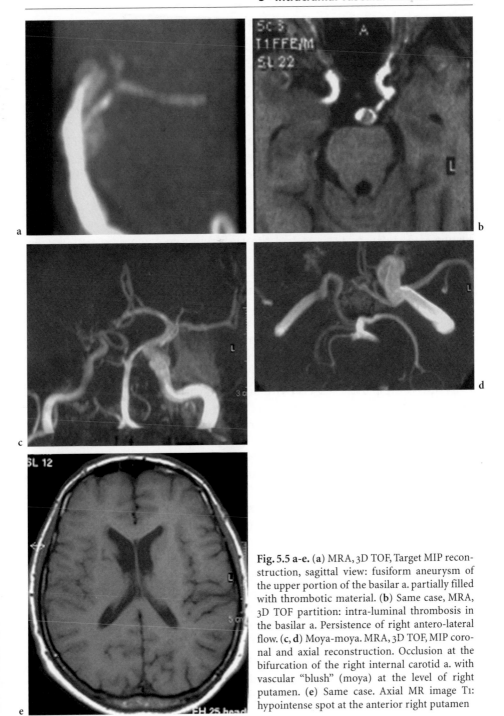

Fig. 5.5 a-e. (a) MRA, 3D TOF, Target MIP reconstruction, sagittal view: fusiform aneurysm of the upper portion of the basilar a. partially filled with thrombotic material. (b) Same case, MRA, 3D TOF partition: intra-luminal thrombosis in the basilar a. Persistence of right antero-lateral flow. (c, d) Moya-moya. MRA, 3D TOF, MIP coronal and axial reconstruction. Occlusion at the bifurcation of the right internal carotid a. with vascular "blush" (moya) at the level of right putamen. (e) Same case. Axial MR image T1: hypointense spot at the anterior right putamen

al MR images provides important diagnostic elements of proof (Fig. 5.5c-e). The use of contrast agents can also be useful in reducing the saturation effects caused by the slow flow in the collateral circulation [17].

5.2.3 Vascular malformations

Vascular malformations derive from amartomatous development of the meso-dermal vascular components and are classified into 4 subgroups: Artero-Venous Malformations (AVM), Venous Angiomas (VA), Cavernous Angiomas (CA) and Capillary Telangiectasias (CT). The AVM can be located at pial or intra-parenchymal level (AVM strictly speaking) or may involve dural vessels [dural artero-venous shunts, usually addressed to as Dural Artero-venous Fistula (DAF)]. In reality, most of the DAF represents acquired pathologies. Vascular malformations can also be distinguished into forms that are angio-graphically detectable (AVM, DAF, and VA) and forms that are occult (CA, CT, and AVM completely occluded as a consequence of thrombosis) [18]. AVM are the only ones that can be studied with MRA.

The VA will be discussed in Paragraph 5.3.

AVM are today considered the result of anomalous regulation of angio-genetic processes, most often occurring at the supra-tentorial level. They consists of 1) mature nutritive arterial vessels with aneurysmatic dilatations, 2) a nidus of dysplastic vessels (with no interposition of the capillary bed nor of the normal cerebral parenchyma) with aneurysmatic dilatations and artero-venous fistulas, 3) superficial or deep draining dilated veins. In 50% of cases an hemorrhagic ictus is the presenting symptom, while epilepsy or focal neurological signs are observed in 25%.

Treatment can be surgical, endovascular, radio-surgical or combined [19].

To date, arterial DSA still remains the most useful diagnostic tool, espe-cially in view of surgical or endovascular treatment; however, MRA provides useful information and plays a very important role in view of radio-surgical therapy and in posttreatment follow-up [20].

In their evaluation by MRA, it is recomended to use both TOF and PC sequences because it is useful to evaluate separately the afferent arteries, the efferent veins, and the nidus when present.

The 3D TOF allows a good identification of the afferent arteries and nidus, while the efferent vessels remain less visible due to spin saturation phenomena, except for high flow AVM (Fig. 5.6a,b).

It is also possible to have selective information on the origin of the indi-vidual feeding arteries of the AVM by properly positioning the presaturation bands and repeating the sequences, but this is a time consuming process. The reconstruction with target MIP algorithms eliminates overlapping vessels that are not involved, providing better diagnostic images [21, 22] (Fig. 5.6c).

When sub-acute intraparenchymal hemorrhage is present, met-hemoglo-bin overlaps the flow signal, making the identification of the AVM vessels dif-

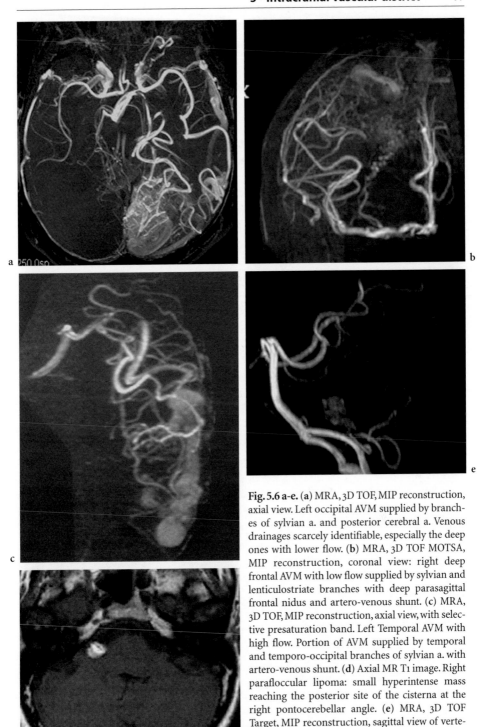

Fig. 5.6 a-e. (a) MRA, 3D TOF, MIP reconstruction, axial view. Left occipital AVM supplied by branches of sylvian a. and posterior cerebral a. Venous drainages scarcely identifiable, especially the deep ones with lower flow. **(b)** MRA, 3D TOF MOTSA, MIP reconstruction, coronal view: right deep frontal AVM with low flow supplied by sylvian and lenticulostriate branches with deep parasagittal frontal nidus and artero-venous shunt. **(c)** MRA, 3D TOF, MIP reconstruction, axial view, with selective presaturation band. Left Temporal AVM with high flow. Portion of AVM supplied by temporal and temporo-occipital branches of sylvian a. with artero-venous shunt. **(d)** Axial MR T1 image. Right parafloccular lipoma: small hyperintense mass reaching the posterior site of the cisterna at the right pontocerebellar angle. **(e)** MRA, 3D TOF Target, MIP reconstruction, sagittal view of vertebro-basilar arteries: hyperintense formation near to the right postero-inferior cerebellar a. that mimics an abnormal AVM-like flow

ficult. Conversely, tissues with short T1 can cause false positives (Fig. 5.6d,e). In these cases the PC sequences are useful since the subtraction of stationary tissues – lipoma and hemorrhage included – allows us to obtain completely flow-related images. The most used PC sequence is the 2D with appropriate VENC (60-80 cm/sec). Even if the 2D images can be visualized only in the acquisition plane, they can be oriented on different planes in short time, providing selective information on the small feeding arterial branches [23, 24].

Identifying the efferent venous vessels is extremely important also for prognostic purposes, as the presence of venous ectasia or deep venous drainages is associated with higher risk of bleeding and with increased surgical risk [25]. If the AVM has low flow velocity, the most suitable TOF sequence is 3D, while 2D is more indicated for high flow artero-venous fistulas.

The PC technique with low VENC (20-30 cm/sec) is also employed in the study of the efferent veins. In the 2D sequence the slice must be positioned at the level of the AVM, both on the sagittal and on the axial plane, as the latter is the most appropriate for visualizing deep venous drainage (Fig. 5.7a).

Gadolinium administration increases the contrast and thereby allows a better identification of small vessels with both TOF and PC techniques, even if the TOFs are negatively affected by stationary tissue enhancement and by the low selectivity of the method (Fig. 5.7b).

Three-dimensional MRA sequences after intravenous contrast agent bolus administration (CEMRA) are extremely useful in the evaluation of AVM. In this sequence, K-space is filled with an ellipsoidal or spiral trajectory, so that it is possible to acquire the main anatomical information in a very short time interval. If acquisition is started when the contrast agent reaches the selected vascular district, images will display the first pass of the contrast agent through the vascular structure. Furthermore, the acquisition can be

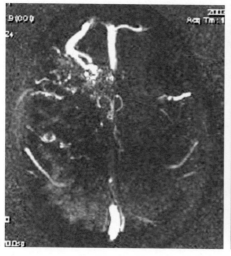
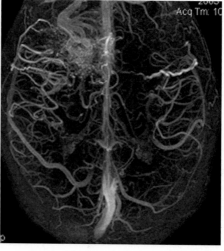

a

b

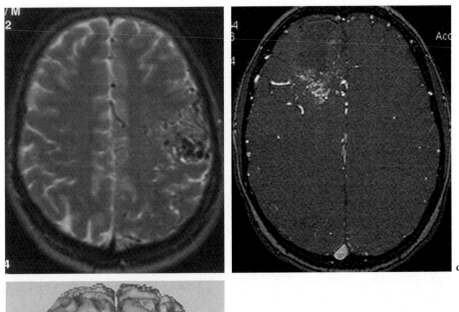

c

d

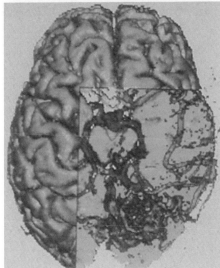

e

Fig. 5.7 a-e. (a) MRA, 2D PC, CDP VENC 40. Right frontal parasagittal AVM. Excellent representation of a superficial venous drainage. (b) Same case, MRA, 3D TOF + contrast agent, MIP reconstruction, axial view. Well defined borders, also of the small vessels but overlapping of arteries, veins, and angiomatous nidus. (c) Axial RM image FSE T2-weighted. Left frontal prerolandic AVM: hypointense cortical-subcortical angiomatous nidus. (d) Same case of a) and b). Partition of MRA, 3D TOF. Well evidenced flow signal deriving from the angiomatous nidus. (e) Volumetric reconstruction of encephalic parenchyma and of the vessels in AVM supplied both by the sylvian a. and by left posterior cerebral a. with the nidus deeply located in the occipital lobe

repeated in a multiphase approach such as the arrival, filling and washout of the contrast agent at the level of the target vessel.

The off-line reconstruction and analysis of all phases, with the Maximum Intensity Projection (MIP) algorithm for example, can allow the detection of the afferent and efferent vessels related to the AVM nidus (Fig. 5.8a-d). In reality, this is only partially true. Sometimes, the speed of the flow is so high and the persistence of the contrast agent within the nidus and in the related vessels is so prolonged, that it is impossible to identify the single phases. This is, however, possible with DSA.

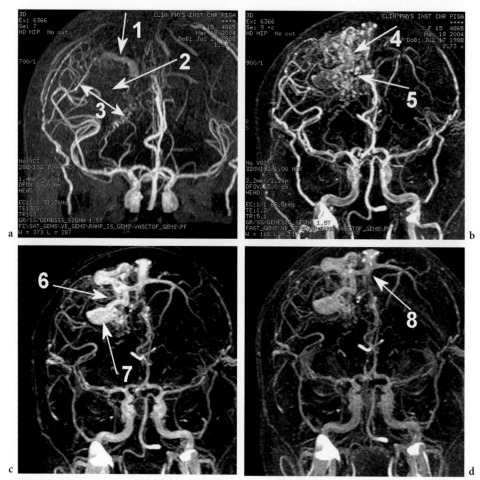

Fig. 5.8 a-d. Frontal artero-venous malformation. (a) Antero-posterior projection from MIP algorithm reconstructions of images acquired in MOTSA. With this technique the vascular nidus is barely visible due to the high flow relative to arterial afferents. (b, c, d) CEMRA images were acquired in three phases following the bolus injection of the contrast agent: early [arterial, (b)], intermediate [capillary-venous, (c)] and late [(venous, (d)]. Arrow 1: dilated draining vein; Arrow 2: absence of direct signal from artero-venous nidus. Arrow 3: arterial supply of AVM (sylvian and lenticulo-striate branches). Arrow 4 and 5: direct enhancement of A-V nidus. Arrow 6: draining veins afferenting to the septal longitudinal sinus. Arrow 7: varicous enlargement of a draining vein. Arrow 8: direct collection of some veins into the superior sagittal longitudinal sinus

The angiomatous nidus must be analyzed precisely regarding its size and its location related to the cerebral eloquent areas so that the physician can plan the correct surgical or radio-surgical approach to preserve such structures as much as possible. Structural MR images can be sufficiently adeguate for this aim [26], however the vascular or parenchymal (hypointense) calcifications may mimic anomalous vascular structures, leading to errors of overestimation of the size of the nidus.

More reliable information can be obtained from the source images of a 3D

TOF sequence (Fig. 5.7c, d), which can be rebuilt also in different planes from the axial one, allowing a 3D view of the nidus. In fact, we can obtain also volumetric and surface reformations that simultaneously show the vessels and the encephalic parenchyma, hence locating the AVM nidus in relation to the cortical topography (Fig. 5.7e).

The MRA techniques are recommended in the follow-up of treated AVM and are the reference point for further decisions on more-invasive procedures.

PC sequences allow the acquisition of data related to velocity and quantity of flow of an AVM. Just by employing 2D Complex Difference Processing (CDP) sequences with a different VENC we can already get an idea, although approximate, on flow velocity, while by using the single section cine PC Phase Difference Processing (PDP) orthogonally oriented to the flow of the main arterial afference, the changes in flow amount can be quantified in comparison to the contralateral unaffected artery [27] and also quantify the reduction of flow as consequence of treatment.

The DAFs are formed by a group of microfistulas located between arterial dural branches coming from the internal and/or external carotid and the dural wall of a venous sinus. Most DAFs are acquired, due to traumas or venous thrombosis, with pathological activation of neo-angiogenesis.

The diagnostic modality of choice of DAFs is DSA. MRA is often normal, especially in the small-sized or low flow forms. If abnormal features are present, these are gross and partial, they do not delimit the angio architecture in detail and require the further employment of DSA, which extensively and selectively documents the feeding arteries, the venous thromboses, and the venous drainages – in particular the cortical ones that are associated with a higher risk of hemorrhage [28].

The MRA evaluation of the DAF can be performed by using both PC with low VENC, and 3D TOF – pulse sequences. The analysis of the single partitions has proven to be very useful because it better shows the small areas of flow signals near dural sinus and sinus thrombosis [29]. The MIP reformation can evidence the DAF supply coming from the internal and external carotid, the iuxta-sinusal anomalous network, the possible occluded venous sinus and cortical or deep drainages (Fig. 5.9a-d).

A particular type of fistula is the Direct Carotid-Cavernous Fistula (DCCF). This is not considered a true DAF; it is of traumatic origin and ensues after laceration of the wall of the intra-cavernous carotid siphon which causes arterial hemorrhage in the cavernous sinus and increases the intra-cavernous pressure inverting the flow in the superior ophthalmic veins [30].

The diagnosis of DCCF is also possible with structural MRI. MRA 3D TOF techniques evidence flow signal around the intra-cavernous carotid siphon and in the superior ophthalmic vein. Source-image analysis helps in defining the peri-arterious high signal of the venous blood, which can be suppressed by a properly positioned presaturation band (Fig. 5.9e,f).

Nevertheless, the diagnostic method of choice for DCCF is still DSA, especially in view of endovascular treatment [31].

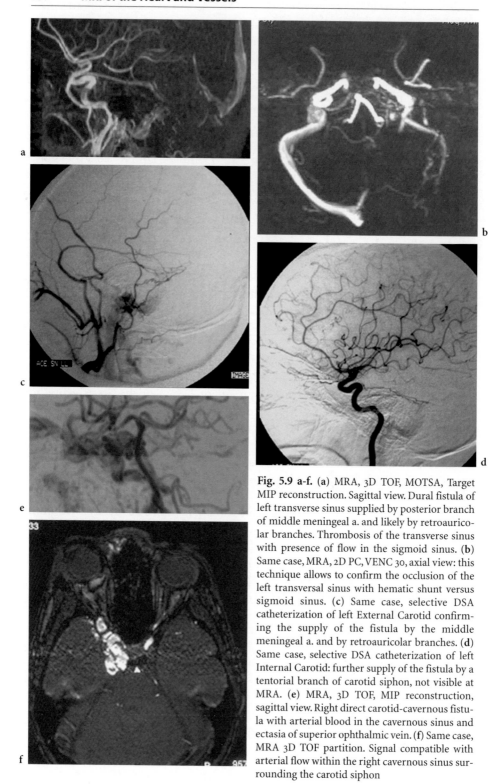

Fig. 5.9 a-f. (a) MRA, 3D TOF, MOTSA, Target MIP reconstruction. Sagittal view. Dural fistula of left transverse sinus supplied by posterior branch of middle meningeal a. and likely by retroauricolar branches. Thrombosis of the transverse sinus with presence of flow in the sigmoid sinus. **(b)** Same case, MRA, 2D PC, VENC 30, axial view: this technique allows to confirm the occlusion of the left transversal sinus with hematic shunt versus sigmoid sinus. **(c)** Same case, selective DSA catheterization of left External Carotid confirming the supply of the fistula by the middle meningeal a. and by retroauricolar branches. **(d)** Same case, selective DSA catheterization of left Internal Carotid: further supply of the fistula by a tentorial branch of carotid siphon, not visible at MRA. **(e)** MRA, 3D TOF, MIP reconstruction, sagittal view. Right direct carotid-cavernous fistula with arterial blood in the cavernous sinus and ectasia of superior ophthalmic vein. **(f)** Same case, MRA 3D TOF partition. Signal compatible with arterial flow within the right cavernous sinus surrounding the carotid siphon

5.2.4 Aneurysms

The aneurysmatic dilations are classified into saccular, fusiform and blister-like. The fusiform aneurysms have already been described and the blister-like ones are too small to benefit from MRA in the diagnostic path. Septic or mycotic aneurysms most likely have a saccular shape and develop along the course of more distal arterial branches.

Uncommon forms defined as "serpentine" aneurysms [32, 33] are the segmental ectasia of an arterial branch, which appears extremely tortuous. Distally, the affected vessel regains its normal shape and supplies the district of competence as normally. Seen with angiography and MRA, they are very similar to fusiform aneurysms but in 50% of cases they affect the sylvian a. and its branching, and occur in young individuals (Fig. 5.10a).

Saccular Aneurysms (SA) are much more frequent; they affect about 11% of the population, mainly women (3/2), rarely children, and are multiple in 20% of cases. At present, it is believed that a number of factors contribute to their development: genetic (they can be found in the Ehlers-Danlos syndrome, in fibromuscular dysplasia, in the autosomal-dominant form of polycystic kidney disease and can be found in several members of the same family), biomechanical (abnormalities in arterial dynamics, vessel wall alterations), etc. [34].

SAs generally arise at the level of arterial bifurcations where there is a defect in the continuity of the tunica media, and focal outpouching of the intima can occur through a localized defect in the internal elastic lamina. In 90% of cases they affect the internal carotid, most often the anterior communicating a. SAs are divided by size into small (up to 12 mm), large (from 12 to 25 mm) and giant (over 25 mm). Their first most common clinical sign is subarachnoid hemorrhage by breaking of the aneurismal sac, with hematic spreading in the pericerebral and intraventricular cerebrospinal fluid. However, in 2-9% of autoptic findings, non-ruptured aneurysms are found [35]. Giant SAs can manifest by focal neurological deficit from brain compression or distal embolism [36].

DSA represents the diagnostic gold standard. When the diagnostic evaluation is performed in the acute phase during subarachnoid hemorrhage, it is also an indispensable tool for chosing the most favorable therapeutic strategy between the endovascular and microsurgical approach.

Despite recent works declaring its usefulness [37], the role of MRA in meningeal hemorrhages seems, to date, still limited in the acute setting (Fig. 5.10b-d) because it is burdened by false negatives, and is unable to evidence vasospasm in a reliable way. Moreover false positives may be due to the presence of peri-aneurysmatic hemorrhage [38].

Conversely, MRA is an important tool in the screening of non-bleeding SAs and is reliable in the search of SAs larger than 3 mm, as the smaller ones cannot be detected due to problems concerning image spatial resolution (Fig. 5.11a-c). Therefore, it is generally used to confirm or exclude uncertain findings of structural MR, in the evaluation of subjects at risk, in the follow-up of non-treated carriers, and in postsurgical or endovascular treatment follow-up [39] (Fig. 5.11d-f). Obviously, patients who have undergone

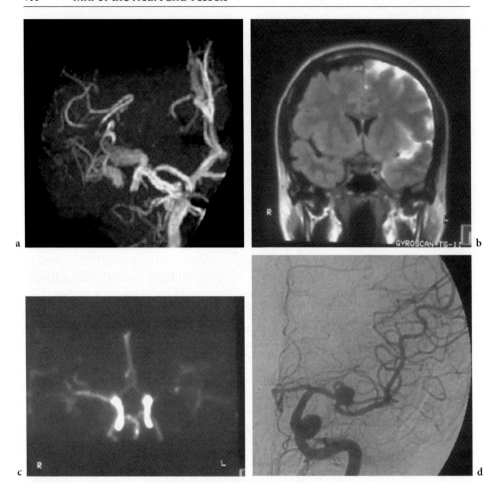

Fig. 5.10 a-d. (a) MRA, 3D TOF, Target MIP reconstruction, coronal view. Serpentine aneurysm of horizontal segment of right sylvian a,: focal fusiform ectasia of M1 and M2 with normal size of arterial branches downstream. (b) MRI, FLAIR sequence, coronal view. Acute hemorrhage: hyperintense material within the left peri-hemispheric subarachnoid space. There is also an hypointense lesion within left sylvian cistern suggesting saccular aneurysm of the middle cerebral a. (c) Same case, MRA, 3D PC, MIP reconstruction, axial view, without conclusive diagnostic features. (d) Same case, DSA with selective catetherization of the left internal carotid: in this image the saccular aneurysm is diagnostically well defined

Fig. 5.11 a-f. (a) MRA, 3D TOF MOTSA, Target MIP reconstruction, axial view. Small saccular aneurysm at the right sylvian bifurcation. (b) MRA, 3D TOF, MIP reconstruction, sagittal view: large saccular aneurysm of carotid-ophthalmic level. The aneurysm has grown superiorly. (c) MRA, 3D TOF MOTSA, Target MIP reconstruction, oblique view: bilobate giant saccular aneurysm of left carotid bifurcation. Extensive thrombosis inside the inferior lobe. (d) MRA, 3D TOF MOTSA, Target MIP reconstruction, parasagittal oblique view: saccular aneurysm of the apical segment of basilar a. In this case the aneurysm has grown posteriorly. (e) Same case, MRA, 3D TOF MOTSA, Target MIP reconstruction, parasagittal oblique view. Two year follow-up: size increase of the saccular aneurysm. (f) MRA, 3D TOF partition. Area void of signal near the posterior wall of the left carotid siphon. The lack of signal is due to the presence of Guglielmis' spirals in saccular aneurysm of the posterior communicant a. which is totally occluded

$\longrightarrow$

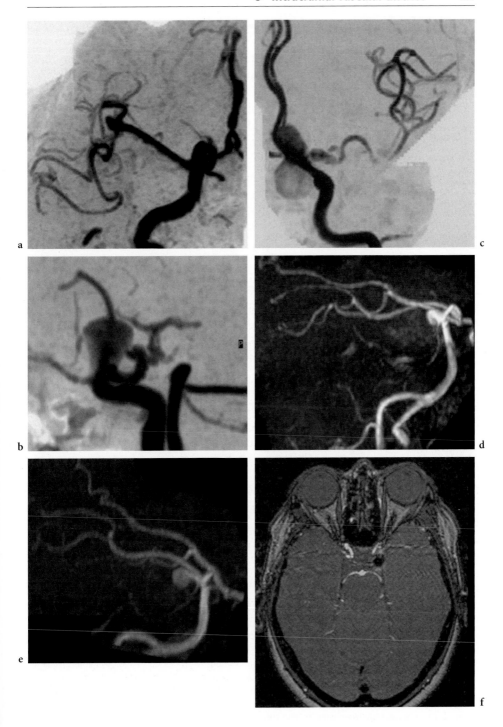

surgical clipping can have MRA only if the material used is magnetically compatible.

Among all the MRA techniques mentioned, the most informative and most used method is the 3D TOF. The need for obtaining images with high spatial resolution that reduce false negatives to the minimum, entails the use of a high matrix and of thin widely overlapped slabs (MOTSA) to study a sufficient volume. Magnetization Transfer (MT) and Fat Suppression (FS) must be used to minimize the signal from stationary tissues. The MOTSA sequences provide the advantages of both 2D and 3D TOF and can thus also evidence slow flow aneurysmatic dilatations with a good spatial resolution [40].

Once the presence of a SA has been established, it is necessary to accurately define its location, the relationship with its parent vessel and with the neighboring anatomical structures, the shape and size of the neck (Fig. 5.12a). For these purposes it is necessary to have selective reconstruction of each vessel to avoid overlapping, and to have an accurate analysis of the single partitions to rule out the presence of multiple SAs.

In the giant forms, intraluminal thrombi are frequently found. When these are not recent, they contain met-hemoglobin, which generates a signal that may be confused with that of arterial flow, causing an overestimation of the intra-aneurysmal lumen, in the TOF sequences. More recent thrombi show intermediate signal on T1 pulse sequences; so MRA 3D TOF images can bring to underestimate the size of the aneurysmal sac (Fig. 5.12b, c).

Therefore, it can also be useful to employ PC techniques, which allow the operator to evidence by choosing different VENC the different flow velocities inside the sac, differentiating them from the endo-saccular thrombus (Fig. 5.12d,e). However, the use of this method is limited to few selected cases due to a number of drawbacks, the main being:

a) the 3D PC sequence, the images of which can be reconstructed on the different planes, is time-consuming because it has to be repeated by chosing different VENCs. In fact, a low encoding velocity allows to evidence exclusively low flow, while high flow is evidenced with higher encoding velocities
b) the selected VENC does not always provide a good visualization of the related vessel.

Fig. 5.12 a-f. (a) MRA, 3D TOF, Target MIP reconstruction, coronal oblique view. Large saccular aneurysm of right vertebral a. at the level of the origin of the postero-inferior cerebellar a. (b) MRA, 3D TOF, Target MIP reformation, coronal view: small saccular aneurysm of distal segment of the basilar a. (c) Same case, MRA, 3D TOF partition. The aneurysm is considered as a large one because of the endoluminal thrombosis which is not visible in the postprocessed image. (d) Same case as a) MRA, 2D PC CDP, axial, VENC 20. Inside the aneurysmatic sac only the slow peripheral flow is evidenced. (e) Same case as a) MRA, 2D PC CDP axial view, VENC 60. Within the saccular aneurysm the fast haematic flow is also evident. (f) Same case as a) MRA, 2D PC PDP, axial view, VENC 40, direction of flow gradient antero-posterior: entering haematic flow along the left wall of the sac (hyperintense: same direction of the gradient); exit flow along the right wall of the sac (hypointense: opposite direction to the gradient)

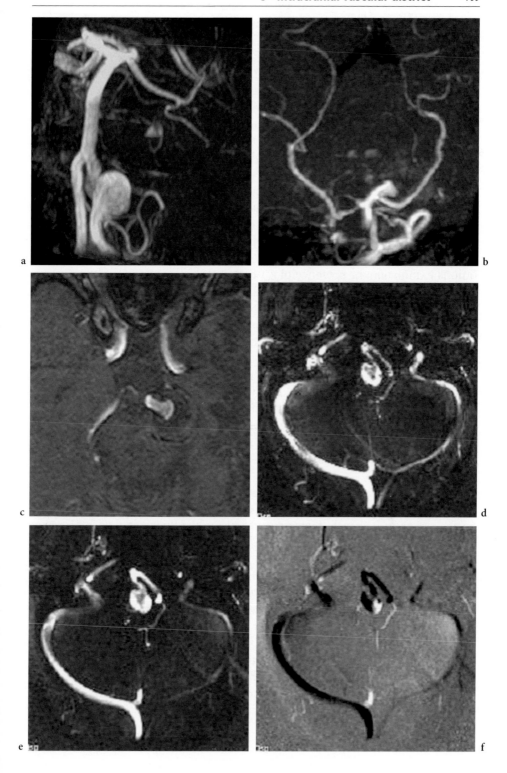

In experimental models it has been demonstrated that the blood flow, in lateral aneurysms (the ones implanted orthogonally to the major axis of the vessels from which they originate) enters the sac at the distal (downstream) aspect of the neck, and exits proximally sliding along the wall. Therefore, the point subject to most dynamic stress, which is also the most likely to rupture, is the distal wall of the aneurysmal neck and not the dome, as was believed in the past [42]. This has been confirmed also in vivo with angiographic PC sequences, which separately evidence the various components of flow inside large lateral aneurysms [43] (Fig. 5.12f): a high VENC reveals the so-called "inflow jet", while a lower VENC evidences the vorticous flow throughout the sac.

MRA can sometimes be used to solve diagnostic problems that arise from analyzing traditional MR images. For example, abnormal pneumatization of an anterior clinoid process at MRI induces an oval lack of signal near to the supra-clinoid segment of carotid siphon, mimicking an aneurysmatic dilatation. The doubt can be solved with CT or MRA. Because it is non-invasive and inexpensive as compared to DSA, MRA has become a sufficiently sensitive and specific screening tool in subjects at risk with familiarity or pathologies of which the SA can be part of, such as the polycystic kidney, the arterial sub-intimal dysplasia, cerebral AVM, aortic coarctation, several connective tissue disorders.

Therefore using MRA 11,7% prevalence of SA has been demonstrated in patients affected by polycystic kidney, and asymptomatic aneurysms have been found in 17,9% of blood-relative to sub-arachnoid hemorrhage [44, 45].

5.2.5 Neurovascular conflict

The Neurovascular Conflict (NVC) is among the most frequent causes of trigeminal neuralgia and facial nerve spasm; NVC is due to the compression by arterial or, more rarely, by venous vessels on the trigeminal or facial nerve at the level of the nerve root exit zone, where there is no myelin sheath [46]. The most frequently involved arteries are the vertebral at the vertebro-basilar junction, the postero-inferior cerebellar, and the antero-inferior cerebellar [46]. MRA is the most informative tool in the assessment of NVC. The analysis of the partitions allows us to confirm or exclude the existence of NVC at the level of a specific nervous emergence, while MIP reconstruction identifies the involved artery. In order to better document the anatomical features, it is advisable to perform Multiplanar Reconstruction (MPR) of the partitions, which provides images of high contrast between the arterial vessel (high signal), the nervous emergence or parenchymal structure (intermediate signal) and the cerebro-spinal fluid (low signal) on different planes [47] (Fig. 5.13a,b).

5.2.6 Expansive lesions
(dislocations and neoformed vascularizations)

In cases of intracranial tumours, MRA – following MRI – provides additional diagnostic elements useful in planning of surgery or stereotassic approach.
The most relevant features concern their relationship to arterial vessels: arterial dislocations caused by mass effect and arterial "blush" in neo-vascular-
rized tumors (Fig. 5.13c-f).

5.3 Venous compartment

Although MRA underwent a great development with the study of arterial
pathology, today it has an important role also in the diagnostic balance of the
intra-cranial venous system pathology, together with MRI.

5.3.1 Occlusive pathology

It is believed that about 1% of severe strokes are caused by Cerebral Venous
Thrombosis (CVT). The clinical symptoms, especially at early stages, are
blurry and non-specific, therefore the diagnosis can be delayed with consequences on the therapeutical decisions: because the pharmacological throm-
bolysis must be established as soon as possible.

There are many causes for venous occlusion. The most common are traumas, infections, pregnancy, oral contraceptives, some metabolic unbalances
(dehydration, hyperthyroidism, hepatic cirrhosis), several coagulopathies,
some collagen diseases and vasculitis (such as Behçet disease).

Usually the thrombus develops in a venous sinus, increasing venous pressure and hindering the functioning of arachnoid villi: hence the first symptom is endo-cranial hypertension. Afterwards, the thrombous extends to the
deep and cortical affluent veins; upstream venous pressure increases affecting the encephalic parenchyma and originating focal neurological signs (50%
of cases) [48].

DSA has been widely employed with excellent results in the diagnosis of
CVT, but at present the combined use of structural MR and MRA provide a
diagnostic accuracy of approximately 100% as it allows the identification of
both the occluded venous vessel and the possible parenchymal damage.

At the MR exam in the acute phase [49], the fresh thrombus inside the
venous sinus is isointense to the brain in the T1-weighted Spin Echo images
(Fig. 5.14a), while it appears hypointense on T2-weighted images. In fact the
red blood cells contain oxy-hemoglobin, lacking the magnet susceptibility
effect on T1 while inducing loss of signal intensity on T2. Hence, the signal of

the acute thrombus is undistinguishable from that of circulating blood. The blood flow on T1 has a variable signal depending on the speed and the orientation of the slices in respect to the direction of the venous vessel, however it can be hypointense or hyperintense. Hence, the fundamental diagnostic element is the isointensity on T1 that can be revealed on all planes [50].

MRA confirms the diagnostic suspicion and better shows the extension of the thrombotic process from the venous sinus to the afferent veins. The 2D TOF sequence with presaturation of the arterial flow is generally used because it better highlights slow flow [51].

The endoluminal thrombus appears as a zone of signal void. To obtain details in cases requiring an accurate study of the venous system, the most suitable sequence is the 3D TOF sequence after Gd administration. The 2D-PC sequence with low VENC (5-15 cm/sec) is employed when rapid information on the patency of a venous sinus is needed (as in the case of poorly cooperative patients) (Fig. 5.14b). Also with this technique there is no flow signal in the occluded vessel.

During the sub-acute phase (after 2-3 days) the hemoglobin inside the venous thrombus changes to met-hemoglobin. As this form causes a magnetic susceptibility effect on both T1 and T2, the thrombotic venous sinus appears hyperintense on T1 and T2 (Fig. 5.14c).

The signal change on T1 must be confirmed in all planes in order to be distinguished from the inflow effect that appears as hyperintensity in the first images acquired orthogonally to the direction of the vessel. Because misinterpretation may also arise from the phenomenon of signal enhancement in T1 given by the slow flow, hyperintensity should be confirmed on T2-weighted images in all cases [50].

Met-Hb inside trombus may show similar signal intensity to the normal flow on MRA TOF images, causing important problems of interpretation. In such cases it is very helpful to apply PC sequences with low VENC, which are not biased by the signal from stationary tissue. The collateral channels can be identified employing phase subtraction, which provides information on flow direction [52].

Both traditional MR and MRA are indispensable for monitoring vascular re-habitation (Fig. 5.14d-f).

Fig. 5.13 a-f. (a) MRA, 3D TOF, target MIP reformation. Vertebro-basilar arteries: tortuous right postero-inferior cerebellar a. (PICA) possible cause of neuro-vascular conflict with the acustic-facial nerve. (b) MPR of the partitions in the coronal oblique plane: contact between the loop of the PICA a. and the emergency acustic-facial nerve. (c) MRI, FLAIR sequence, coronal view: large size meningioma in the right middle cranial fossa. (d) Same case, MRA 3D TOF Target MIP reconstruction, coronal view: cerebral anterior aa. are dislocated toward the left side and the right sylvian horizontal tract is pushed up and medially. (e) MRA, 3D TOF, Target MIP reconstruction, sagittal view. Right Tympano-giugular glomangioma: vascolar "blush" supply by ascending pharingeal a. (f) Same case, MRA 3D TOF, partition: confirmation of tumoral neovascularization with confluencing of hyperintense areas in the tympanic region and the right posterior foramen lacerum

$\longrightarrow$

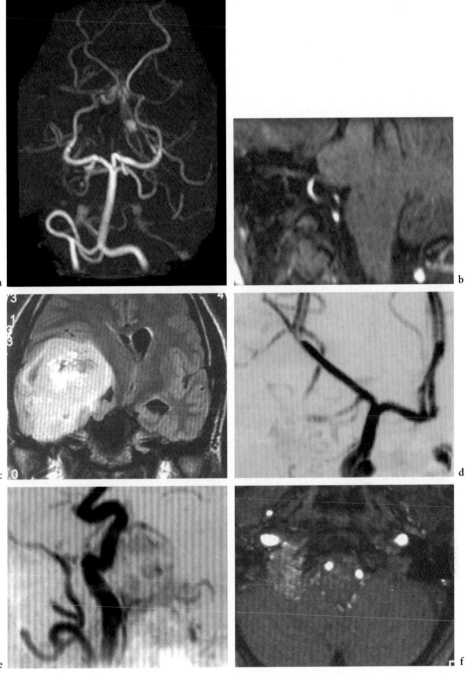

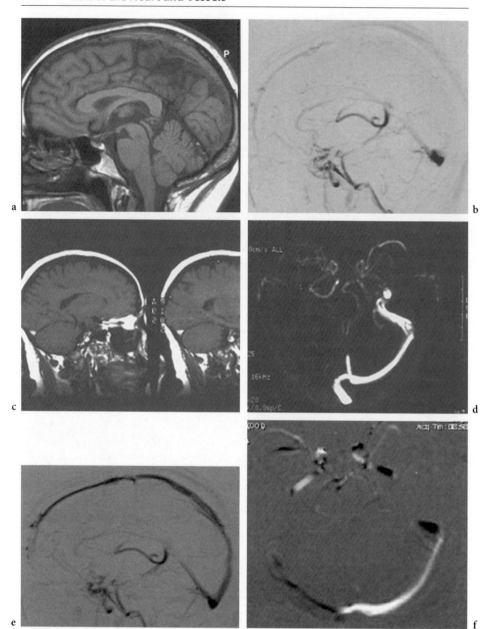

Fig. 5.14 a-f. (a) MR T1 image, sagittal view. Acute thrombosis of the sagittal sinus: intermediate signal of the superior longitudinal sinus. (b) Same case, MRA 2D PC, VENC 40, sagittal view: lack of signal within the superior longitudinal sinus and the rectus sinus. (c) contiguous RM T1 images, sagittal view. Sub-acute thrombosis of the right lateral sinus: hyperintensity of sinus lumen. (d) Same case, MRA 2D PC, VENC 40, axial view: lack of signal within the right transverse sinus. (e) Same case as a), MRA, 2D PC, VENC 40, sagittal view, follow-up after treatment: rehabitation of the sinus lumen. (f) Same case of c), MRA, 2D PC, PDP, VENC 40, axial view, right to left direction of flow gradient: rehabitation of lateral sinus with orthodromic flow direction (hypointense because directed from left to right)

5.3.2 Venous angiomas

Venous Angiomas (VA) are also defined venous dysplasias, because they are not true malformations but rather venous vessels angiogenically mature and morphologically dysplastic. Often they remain asymptomatic and are occasionally found upon MRI. The association of cavernous malformation to VA is well known, and is often complicated by bleeding. Structural MRI is sufficient for diagnostic purposes [53], while MRA is limited to cases of uncertain diagnosis.

To study VAs that show slow flow, the most suitable sequences are the 2D TOF with saturation band for the arterial flow and PC sequences with low VENC. Also the 3D TOF can be used after the administration of a contrast agent to reduce the circulating blood T1 signal.

Within 3D angiograms it is possible to evidence thin dysplastic medullary veins with radiated appearance (like a "caput medusae") that converge in an enlarged transcortical or subependymal collector vein. Sometimes the drainage is double and in some cases the VA are multiple [54].

5.3.3 Tumors (relationship with main venous structures: surgical planning)

The study of the intracranial venous system is very useful in the presurgical assessment of the tumors for a correct planning of surgical approach.

In traditional surgery of intra-axial tumors it is recommended that the surgeon know in advance the relationship between the tumor and the cortical veins in order to prevent lesions of the normal surrounding tissue [55].

In the traditional surgical approach to para-sagittal menigiomas it is mandatory to know whether the tumor has infiltrated or compressed the superior longitudinal sinus. In particular this information is needed in the case of retro-coronal menigiomas, since the intermediate-posterior segment of superior longitudinal sinus cannot be ablated without causing severe parenchimal lesions – unless obviously the sinus is completely obstructed by the tumor and compensatory circles have developed. Therefore, if the meningioma completely obstructes the sinus, the total ablation can be performed, but if the sinus is even only in part patent, the neurosurgeon has to choose between the subtotal ablation or delaying the operation until obstruction has become complete.

In these cases the intravenous Gd administration has proven to be useful on the 3D TOF since the tumor enhancement appears together with the venous sinus [56] (Fig. 5.15a-c).

In the stereotassic approach to tumoral pathology, it is extremely useful to obtain presurgery images of both the arterial and venous peritumoral circle and any relationships of the vessels with the lesion, since the access to the

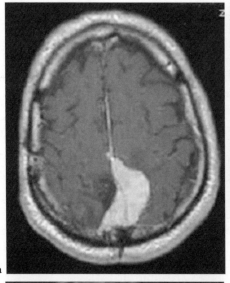

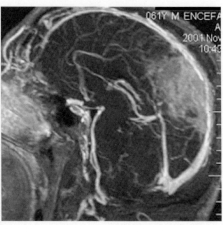

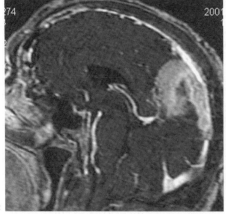

Fig. 5.15 a-c. (a) RM T1 + contrast agent image, axial view. Left parasagittal meningioma infiltrating the falx and crossing on the other side. (b) Same case, MRA, 3D PC VENC 40 + contrast agent, sagittal view: infiltration of the intermediate third of superior sagittal sinus. (c) Same case, MRA, 3D PC, VENC 40 + contrast agent, sagittal partition: superior sagittal sinus is occluded at its posterior third because of meningiomatous infiltration

brain is reduced in size and the operating field is not exposed. The volumetric and surface reconstructions in these cases can result extremely useful in the choice of the least invasive way of access [57].

References

1. Riggs HE, Rupp C (1963) Variation in form of circle of Wills. Arch Neuril 8:24-30
2. Fisher CM (1965) The circle of Willis: Anatomical variations. Vasc Dis 2:99-105
3. Pearse Morris P, In: Sup Choi (1996) Cerebral vascular anatomy. Neuroimaging Clin N Am 6:541-560
4. Truwit CL (1994) Embryology of the cerebral vasculature. Neuroimaging Clin N Am 4:663-669

5. Ballotta E (2000) Carotid plaque gross morphology and clinical presentation: a prospective study of 457 carotid artery specimens. J Surg Res 89:78-84

6. Marzewski DJ, Furlan AJ, St. Louis P et al (1982) Intracranial internal carotid artery stenosis: longterm prognosis. Stroke 13:821-834

7. Heiserman JE, Drayer BP, Keller PJ et al (1992) Intracranial vascular stenosis and occlusion: evaluation with three-dimensional time-of-flight MR angiography. Radiology 185:667-673

8. Spritzer CE, Pelc NJ, Lee JN et al (1990) Rapid MR imaging of blood flow with a phase sensitive, limited-flip-angle, gradient recalled pulse sequence: preliminary experience. Radiology 176:255-262

9. Jung HW, Chang KH, Choi DS et al (1995) Contrast-enhanced MR angiography for the diagnosis of intracranial vascular disease: optimal dose of gadopentetate dimeglumine. Am J Roentgenol 165:1251-1255

10. Hankey GJ, Warlow CP (1991) The role of imaging in the management of cerebral and ocular ischemia. Neuroradiology 33:381-390

11. Heiserman JE (1992) The role of magnetic resonance angiography in the evaluation of cerebrovascular ischemic disease. Neuroimaging Clin N Am 2:753-767

12. Siewert B, Patel MR, Warach S (1995) Stroke and ischemia. Magn Reson Imaging Clin N Am 3:529-540

13. Ross MR, Pelc NJ, Enzmann DR (1993) Qualitative phase contrast MRA in the normal and abnormal circle of Willis. Am J Neuroradiol 14:19-25

14. Harris KG, Tran DD, Cornell SH et al (1994) Diagnosing intracranial vasculitis: the roles of MR and angiography. Am J Roentgenol 15:317-330

15. Heiserman JE, Bird CR (1994) Cerebral aneurisms. Neuroimaging Clin N Am 4:799-822

16. Jager HR (2000) Contrast-enhanced MR angiography of intracranial giant aneurysms. Am J Neuroradiol 21:1900-1907

17. Yamada I, Matsushima Y, Suzuki S (1992) Moyamoya disease: diagnosis with three-dimensional time-of-flight MR angiography. Radiology 184:773-778

18. Chaloupka JC, Huddle DC (1998) Classification of vascular malformations of the central nervous system. Neuroimaging Clin N Am 8:295-321

19. Berman MF (2000) The epidemiology of brain arteriovenous malformations. Neurosurg 47:389-397

20. Warren DJ (2001) Cerebral arteriovenous malformations: comparison of novel magnetic resonance angiographic techniques and conventional catheter angiography. Neurosurgery 48:973-983

21. Kesava P, Baker E, Metha M et al (1996) Staging of arteriovenous malformations using three-dimensional time-of-flight MR angiography and volume-rendered displays of surface anatomy. Am J Roentgenol 167:605-609

22. Metha MP, Petereit D, Turski P et al (1993) Magnetic resonance angiography: a three-dimensional database for assessing arteriovenous malformations. Technical note. J Neurosurg 79:289-293

23. Marks MP, Lane B, Steinberg GK et al (1990) Hemorrhage in intracerebral arteriovenous malformations: angiographic determinants. Radiology 176:807-813

24. Korosec F (1992) Development and evaluation of acquisition techniques for magnetic resonance angiography. In: Medical Physics. Madison, University of Wisconsin

25. Spetzler RF, Martin NA (1986) A proposed grading system for arteriovenous malformations. J Neurosurg 65:476-483

26. Guo WY, Lindquist C, Karlsson B et al (1993) Gamma knife surgery of cerebral arteriovenous malformations: serial MR imaging studies after radiosurgery. Int J Radiat Oncol Biol Phys 25:315-323

27. Wasserman BA, Lin W, Tarr RW et al (1995) Cerebral arteriovenous malformations: flow

quantitation by means of two-dimensional cardiac-gated phase-contrast MR imaging. Radiology 194:681-686

28. Malek AM, Halbach VV, Dowd CF et al (1998) Diagnosis and treatment of dural arteriovenous fistulas. Neuroimaging Clin N Am 8:445-468

29. De Marco JK, Dillon WP, Halbach VV et al (1990) Dural arteriovenous fistulas: evaluation with MR imaging. Radiology 175:193-199

30. Lewis AI, Tomsick TA, Tew JJ (1995) Management of 100 consecutive direct carotid-cavernous fistulas: results of treatment with detachable balloons. Neurosurgery 36:239-245

31. Panasci DJ, Nelson PK (1995) MR imaging and MR angiography in the diagnosis of dural arteriovenous fistulas. Magn Res Imaging Clin N Am 3:493-508

32. Setton A, Davis AJ, Bose A et al (1996) Angiography of cerebral aneurysms. Neuroimaging Clin N Am 6:705-738

33. Kobayashi S (1999) Blisterlike aneurysms. J Neurosurg 91:164-166

34. Stehbens WE (1989) Etiology of intracranial berry aneurysms. J Neurosurg 70:823-831

35. Locksley HB (1966) Report on cooperative study of intracranial aneurysms and subarachnoid hemorrhage: section V. Natural history of subarachnoid hemorrhage, intracranial aneurysms, and AVMs, based on 6368 cases in the cooperative study. J Neurosurg 25:219-236, 321-369

36. Drake CG (1979) Giant intracranial aneurysms: experience with surgical treatment in 174 patients. Clin Neurosurg 26:12-95

37. Anzalone N, Triulzi F, Scotti G (1995) Acute subarachnoid hemorrhage: 3D time-of-flight MR angiography versus intra-arterial digital angiography. Neuroradiology 37:257-261

38. Atlas SW (1993) MR imaging is highly sensitive for acute subarachnoid hemorrhage......not! Radiology 186:319-322

39. Derdeyn CP, Graves VB, Turski PA et al (1997) MR angiography of saccular aneurysms after treatment with Guglielmi detachable coils: preliminary experience. Am J Neuroradiol 18:279-286

40. Korogi Y, Takahashi M, Mabuchi N et al (1996) Intracranial aneurysms: diagnostic accuracy of MR angiography with evaluation of maximum intensity projection and source images. Radiology 199:199-207

41. Houston J, Rufenacht DA, Ehman RL et al (1991) Intracranial aneurysms and vascular malformations: comparison of time-of-flight and phase-contrast MR angiography. Radiology 181:721-730

42. Strother CM, Graves VB, Rappe A (1992) Aneurysm hemodynamics: an experimental study. Am J Neuroradiol 13:1089-1095

43. Meyer FB, Huston J, Riederer SS (1993) Pulsatile increases in aneurysm size determined by cine phase-contrast MR angiography. J Neurosurg 78:879-883

44. Wiebers DO, Torres VE (1992) Screening for unruptured intracranial aneurysms in autosomal dominant polycystic kidney disease. N Engl J Med 327:953-955

45. Ronkainen A, Puranen MI, Hernesniemi JA et al (1995) Intracranial aneurysms: MR angiographic screening in 400 asymptomatic individuals with increased familial risk. Radiology 195:35-40

46. Jannetta PJ, Abbasy M, Maroon JC et al (1977) Etiology and definitive microsurgical treatment of hemifacial spasm. Operative techniques and results in 47 patients. J Neurosurg 47:321-328

47. Adler CH, Zimmerman RA, Savino PJ et al (1992) Hemifacial spasm: evaluation by magnetic resonance imaging and magnetic resonance tomographic angiography. Ann Neurol 32:502-506

48. Lee SK, Kim BS, Terbrugge KG (2002) Clinical presentation, imaging and treatment of cerebral venous thrombosis. Intervent Neuroradiol 8:5-14

49. Tsai FY, Wang AM, Matovich VB et al (1995) MR staging of acute dural sinus thrombosis: correlation with venous pressure measurements and implications for treatment and prognosis. Am J Neuroradiol 16:1021-1029

50. Macchi PJ, Grossman RI, Gomori JM et al (1986) High field MR imaging of cerebral venous thrombosis. J Comput Assist Tomogr 10:10-15

51. Mattle HP, Wentz KU, Edelman RR et al (1991) Cerebral venography with MR. Radiology 178:453-458

52. Johnson BA, Fram EK (1992) Cerebral venous occlusive disease. Neuroimaging Clin N Am 2:769-783

53. Augustyn GT, Scott JA, Olson E et al (1985) Cerebral venous angiomas: MR imaging. Radiology 156:391-395

54. Kesava PP, Turski PA (1998) MR angiography of vascular malformations. Neuroimaging Clin N Am 8:349-370

55. Yanaka K, Shirai S, Shibata Y et al (1993) Gadolinium-enhanced magnetic resonance angiography in the planning of supratentorial glioma surgery. Neurol Med Chir 33:439-443

56. Zimmerman RA, Bilaniuk LT, Hackney DB et al (1986) Magnetic resonance imaging of dural venous sinus invasion, occlusion and thrombosis. Acta Radiol Suppl (Stockh) 369:110-112

57. Kelly P (1991) Tumor Stereotaxis. WB Saunders, Philadelphia, USA

6 Vessels of the neck

Mirco Cosottini, Maria Chiara Michelassi, Guido Lazzarotti

6.1 Introduction

The study of epi-aortic vessels can be performed with a variety of imaging techniques that provide morphological or functional information and show the vascular lumen of the vessel wall itself. From a technical point of view, these can be sub-grouped into invasive, such as Digital Subtraction Angiography (DSA), and into non-invasive or minimally invasive, such as Echo-Doppler, angio-Computed Tomography (CT), and Magnetic Resonance Angiography (MRA). This latter technique presents some advantages over angio-CT such as that of not using ionizing radiation and iodinated contrast agents, and of being more versatile in its reconstruction techniques thanks to the invisibility of the bone structures located in the field of investigation. Differently from other ultra-sonographic techniques, MRA allows a panoramic and objective view of the vascular district being examined, without the limit of a reduced field of view or of dependence on the operator.

6.2 Imaging techniques

Today, MRA techniques that are based on the principles of blood flow and allow the visualization of vessels without the use of a contrast agent have a limited role in the study of epi-aortic vessels. Contrast Phase (CP) sequence maintains a role in the evaluation of the vascular hemodynamics, while the Time of Flight (TOF) technique has been substituted by Contrast Enhanced MRA (CEMRA).

The diagnostic interpretation of magnetic resonance angiograms has been revolutionized by the ultrafast technique with contrast bolus. Indeed, in the techniques based on flow, the evaluation of the stenosing pathology is based on the effect of blood flow inside the vessel and requires experience in the reading and knowledge of the physical phenomena associated to flow in Magnetic Resonance Imaging (MRI); conversely, in contrast-enhanced techniques the angiogram is interpreted as a luminography, the same way as happens in conventional angiography.

6.3 Evaluation of epi-aortic vessels

MRA is usually performed with a super conductive magnet, preferably equipped with a high field and, necessarily, with high-performance gradients (maximum gradient strength >20 mT/m, slew rate >120 mT/m msec). The sequence utilized for CEMRA acquisition is a 3D fast SPGR on the coronal oblique plane, positioned along the sagittal plane after the acquisition of a scout image. In order to obtain a T1 for blood lower than that of the stationary tissue having a higher signal intensity, the operator must use a quantity of Gd-based contrast agent sufficient to reduce the blood's T1 to values below 280 msec (280 msec is the T1 of fat tissue at 1.5 T). As to the other characteristics of the CEMRA, the reader is invited to go to the chapter on fast sequences. Here, we shall recall that in the case of supraortic vessels, in order to have a better visualization of the terminal branches of small caliber, an elliptic filling of K-space is recommended [1].

The parameters utilized in a typical sequence are: TR/TE 5.7/1.6 msec, FA 30°, NEX 0.5, matrix 192×256, zero filling in slice and frequency direction, bandwidth 62.5 KHz, thickness 1.8, 40 partitions, FOV 24 cm. Generally, this technique employs a phased-array coil dedicated to the neurovascular structures of the neck. Some coils in commerce today allow the contemporary visualization of the carotid-vertebral axes and the epi-aortic vessels emerging from the arc thus allowing the study to be performed in a single acquisition.

The injection with contrast bolus is performed through the use of a MR-compatible automatic injector, using 0.2 mmol/kg of paramagnetic contrast agent that is injected intravenously at a constant rate (e.g. 2 ml/sec).

CEMRA images are then transferred to a dedicated workstation and reformatted by the reconstruction algorithms: Maximum Intensity Projection (MIP) and Multiplanar Volume Reconstruction (MPVR). Similarly, 3D volume reconstructions can be made.

In the case of steno-occlusive pathology of the cerebral ascending vessels, the CEMRA procedure can be preceded by a hemodynamic evaluation with Fast PC axial scannings or cine-PC positioned in the most vertical tracts of the carotid siphons and of the basilar artery. If requested, the CEMRA investigation can be preceded by the MRA of the intracranial vessels (see Chapter 5). When dissection of the carotid a. or of the vertebral a. is suspected or already acknowledged, it is necessary that CEMRA be preceded by T1- weighted axial scanning on the axis of the vertebral carotid, possibly with a spectral fat-saturation pulse to establish the presence of a sub-intimal hematoma.

Some MR machines do not have coils specific for MRA studies of the cerebral ascending vessels; therefore, the anatomic coverage of the emergence of epi-aortic vessels is not properly guaranteed by the coils dedicated to the examination of the neck. In such situations, it is necessary to perform a separate study on the emergence of epi-aortic vessels with surface coils or phased-array coils that are normally utilized for the study of the abdomen and, in this case, positioned at the upper part of the chest. When a non-dedicated coil is used in order to maintain a sufficient spatial resolution, it is suggested to evaluate separately the aortic arc together with the emergence of vessels and in a subsequent acquisition the vertebral carotid axes [2]. For aimed evaluations of the aortic arc and of epi-aortic vessels, the CEMRA protocol may be slightly modified. The tendency is to use a wider field-of-view (36-49 cm) to avoid the *wrap around* of the patient's shoulders. For a study limited to the epi-aortic vessels where the anatomical distribution of the vessels on the coronal plane has a relative depth, a minor number of partitions can be utilized for covering the entire anatomical district under examination. Consequently, in such cases, the scanning time decreases to values that permit acquisitions in apnea. Although the respiratory excursions of the chest cage at the pulmonary apexes are minor and breath-hold is not mandatory, apnea enhances the quality of the images and is suggested for improving CEMRA's diagnostic accuracy for such district [2]. For the study of the subclavian arteries with exclusion of the neck vessels, the controlateral brachial vein of the side having the suspected pathology is connected to the injector; otherwise an alternative access may be attempted from the dorsal surface of the foot.

In the case a functional stenosis of the subclavian is suspected, as in the Thoracic Outlet Syndrome (TOS), the exam can be performed with the patient in a supine position with the affected superior limb in abduction and the head rotated contro-laterally to the affected limb, in order to induce a paraesthesic symptomatology in the arm. Despite the uncomfortable position, the rapidity of acquisition of the CEMRA allows to perform the diagnostic test. The addition of 2D PC sequences with phase reconstruction algorithms, perpendicularly positioned to the inter-transverse tract of the vertebrae, allows to establish whether there is a vertebral steal syndrome in occurrence of a functional stenosis. Conventional T1 and T2-weighted MR topographic scans, can be made to establish the spot of compression on the vascular structures, which is usually located at the level of the scalene muscles.

6.4 Subclavian arteries

The pathologies that affect the epi-aortic vessels include the steno-occlusive diseases of atherosclerotic or inflammatory origin, functional stenoses in patients with TOS, aneurysmatic pathology and arterial-venous malformations. The stenosis of the subclavian a. is cause of claudicatio of the superior limb, paraesthesias, weakness and pain. In the case of subclavian steal syndrome, vertebro-basilar failure can occur.

Atherosclerotic disease is the most frequent pathology in the arterial epi-aortic vascular district. There has been great controversy concerning the degree of stenosis that should be treated; therefore, with the growth of endovascular treatments, the correct grading of the stenosis has taken on an important role from a clinical point of view. In order to determine the success of a Percutaneous Transluminal Angioplasty (PTA) it is, in fact, important to know the site, the length, and the morphology of the lesion [3].

Conventional angiography is the technique of reference for evaluating epi-aortic vessels. The technique implies, however, the ensuing of complications such as thrombo-embolic events and allergic reactions, in addition to nephro-toxicity of the iodinated contrast agent.

The Echo-color Doppler technique offers important information on vascular anatomy and on hemodynamic aspects, but is still operator-dependant and does not allow a panoramic view of the vascular architecture, especially for what concerns the epi-aortic vessels emerging from the arc, where the visualization is hindered by the deep lodging of such structures in the chest.

MR represents a non-invasive alternative to conventional angiography, even if classical MRA techniques (TOF and PC) based on blood-flow have produced a non-optimal visualization of this district due to artifacts caused by respiration, cardiac pulsatility, and by a saturation effect in the cases of slow or turbulent flow.

The diffusion of CEMRA has improved the diagnostic accuracy of MRA in this district, as the use of more powerful gradients allows a rapid acquisition of data, making it possible to obtain an angiogram, also breath-held, during the arterial phase of the passage of the bolus [4]. CEMRA has a high concordance with DSA in both normal and diseased arteries, with a sensitivity and specificity of respectively 92 and 96% in detecting any pathology within this vascular district.

The method identifies correctly the presence of stenoses, with a slight tendency to overestimation: the concordance with conventional angiography for the steno-occlusive disease, on both atheromasic and functional basis is excellent (k=0.85), with a sensitivity of 90%, specificity of 95% and diagnostic accuracy of 93% [5]. The correct picture can be given for both the atheromasic nature of the lesion and the arteritic one. In the case of dilatatative aneurysmatic pathology of vascular malformations, or abnormalities of the emergence of epi-aortic vessels, CEMRA has a perfect correlation with digital angiography. Greater problems arise when assessing an occlusive pathology. In fact, reperfusion of the subclavian in the postvertebral tract brought about by the inverted vertebral flow may cause diagnostic dilemmas in establishing whether there is an overestimation of a narrowed stenosis or an occlusion.

The tendency toward overestimation has been demonstrated in the case of atheromasic stenoses and functional stenoses. In the case of a functional stenosis, overestimation is neither a diagnostic nor a clinical problem. The compression *ab extrinseco* occurs downstream from the vertebral ostium, therefore the opacification downstream cannot be caused by the inverted vertebral reperfusion, but necessarily by an overestimation of functional

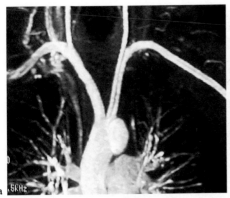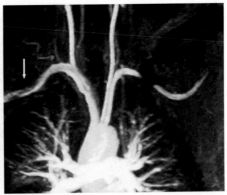

a   b

Fig. 6.1 a, b. The location of the stenosis in the functional stenosis of the subclavian a. can be established by the CEMRA technique, as for TOS. In (a) the patient in supine position, with both superior limbs abducted, has a regular flow at the supraortic vessels. In (b) the controlateral rotation of the head to the side, induces a functional stenosis caused by the Scalene syndrome. The functional stenosis is overestimated (as the residual lumen is not detected). In fact downstream vessel opacification cannot derive from vertebral reperfusion since its ostium is upstream from the stenosis. (b) also evidences the typical artifact by magnetic susceptibility (arrow) induced over the distal tract of the subclavian a. from the high concentration of gadolinium flowing in the right subclavian vein that runs beside the artery. To avoid artifact in the side clinically suspected of being affected by functional stenosis (as resulted!!), a vein of the controlateral arm was utilized to inject the contrast agent

stenoses. Moreover, it is known that treatment of TOS, as other causes of compression on the subclavian artery, does not indicate endovascular treatment and, therefore, the degree of functional stensosis does not influence the therapeutic decision (Fig. 6.1).

In the case of atherosclerotic pathology, due to the tendency of overestimation, it is possible to misinterpret the occluded arteries that are reperfused downstream because of the inverted flow in the vertebral artery. The main limit of CEMRA, compared to DSA, is the scarce temporal resolution that does not allow to appreciate of the progressive flowing of the contrast medium into the arterial tree enough to see the reperfusion of the occluded subclavian a. directly through the vertebral artery. Establishing the direction of flow – and its eventual inversion – would be possible by adding PC sequences with phase-difference reconstruction; however, it is also true that flow inversion in the vertebral a. occurs both in occasion of an occlusion of the subclavian a., and in the case of a narrowed stenosis. Hence, the demonstration of a subclavian a. steal cannot be proof of occlusion. Probably the time-resolved techniques will be able to solve the temporal hemodynamics of such situations on advancement, which would open the way to the use of radiological semiotics currently utilized with DSA for diagnosing occlusion of the subclavian a. At present, the sign of occlusion is considered to be the absolute lack of opacity of the vessel in the occluded tract, in association to flow inversion in the homolateral vertebral a. The diagnostic confidence remains in these

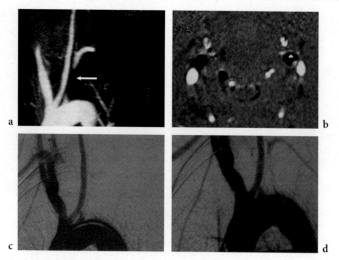

Fig. 6.2 a-d. Occlusion of the left subclavian a. (a) CEMRA evidences the long strip of missing opacification (arrow) in the prevertebral tract. (b) Downstream the vertebral ostium normal opacification of the vessel can be appreciated. The 2D PC sequence with phase difference reconstruction demonstrates an inversion of vertebral flow on the left side. (c, d) Digital angiography confirms the obstruction and the reperfusion of the postvertebral tract by the inverted left vertebral flow. In this case, CEMRA could lead the operator to consider, in addition to an occlusion, an overestimation of the narrowed stenosis, which would explain the limited diagnostic confidence that high-resolution CEMRA has in the diagnosis of occlusion of the subclavian a.

cases limited, conversely to the diagnosis of occlusion in terminal vessels such as the renal arteries, where the lack of opacification downstream surely points to occlusion. Instead, in the occluded prevertebral subclavian a., if the occlusion extends over a short lenght, downstream vessel reperfusion can induce to an erroneous diagnosis of severe stenosis overestimated by CEMRA (Fig. 6.2).

The correct diagnosis of occlusion of the subclavian a. is important inasmuch as such information changes the therapeutic choice. According to the guidelines for PTA of the Society of Cardiovascular and Interventional Radiology [3], occlusions of the subclavian a. are grouped into different categories in function of their length; in particular PTA is recommended when the occlusion is less than 5 cm, as PTA yields scarce results with occlusions over 5 cm. Therefore, the limits of CEMRA in regards to the evaluation of epiaortic vessels must be in these cases considered relevant.

In regards to vascular malformations, CEMRA is able to easily locate and visualize the main arterial feeders. The afferent vessels of smaller size are not clearly distinguishable due to the technique's limits of spatial resolution. Its use is therefore linked to the panoramic visualization of the pathology, with the end purpose of obtaining a preliminary evaluation for digital angiography, which maintains its principle diagnostic and therapeutic role.

Among the main problems in the execution of the CEMRA exams in this vascular district, noteworthy are the patient's compliance – especially for breath-holding – and the correct injection time of the bolus contrast, which remains the pivotal factor for the good outcome of all exams with contrast bolus. In reference to this, we shall recall that whenever an automatic or an interactive detection method is not available, a bolus test must be performed. This test is necessary in order to overcome the variations in circulation time, particularly relevant in patients with cardiac pump failure, in those with aneurysmatic disease of the aorta, and in subjects in whom venous access is practised in the veins of the foot dorsum rather than in the antecubital veins of the arm. Access from the foot is sometimes required for overcoming a typical artifact that occurs in the study of the subclavian arteries: the high concentration of contrast agent in the veins of the arm during the injection of the contrast agent induces an effect of magnetic susceptibility in the surrounding tissues. In relation to the particular anatomic location of the subclavian artery and vein, such distortion of the magnetic field induced by the paramagnetic contrast medium determines a loss of signal in the subclavian artery, which becomes more enhanced the more the aorta and vein overlap. One way of reducing the artifact caused by magnetic susceptibility, although not feasible in routine diagnosing, is to diminish the concentration of the contrast in the vein and to shorten the TE. Another method is to use a venous access contralateral to the side suspected of being affected (see Fig. 6.1). When there is a suspicion of a pathology of the bilateral subclavian aa., the artifact can be completely eliminated by using a venous access in the inferior limbs such as a dorsal vein of the foot which is afferent to the inferior caval system and avoids accumulation of the contrast in the subclavian vein. Although it is known that the atherosclerotic stenoses of the subclavian a. preferentially affects the prevertebral tract, and the overlapping of the vein and artery occurs in the distal tract of the subclavian a., the presence of the susceptibility artifact can create diagnostic difficulties by hindering the visualization of the distal tract of the subclavian a. Therefore, it is advised to search an access to the vein, in consideration of the diagnostic query and, if possible, an afferent access through the inferior caval system, which does not cause a reduced opacification of the arterial tree by dilution.

6.5 Carotid and vertebral arteries

6.5.1 Atherosclerotic steno-occlusive disease

To date, acute cerebral ischemic disease is one of the largest issues in healthcare, not only in clinical terms but also in terms of the financial burden of the high cost of treatment for patients who survive this disease. Atherosclerosis is the most frequent arterial pathology, often with a thrombo-embolic mechanism, and represents the most common cause of cerebral ischemia among the older population.

The risk of cerebral ischemia can be significantly reduced by Thromboendoarterectomy (TEA) in both symptomatic and asymptomatic patients with severe carotid stenosis over 70% of the vessel lumen [6]. Recently, the NASCET study (North American Symptomatic Carotid Endoarterectomy Trial Collaborators) has demonstrated the benefit of surgical treatment also in selected patients with a carotid stenosis above 50% [7]. The accurate grading of the stenosis is thus an important objective, achievable by preoperation imaging techniques, and which should be pursued for a proper planning of the thromboendoarterectomy.

The assessment of a carotid stenosis is mainly performed by digital angiography (DSA) because of its high diagnostic accuracy; it is also accepted as a preoperating technique for establishing the presence of a severe carotid stenosis requiring surgical treatment through thromboendoarterectomy. In reality, DSA is an invasive technique not free from procedural risks; moreover, it has been established that the angiographic exam may lead to a risk of cerebral ischemia in 0.7-1% of cases.

An accurate non-invasive imaging protocol void of severe complications could thus increase the benefit of surgical treatment and is greatly auspicated by physicians and surgeons. Because of the consequences of procedural risks involved in DSA, many vascular surgeons have performed endoartectomies on the basis of results from non-invasive imaging techniques. Therefore, non-invasive evaluation techniques such as spiral CT, MRA and Echo-Doppler have become widespread.

Angio-CT received a boost with the introduction of spiral tomographers and later on with the multidetector tomographer. The axial images obtained can be utilized in the measurement of the percentage reduction in the cross-section area of the vessel or in the measurement of the densities forming the atheromasic plaques, in the aim of establishing fatty, calcified, or fibrous components of the plaque itself. Because of the necessity of segmenting the various components of the structures being examined, two- and three-dimensional reconstructions are extremely laborious, yet they allow an angiographic-like visualization that has an excellent correlation with conventional angiography and the best spatial resolution among all non-invasive techniques [8]. The limits of CT with single-layer tomographers are a reduced field of view, the exposure to ionizing radiation, and the iodinated contrast agents – the latter also used in the new multiplayer tomographers.

Echo-Doppler allows the collection of information on the degree of the carotid stenosis and on the characteristics of the stenosing plaques. The similarity between results obtained by Echo-Doppler and DSA is about 70% [9], and along with the high predictive value of this non-invasive exam, it makes an ideal screening for patients who are at high risk of cerebral ischemia. The limits of this technique remain the dependency on the operator and the incomplete visualization in the case of calcified plaques, especially in the intracranial portions of the cerebro-afferent vessels. In the case of sub-occlusion, the use of contrast agents (microbubbles) seems to increase the diagnostic accuracy of the technique.

Classical MRA methods based on the properties of blood flow are frequently used in the non-invasive evaluation of carotid stenosis. 2D TOF sequences are sensitive to slow flow, even if in situations of narrowed stenosis the appearance of saturation artifacts can provoke the loss of the MR signal, which consequently leads to an overestimation of the stenosis or even to a mistaken diagnosis of occlusion, especially in the preocclusive forms. The sensitivity of MRA with conventional techniques in comparison to the gold standard of digital angiography varies in literature from 75% to 100%, while specificity varies from 59% to 99%. The major limit within these MRA techniques remains, however, the phase dispersion inside the voxel in the case of turbulent flow. Among the other limitations worthy of note are: the motion artifacts caused by long acquisition times – especially when patients are not too cooperative; saturation artifacts on the plane that in the case of tortuous cerebro-afferent vessels can lead to a mistaken diagnosis of stenosis; the limited field of view that eliminates the possibility of evaluating satellite stenoses.

The advent of CEMRA has drastically improved MRA's diagnostic accuracy in many vascular districts. Although the exact role of MRA in the diagnostic protocol of patients with carotid stenosis has not been completely established, the Echo-Doppler screening added to CEMRA appears to form a relevant alternative to DSA [10]. Several authors have reported interesting results in the evaluation of epi-aortic vessels, especially those in the carotid district, even if using low field magnets. The diffuse acceptance of this MRA technique by surgeons is due to the high sensitivity and specificity, the high diagnostic accuracy and, especially, the better representation of the morphology of the stenosis as compared to the angiographic flow-based methods, and on the panoramic potential of the evaluation (Fig. 6.3).

For what concerns the evaluation of the vertebro-basilar district, CEMRA has taken the place of TOF techniques, which are notoriously poorly reliable in the study of the vertebral ostium because of breath-motion artifacts, and in the study of the superior cervical tract, where the tortuous coursing of the vertebral a. is burdened by on-plane saturation artifacts that eventually cancels flow signal. CEMRA can reveal a vertebral stenosis over 50% with an accuracy of 98-100% and reveal occlusions with an accuracy of 100%. A greater number of studies have been undertaken on the carotid circle. In our experience on 97 patients, the comparison between CEMRA and DSA has revealed a high concordance between the two angiographic methods for the evaluation of the internal carotid (K=0.87). Sensitivity and sensibility were respectively 97 and 82% with a positive predictive value of 93% and a negative predictive value of 92%. The diagnostic accuracy was 92.5%. The intraobserver and interobserver concordance were respectively 0.94 and 0.90 [11].

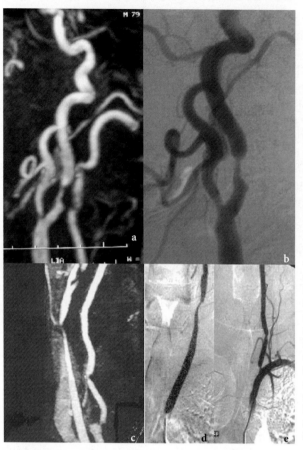

Fig. 6.3 a-e. The panoramic nature of CEMRA is useful in grading atherosclerotic disease of the cerebro-afferent vessels. Example of stenosis of the eccentric plaque of the internal carotid a. Here the excellent correlation of the degree of stenosis between CEMRA (**a**) and conventional angiography (**b**) can be appreciated. Also the basilar vertebral circle, which is difficult to explore with non-invasive techniques can be excellently visualized by CEMRA. In (**c**) a narrowed stenosis of the common carotid a. and the presence of a double stenosis of the vertebral artery. The angiography obtained with selective catheterism of the common carotid (**d**) and of the left subclavian a. (**e**) confirm the carotid stenosis before the bifurcation and the stenosis of the ostium and the intra-transversal vertebral tract

The high diagnostic accuracy of CEMRA in evaluating carotid stenoses over 70% is documented in literature by comparative studies, with DSA being variable ranging from 67 to 94%. Yet, despite these data, some authors have documented the tendency of CEMRA to overestimate stenosis [12] (Fig. 6.4). The main cause of overestimation is the mistaken timing between peak-contrast concentration within the vessel and the filling of the center of K-space, which is considered an intrinsic limit of CEMRA. It is known that the variation in infusion time influences arterial opacification. The center of K-space, and hence the area with low spatial frequencies, contributes to the contrast of the image, while the borders of K-space, hence the high spatial frequencies, contribute, to spatial resolution. The maximum signal intensity with the least artifacts is achieved when the synchronization of time of infusion allows to match the sampling of the center of K-space with peak-contrast concentration in the artery. In practice, if the center of the K-space is not acquired during peak-contrast concentration, the presence of artifacts such as ringing or blurring can cause a marked reduction of the vessel's

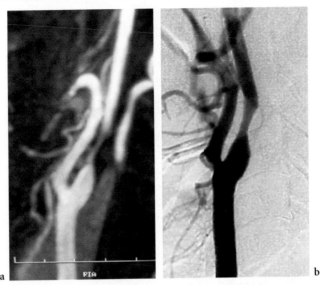

a   PIA   b

Fig. 6.4 a, b. The tendency of CEMRA to overestimate the stenosis is an important issue to consider each time there is an attempt to quantify a carotid stenosis. Although CEMRA has a low frequency for erroneous stenosis grading, an overestimation can expose the patient to a needless surgical risk. In this example CEMRA (**a**) overestimates the carotid stenosis as compared to conventional angiography (**b**), yielding an erroneous radiological indication for thromboendoarterectomy. Hence, it is suggested the surgeon obtain a concordance between Echo-color Doppler and CEMRA techniques in order to avoid conventional preoperatory angiography

lumen [13]. Another factor contributing to overestimation is given by the spin intravoxel dephasing in CEMRA. As extensively reported in literature, CEMRA is based on the shortening of blood's T1 after the infusion of a contrast bolus. This initially was considered to be a technique that was not influenced by in-flow phenomena. Recently, however, intravoxel dephasing induced by blood velocity has also been shown in CEMRA. Moreover, dephasing causes a loss in signal (which has been calculated) that depends on the medium velocity of flow when the vessel is located in a voxel [14]. In clinical practice however, this kind of artifact has a limited role with voxels currently utilized in CEMRA. In addition, the reduction of voxel-size, which should reduce the dephasing effect, translates into a better demarcation of vessel margins. Nevertheless, it does not imply a diagnostic tradeoff in the grading of the carotid stenosis according to the NASCET criteria [15]. The reduction in voxel size is hence desirable, and probably an additional size reduction would reduce intravoxel dephasing, although this potential benefit is limited by a much too weak Signal-to-Noise Ratio (SNR). Another factor towards the overestimation by CEMRA may derive from the phenomenon of magnetic susceptibility. In high-graded stenoses of the internal carotid, high contrast medium concentrations might contribute to signal loss in frail residual patent lumens.

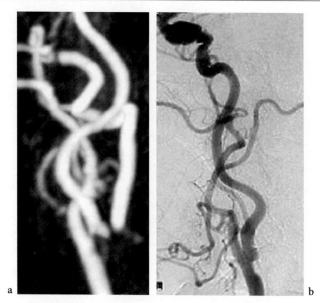

a   b

Fig. 6.5 a, b. CEMRA's tendency to overestimation is amplified by the comparison between a 3D technique and the conventional angiographic technique of reference in 2D. In this example it is clear how the narrowed stenosis visible at CEMRA (**a**) can be underestimated by conventional angiography (**b**), where the limited number of projections does not allow to obtain a correct prospective for visualizing the stenosis

The grading of a carotid stenosis is correlated to the gold standard of digital angiography, a two-dimensional technique that is at the base of the NASCET studies. Probably the introduction of rotational digital angiography will change the approach to the grading of carotid stenoses; the overestimation of stenosis by MRA discussed above is affected by the comparison between a technique based on 3D acquisitions and the 2D digital angiographic reference. It is demonstrated that the tendency of CEMRA to overestimation decreases when MRA is compared to angiograms obtained through rotational angiography of the same patients, rather than with conventional digital angiography. Likewise, the high number of projections obtainable with CEMRA is more comparable to the projections of rotational angiography than to the classic projections of conventional 2D angiography. Hence, some authors hypothesize that 2D angiography is cause for underestimation of stenosis rather than CEMRA being the cause for overestimation [16], questioning the role of conventional digital angiography as a method of reference (Fig. 6.5). Furthemore, because the surgical indications to endoarterectomy are based on conventional angiographic criteria, physicians must follow these indications in clinical practice, yet considering the possibility that CEMRA may overestimate the carotid stenosis.

Despite the fact that data report a high diagnostic accuracy for CEMRA, we must establish CEMRA's diagnostic capacity within the decision on surgical revascularization. In other words, the technique must demonstrate its capability of yielding a correct surgical indication through a correct grading of stensosis for each patient. It has recently been evaluated whether DSA modifies the decision of surgical revascularization over Echo-color Doppler and MRA in clinical practice [17]. The frequency of erroneous Echo-Doppler indications was 28%, and of that percentage 18% were for MRA alone. In the cases where the two non-invasive methods utilized were in agreement, the rate of erroneous indications toward revascularization treatment decreased to 7.9%. The authors conclude that the surgical decision of revascularization based on non-invasive methods must be taken cautiously. It is important to notice that only 1% of MRAs were performed with the ultrafast bolus contrast technique and that the vast majority of patients were evaluated by flow-based MRA.

The indication to thromboendoartectomy is based on clinical and radiological criteria as recommended by the Guidelines for carotid arterectomy [18]. A stenosis of the carotid of over 70% is considered as a surgical indication for revascularization in symptomatic and asymptomatic patients. The presence of an occlusion of the internal carotid a., or of a severe satellite stenosis of the internal or common carotid aa. is considered a radiological contraindication to revascularization.

According to our experience, the frequency of erroneous classification of the stenoses leading to a misjudged radiological indication for revascularization is 3.1% [11]. This is the lowest value for what concerns non-invasive techniques. Other studies [19] have found a much higher percentage of cases in which CEMRA has lead to erroneous indications for surgical revascularization (24%), and therefore suggest to associate CEMRA to Echo-Doppler results: if the two results agree, the erroneous indications of the combined two non-invasive methods decrease significantly. The performance of an endoarterectomy on the bases of false positive exams exposes the patient to a needless surgical risk; conversely, non-invasive exams that provide a false negative exclude the patient from the potential benefits of revascularization treatment. It is likely that non-invasive false exams, which increase the risk for cerebral infarction in patients who are deprived of the potential benefit of a surgical intervention, balance the procedural risk involved in conventional angiography: this means that a non-invasive procedure is necessarily safer than an invasive technique [20]. As we have not found surgical stenoses that have been underestimated as non-surgical, we suppose that CEMRA does not constitute a font of false negatives that deprive patients of surgical benefits. Conversely, CEMRA tends to overestimate moderate stenoses grading them as more severe than 70%, which leads to an unnecessary and useless exposure of the patient to surgical risk. The real matter that needs to be approached in detail is, hence, whether the surgical risk induced by noninvasive false positive exams balances the procedural risks of conventional angiography.

For surgeons, the presence of satellite stenoses associated with stenoses of the internal carotid a. of the neck significantly influences the decision on intervention. A severe stenosis distal to the internal carotid a. or a stenosis proximal to the common carotid a. is considered a radiological contraindication to surgery. Although the presence of satellite stenoses rarely influences in clinical practice the surgeon's decision to revascularize the patient, the additional information may have important implications for long-term treatment in symptomatic patients. Since, unfortunately, the rate of erroneous detections of such lesions is relevant, the pursuit of this information should be the main aim of non-invasive techniques. It is therefore noteworthy to underline how the stenoses of the petrousus tract of the internal carotid a. (that can be satellites to the stenoses of the neck) are revealed by CEMRA. The classical MRA techniques based on blood flow that do not use contrast media reveal only 56% of the satellite lesions [17]; this means that the introduction of CEMRA has greatly increased the possibility of the non-invasive techniques to detect satellite stenoses.

Another important observation is that the benefit from endoarterectomy does not depend on the degree of the stenosis alone, but also on the surface morphology of the stenosing plaque. While the classical MRA techniques do not provide any information on plaque configuration, CEMRA has a high sensitivity in detecting a plaque ulcer up to 100%.

One of the most important presurgical notions of the evaluation of patients with carotid stenosis is the identification of preocclusive stenosis, since endoaterectomy is suggested in preocclusive stenoses presenting a "mouse tail" at conventional angiography. It is in fact demonstrated that perioperatory complications do not increase in respect to severe stenoses showing no "mouse tail". In the past, the diagnosis of carotid occlusion collected with non-invasive techniques needed to be confirmed by digital angiography in order to exclude pseudo-occlusion, although the combination of DSA procedural risks and the surgical risk of TEA in the pseudo-occlusion would significantly increase the risk of cerebral failure.

CEMRA, conversely to other classic MRA techniques based on properties of flow, is considered accurate in distinguishing an occlusion from a pseudo-occlusion [21]. Its accuracy in diagnosing occlusions is 100%, and 77-100% for pseudo-occlusions. (Fig. 6.6). The improvement of the diagnostic accuracy in the evaluation of cerebral ascending vessels obtained by CEMRA in comparison to 2D and 3D TOF has been demonstrated as CEMRA does not have saturation effects and dephasing is limited.

For the reasons above CEMRA can be considered an accurate non-invasive technique for evaluating carotid arteries; in addition, the non-exposure to ionizing radiation and the safety in the use of paramagnetic contrasts let us to predict an ever-growing utilization of MRA. The overcoming of the long acquisition times of classic MRA advises the use of CEMRA also with less collaborative patients, as in the case of acute or sub-acute cerebral infarction. Despite the high negative predictive value of the technique, CEMRA cannot be considered a screening technique like Echo-Doppler, because of its high

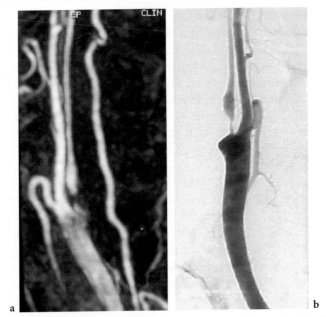

a   b

Fig. 6.6 a, b. CEMRA has surpassed the flow-based MRA techniques, particularly in the evaluation of preocclusive stenosis, which is an important watershed for the patient's eligibility for operation. With CEMRA the absence of saturation effects and the shortening of T_1 by the paramagnetic contrast agent allow the opacification, also of a frail residual lumen (**a**), allowing the radiologist to use the same semiologic criteria used for conventional angiography (**b**) in the diagnosis of preocclusion

costs and the scarce diffusion of the equipment. The main limit of CEMRA, especially in respect to digital angiography, remains the limited time-resolution, which conditions the correct evaluation of compensations at the level of the circle of Willis, and the retrograde opacification of the vessels, as may happen for example in the steal of the subclavian a.

The combination of the data obtained by Echo-Doppler and CEMRA can be exploited in a much more efficient manner by surgeons in the presurgical evaluation of the carotid stenosis. CEMRA is in fact able to satisfy the main surgical questions: whether the stenosis is detectable; its size; how far it has extended; whether it is a preocclusion or occlusion; and the presence of satellite stenoses. The unresolved surgical issues are the location of the stenosis as to the cervical metamers and the hemodynamic functional information on the intracranial circulatory compensation, that remain a prerogative of digital angiography. Probably the association of CEMRA with MRA of the intracranial vasculature and MRA perfusion studies of the encephalic parenchyma will play a determinant role in the coming years for revealing the functional aspects of the cerebral vasculature, which is indispensable information for a correct presurgical approach to the patient with carotid stenosis.

MR also allows an integrated approach of MRA and MRI. The exam can be implemented with PC sequences with phase-difference reconstruction in order to have hemodynamic information on the flow downstream the carotid stenosis (Fig. 6.7); otherwise it can be implemented with TOF MRA sequences for the evaluation of intracranial vessels. Recently, the use of specific coils allowed a good enough spatial resolution to perform a study of the atheromasic plaque with conventional sequences (T1, T2, DP) or angio, both by black blood and white blood techniques, which allow not only to measure vessel wall thickness, but also to cheracterize the components of the atherosclerotic plaque including the lipidic core, the fibrous hood, the calcified and thrombotic components [22] (Fig. 6.8). Many techniques for evaluating the plaque have the disadvantage of being invasive, as is the case for conventional angiography, intravascular Echo-Doppler and angioscopy. Non-invasive techniques such as ultrasonography and CT allow an evaluation of the size of the plaque but have a limited role in evaluating the single components of the atherosclerotic plaque. MRI allows both the evaluation of the components of the plaque and the monitoring of its changes in size in a non-invasive fashion, given the close correlation between in vitro and in vivo measurements. Moreover, attempts have been made to evaluate plaque vulnerability by measuring the thickness of the fibrous cap and evaluating an eventual rupture. Further information on plaque vulnerability can derive from the use of paramagnetic contrast agents, since the fibrous cap, which has inflammatory components shows a much higher uptake of the contrast agent than the stable fibrous cap. Studies on animal models are investigating the role of superparamagnetic contrast agents that are phagocyted by the macrophages of the atherosclerotic plaque.

6.5.2 Non-atherosclerotic pathology

The non-atherosclerotic pathology of the carotid-vertebral vessels is much less frequent than the atherosclerotic one, but is however an important cause for cerebrovascular disease especially among younger patients.

The dissection of the cerebro-afferent arteries is the main cause for cerebral infarction among younger individuals [23], causing 10% of the cerebral infarctions among individuals under 20 years of age, 20% of those under 30 years, and 2% of overall cerebral infarctions (Fig. 6.9). The first cause of artery dissection is trauma, while all remaining cases of dissection occur spontaneously. The pathogenesis of dissection still remains unknown but it has been hypothesized that a generic arteriopathy may be responsible for the intrinsic weakness of the vessel wall. The hypothesis is based on the association between dissection and predisposing pathologies, such as fibro muscular fibrosis (a hereditary disease of the connective tissue), Ehlers-Danlos type IV, Marfan syndrome, Osteogenesis Imperfecta, and Pseudoxantoma Elasticum. It has recently been reported that cutaneous biopsies from patients with no clinical signs of connective tissue disease show an association of ultra structural abnormalities of the connective tissue associated with dissection of the

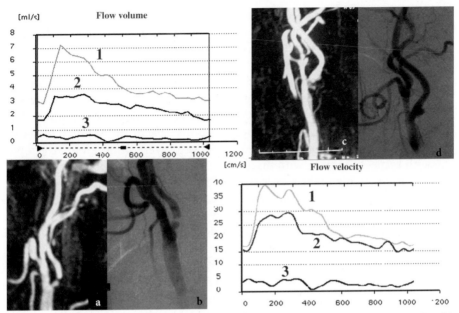

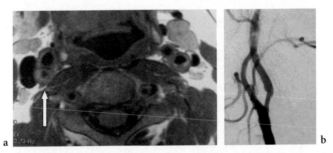

Fig. 6.7 a-d. (**a**) MRA, morphological evaluation of severe stenosis of the internal carotid a. (**b**) Same case, DSA control. (**c**) Same patient, MRA morphological evaluation of ulcerated plaque in the controlateral internal carotid a. (**d**) Same case, DSA control. The cine-PC or Fast PC sequences allow to map velocity (graphic at lower right) and flow (graphic at upper left) during the cardiac cycle in each of the vessels afferent to the brain. The example shows the marked reduction of the haematic flow downstream a severe carotid stenosis (curve 3) compared to the controlateral carotid a. where, despite an ulcerated plaque, the stensosis is not hemodynamically significant (curve 1). The flow on the stenotic side is reduced to values below those measurable in the basilar trunk (curve 2)

Fig. 6.8 a, b. MRA can be integrated by conventional MR images. The introduction of coils dedicated to the evaluation of the plaque allows the direct visualization of the stensoing plaque and its components also in vivo. (**a**) shows an axial high-resolution T1-weighted image that allows to evaluate, in addition to the grade of the stenosis on the transversal plane, also the components of the atheromasic plaque (arrow). (**b**) shows the corresponding digital angiography for stenosis of the right internal carotid a.

ascending cerebral arteries. Such abnormalities, found in 55% of patients with dissection and 100% of patients with recurring dissection, suggest that dissection represents a manifestation of genetic predisposition toward an intrinsically weak vascular phenotype.

Carotid dissection can occur at the level of the sub-intima, characterized by a consequent dissected angiographic pattern, or may occur at the level of sub-adventitious with a consequent aneurysmatic angiographic pattern. The aneurysmatic form of dissection makes up for 43% of the spontaneous dissections and seems to be supported by a more severe underlying arteriopathy with respect to forms with dissection. Within the dissection, the intramural hematoma determines a reduction of the internal lumen and an increase of the total diameter of the dissected vessel, a finding which translates at MRI into a reduction of the centroluminal flow and in an increase of vessel caliber. These are the only findings that lead to the diagnosis of dissection when the intramural hematoma in the acute phase (1-4 days) has a low signal both in T_1- and T_2-weighted images. Successively, during the sub-acute phase, when the intramural hematoma is characterized by the presence of metahemoglobin, conventional MRI allows a direct visualization of the hematoma as a hyperintense structure, often with a helicoidal coursing in contiguous scannings [24].

Flow-dependent MRA techniques are considered a useful non-invasive method for detecting the carotid dissection and posttreatment follow-up, especially when they are integrated with T_1-dependant axial tomographic scannings. Yet, the main limit to this technique remains the evaluation of the vessel wall morphology (as in cases of muscular fibrodysplasia), and the evaluation of the aneurismal dissection pattern.

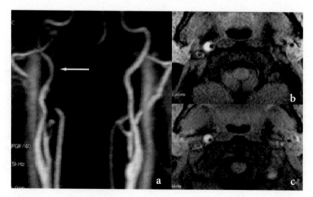

Fig. 6.9 a-c. A case of the carotid dissection. CEMRA (**a**) evidences, as in conventional angiography, a progressive narrowing of the caliber of the right internal carotid a. in its extra-cranial segment (arrow). The axial T_1-weighted scannings with spectral saturation of fat (**b, c**) evidence an intra-parietal hyperintense ring of met-hemoglobin with helicoidal disposition indicative of dissection of the sub-intima

Reports on data concerning dissecting disease of the ascending cerebral vessels obtained by CEMRA are few even if literature reports some encouraging experiences of the combined use of CEMRA and conventional imaging [25]. In theory, CEMRA should improve the evaluation of the vessel wall in cases of muscular fibro-dysplasia and of aneurysmatic patterns of the dissection. Recently, CEMRA has proven to be a powerful technique in the dissection of arterial vessels of the neck also with pseudo-aneurysmatic patterns [26]. Because digital angiography is an invasive method, it is unsuitable for repeated investigations as for monitoring recurring asymptomatic dissections, where CEMRA would instead be more indicated.

Fibro muscular dysplasia, which is a predisposing factor for dissection, is a disease with unknown etiology characterized by the proliferation of the media and intima, affecting the internal carotid a. and vertebral aa. It is cause of vascular disease among young individuals, especially in women. Although rare compared to the localization of the renal aa., it may occur that a carotid localization affects the middle third of extra-cranial internal carotid, saving the bifurcation, with the typical aspect given by the alternation of narrowings and sacciform dilatations (Fig. 6.10). It may be mono- or bi-lateral (60-75% of

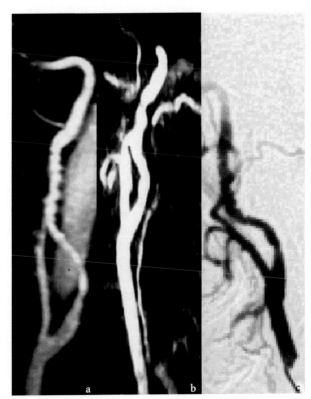

Fig. 6.10 a-c. CEMRA images are interpreted as a luminography, similar to conventional angiography. This property of CEMRA is exemplified by this case of carotid a. fibrodysplasia. In (a) CEMRA allows the appreciation of fine wall irregularities with a bead thread aspect of the carotid tract at the neck with preservation of the carotid bifurcations. In (b) the TOF technique does not allow a correct diagnosis. In (c) the digital angiography confirmation corresponds perfectly to the picture by CEMRA

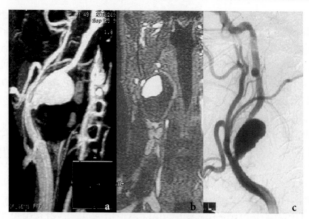

Fig. 6.11 a-c. The role of CEMRA in the aneurysmatic pathology or in carotid pseudoaneurysm is important as the limited intravoxel dephasing effect and the opacification due to the contrast agent, especially in the dilatations of greater sizes, allow a complete visualization of the aneurysmatic sac and of its neck, where present (**a**). In the single partitions of the volume acquired with CEMRA, it is also possible to visualize the endoluminal thrombotic component (**b**) increasing the information obtainable by digital angiography (**c**)

cases) and contemporarily involve the vertebral arteries (15-25% of cases). Further, it is associated with a higher incidence of intracranial aneurysms.

Other forms of obliterating arteriopathies of non-atherosclerotic nature that involve the vessels of the neck are some autoimmune and cell-mediated forms of arteritis, such as the arteritis of Takayasu or the radiation-induced arteritis. This is brought by late sequels of radiation therapy for neck tumors and appears as long stenotic tracts of the internal carotids. Although these pathologies have no typical angiographic characteristics, they could be thoroughly evaluated by a non-invasive technique such as CEMRA in virtue of its capacity of evaluating the morphology of the vessel wall in an indirect way.

Mention should also be given to carotid aneurysmatic formations of possible posttraumatic or postmycotic genesis. In such pathologies CEMRA could cover an important role in the presurgical evaluation or in view of an endovascular treatment since the filling of the aneurysmatic sac with paramagnetic fluid allows to overcome the typical problems of classic MRA techniques caused by turbulent and slow flow inside the vascular ectasia. Moreover, the analysis of the single partitions acquired by CEMRA allows to evaluate also the real dimensions of the aneurysmatic sac independently from the amount of stratified thrombotic material inside the aneurysm. In this context CEMRA provides more complete information than conventional angiography (Fig. 6.11).

A role that still must be defined is the one concerning vascular malformations. Time resolved CEMRA has shown to be a useful complement to con-

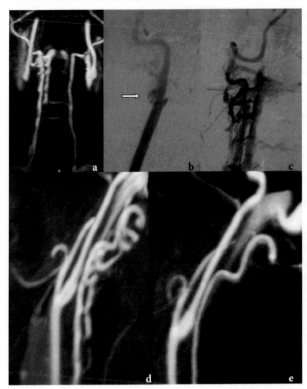

Fig. 6.12 a-e. In this example the abnormal and early opacification of the epidural venous plexa is visible during the arterial phase of the angiogram (**a**), indicative of an extradural spinal malformation (vertebral-epidural fistula). The small fistula (arrow) visible in conventional angiography (**b, c**) cannot be appreciated with CEMRA because of the technique's limited spatial resolution. Compared to the initial exam (**d**), after endovascular treatment of the fistula, CEMRA allows to establish the success of the treatment confirmed by the disappearance of the abnormal epidural enhancement (**e**)

ventional MRA techniques in the study of spinal vascular malformations [27] and could have a role in that of extradural spinal malformations involving the cerebral ascending vessels (Fig. 6.12).

References

1. Wutke R, Lang W, Fellner C, et al (2002) High-resolution, contrast-enhanced magnetic resonance angiography with elliptical centric k-space ordering of supra-aortic arteries compared with selective ray angiography. Stroke 33:1522-1529
2. Wetzel S, Bongartz GM (2000) Carotid and vertebral arteries in magnetic resonance angiography. Springer Verlag Berlin, pp 217-234
3. Standards of practice committee of the society of cardiovascular and interventional radiology (1990) Guidelines for percutaneous transluminal angioplasty. Radiology 177:619-626
4. Prince MR, Yucel EK, Kaufman JA, Harrison DC, Geller SC (1993) Dynamic gadolinium-enhanced three-dimensional abdominal MR arteriography. J Magn Reson Imaging 3:877-881
5. Cosottini M, Zampa V, Petruzzi P et al (2000) Contrast-enhanced three-dimensional MR angiography in the assessment of subclavian artery diseases. Eur Radiol 10:1737-1744

6. North American Symptomatic Carotid Endarterectomy Trial Collaborators (1991) Beneficial effect of carotid endarterectomy in symptomatic patients with high-grade carotid stenosis. N Engl J Med 325:445-453

7. Barnett HJ, Taylor DW, Eliasziw M et al (1998) Benefit of carotid endarterectomy in patients with symptomatic moderate or severe stenosis. N Engl J Med 339:1415-1425 for the North American Symptomatic Carotid Endarterectomy Trial Collaborators

8. Sameshima T, Futami S, Morita Y et al (1999) Clinical usefulness of and problems with three-dimensional CT angiography for the evaluation of arteriosclerotic stenosis of the carotid artery: comparison with conventional angiography, MRA, and ultrasound sonography. Surg Neurol 51:301-309

9. Steinke W, Kloetzsch C, Hennerici M (1990) Carotid artery disease assessed by Color Doppler flow imaging: correlation with standard Doppler sonography and angiography. AJR 154:1061-1068

10. Patel MR, Kuntz KM, Klufas RA et al (1995) Preoperative assessment of the carotid bifurcation. Can magnetic resonance angiography and duplex ultrasonography replace contrast arteriography? Stroke 26:1753-1758

11. Cosottini M, Pingitore A, Puglioli M et al (2003) Contrast-enhanced three-dimensional magnetic resonance angiography of atherosclerotic internal carotid stenosis as the non invasive imaging modality in revascularization decision making. Stroke 34:660-664

12. Leclerc X, Martinat P, Godefroy O et al (1998) Contrast-enhanced three-dimensional fast imaging with steady-state precession (FISP) MR angiography of supraaortic vessels: preliminary results. AJNR 19:1405-1413

13. Maki JH, Prince MR, Londy FJ, Chenevert TL (1996) The effects of time varying intravascular signal intensity and k-space acquisition order on three-dimensional MR angiography image quality. J Magn Reson Imaging 6:642-651

14. Scheffler K, Boos M, Steinbrich W, Bongartz G (1998) Flow sensitivity of contrast enhanced MRA. MAGMA 6(suppl 1):178

15. Cosottini M, Calabrese R, Puglioli M et al (2003) Contrast-enhanced three-dimensional (3D) MR-angiography (CEMRA) of neck vessels: does dephasing effect alter diagnostic accuracy? Eur Radiol 13:571-581

16. Fellner FA, Wutke R, Lang W (2001) Imaging of internal carotid arterial stenosis: is the new standard non invasive? Radiology 219:858-859

17. Johnston DC, Goldstein LB (2001) Clinical carotid endarterectomy decision making: noninvasive vascular imaging versus angiography. Neurology; 56:1009-1015

18. Moore WS, Barnett HJ, Beebe HG et al (1995) Guidelines for carotid endarterectomy. A multidisciplinary consensus statement from the ad hoc. Committee, American Heart Association. Stroke 26:188-201

19. Johnston DC, Eastwood JD, Nguyen T, Goldstein LB (2002) Contrast-enhanced magnetic resonance angiography of carotid arteries: utility in routine clinical practice. Stroke 33:2834-2838

20. Norris JW, Rothwell PM (2001) Noninvasive carotid imaging to select patients for endarterectomy: is it really safer than conventional angiography? Neurology 56:990-991

21. Remonda L, Heid O, Schroth G (1998) Carotid artery stenosis, occlusion, and pseudo-occlusion: first pass, gadolinium enhanced, three-dimensional MR angiography. Preliminary study. Radiology 209:95-102

22. Choi CJ, Kramer CM (2002) MR imaging of atherosclerotic plaque. Radiol Clin North Am 40:887-898

23. Guillon B, Levy C, Bousser MG (1998) Internal carotid artery dissection: an update. J Neurol Sci 153:146-158

24. Levy C, Laissy JP, Raveau V et al (1994) Carotid and vertebral artery dissections: three-

dimensional time-of-flight MR angiography and MR imaging versus conventional angiography. Radiology 190:97-103

25. Phillips CD, Bubash LA (2002) CT angiography and MR angiography in the evaluation of extracranial carotid vascular disease. Radiol Clin North Am 40:783-798

26. Phan T, Huston J 3rd, Bernstein MA, Riederer SJ, Brown RD Jr (2001) Contrast-enhanced magnetic resonance angiography of the cervical vessels: experience with 422 patients. Stroke 32:2282-2286

27. Mascalchi M, Cosottini M, Ferrito G et al (1999) Contrast-enhanced time-resolved MR angiography of spinal vascular malformations. J Comput Assist Tomogr 23:341-345

7   Heart

7.1 Heart morphology

Massimo Lombardi, Anna Maria Sironi, Lorenzo Monti, Mariolina Deiana, Piero Ghedin

7.1.1 Introduction

Echocardiography is the most commonly employed technique for the study of heart morphology. This technique satisfies most clinical necessities but may present some problems with the acoustic window and produce poor quality images. In such cases, aid may be provided by an additional Magnetic Resonance Imaging (MRI) study. Indeed, MRI has no window limitations, has a large Field of View (FOV), allows to obtain images on any spatial plane and to acquire both static and dynamic images, and provides three-dimensional (3D) images. Furthermore, this technique allows accurate non-invasive assessment of the Right Ventricular (RV) mass and function (quantitative measurements of volumes); their evaluation is limited when using two-dimensional Echocardiography or radionuclide ventriculography because of the required geometric assumptions regarding RV anatomy or overlapping of other cardiac chambers. MRI offers some special advantages over other diagnostic imaging methods (transthoracic and transesophageal Echocardiography, Computed Tomography (CT), Electron Beam Tomography (EBT), catheterization and chest X-ray) since it does not use ionizing radiation and, furthermore, the radio frequency radiation penetrates bone structures and air without attenuation.

Importantly, MRI offers additional diagnostic information on characteristics of tissue and gives images with a high contrast between stationary tissues and circulating blood, in addition to good spatial resolution. In certain circumstances, due to its particular features, MRI allows to characterize and differentiate the tissues with great accuracy and a wealth of histopathological information that would otherwise be obtained only in an invasive manner.

7.1.2 Study of heart morphology

The best morphological images are those obtained with fast techniques, requiring acquisitions in breath-hold, and particularly those in which the patient stops to breath in the middle of expiration in order for the operator to have the best reproducibility. One of the prerequisites for an accurate morphological study of the heart by MRI is an efficient synchronization with ECG and the presence of sinus rhythm or, at least, the absence of uncontrolled arrhythmias. In fact, in presence of a ventricular bigeminism or of an atrial fibrillation with great variability of ventricular response, image quality is inevitably poor and the best solution is to postpone the exam or pretreat the patient with anti-arrhythmic drugs. In cases of arrhytmia breath-holding sequences are unfeasible: when R-R variability exceeds the preset limits (in the "arrhythmia rejection" windows of the scanner software menu), the machines automatically set in standby, lengthening the acquisition time, which eventually reduces patient compliance. Today, the study of the morphology, as well as of other cardiological aspects, is done preferably using specific surface coils that exploit phases-array technology (4-8 channels), which remarkably improve the Signal-to-Noise Ratio (SNR).

7.1.3 Scanning and segment planes of the heart

In general, the images obtained with a rigorous orientation along the body axes (axial plane for example) are indispensable for the topographic images of the cardiac and pericardiac masses, for the evaluation of the pericardium, of the aorta, of the anterior wall of the right ventricle, of the pulmonary veins, of the superior and inferior cava veins and for the study of the mediastinal space (Fig. 7.1a-f). Yet, the axial approach is not suitable for measuring wall thickness and the diameters of the cardiac chambers, since these structures lay on planes oblique to the three spatial planes; therefore, the correct measurements must be taken on planes oriented according to the cardiac axes. Likewise, the sizes of the aorta and of the large vessels must be taken keeping into account their spatial position, and thus on planes orthogonal to the vessel's major local axis.

As recommended by the American Heart Association (AHA), a correct evaluation of heart morphology requires that the images be obtained according to oblique planes along the main axes of the heart [1]. This involves the use of planes passing through the short axis of the left ventricle, and the long vertical and horizontal axes (Fig. 7.2), and oriented in space 90° one to the other. In Echocardiography, these planes correspond respectively to the short parasternal axis, to the apical projection in 2 chambers and 4 chambers.

The cardiac muscle visualized in this manner can be divided into a variable number of segments; in particular MRI can employ from 9 (for clinical use) to 400 segments (for research purposes). However, it is general accepted practice to use 17 segments (Fig. 7.3), 6 of which are basal, 6 mid-cavity, 4 apical, plus 1 that is the so-called true apex (consisting of the apical cap); the third basal segment is located between the mitral annulus and the apex of the

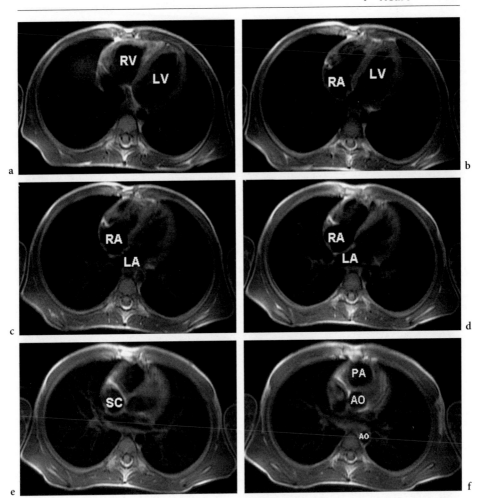

Fig. 7.1 a-f. Spin Echo Images obtained in breath-hold on axial planes parallel one to the other (slice thickness 8mm) in caudal-cranial direction. Abbreviations: RA=Right Atrium, LA=Left Atrium, RV=Right Ventricle, LV=Left Ventricle, PA=Pulmonary Artery, AO=Aorta, SC=Superior Vena Cava

papillary muscles in end-diastole; the third mid-cavity covers the entire length of the papillary; the third apical covers the area that goes beyond papillary muscles to just before the cavity end. The true apex is the area of myocardium located after the end of the left ventricular cavity (along an imaginary line going from the base to the apex).

The true apex can be evaluated from the vertical and horizontal long axis. The division into 17 segments is the most truthworthy, reflecting both the territories supplied by the main coronary arteries and the distribution of the heart mass, which from autoptic studies results to be 42% for the base, 36% for all the medium tract, and 21% for the distal tract + apex: using this tech-

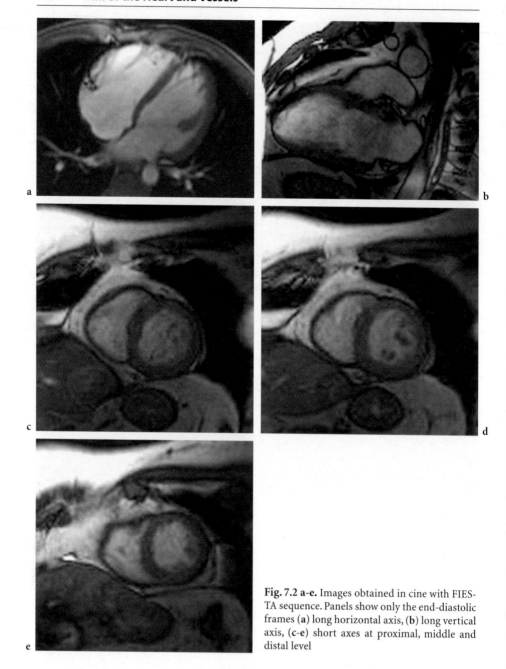

Fig. 7.2 a-e. Images obtained in cine with FIES-TA sequence. Panels show only the end-diastolic frames (**a**) long horizontal axis, (**b**) long vertical axis, (**c-e**) short axes at proximal, middle and distal level

nique a distribution of 35% is assigned to the base and the mid-cavity tract, 30% to the distal region plus the apex. Hence, for assessing of the myocardium and the left ventricular cavity it is recommended to divide the heart into 17 segments.

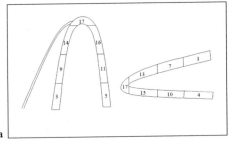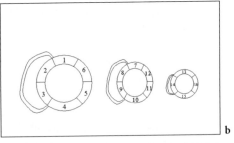

a   b

Fig. 7.3 a, b. Diagram of left ventricle segmentation. Left panel: horizontal (left) and vertical (right) long axis. Right panel: short axis of the left ventricle, proximal (basal), middle and distal (apical) planes (from left to right).

A total of 17 segments are defined:

1 = proximal anterior	7 = middle anterior	13 = apical anterior
2 = proximal antero-septal	8 = middle antero-septtal	14 = apical septal
3 = proximal infero-septal	9 = middle infero-septal	15 = apical inferior
4 = proximal inferior	10 = middle inferior	16 = apical lateral
5 = proximal infero-lateral	11 = middle infero-lateral	17 = true apex
6 = proximal antero-lateral	12 = middle antero-lateral	

The slice thickness used for evaluating myocardial segments (for example, for locating ischemic areas) is generally between 6-8mm, or at least less than 1 centimeter: slices less than 3 mm do not present particular advantages.

In addition to the images along the cardiac axes, we may use sagittal images to visualize the RV outflow tract (as in the study of Arrhythmogenic Right Ventricular Cardiomyopathy (ARVC), congenital heart diseases, etc) and axial images to evaluate pulmonary veins and large vessels.

7.1.4 Strategy of image acquisition

The first unevitable approach for locating the approximate position of the heart and of the large vessels within the chest is to obtain scout images, taking the three main planes of the body (axial, coronal, and sagittal) as reference. Scout images are obtained in Gradient Echo, which have the advantage of being acquired in a few seconds (10-30 depending on the number of images and on heart rate).

In certain circumstances (as in complex congenital cardiopathies), that require more specifically oriented images in terms of spatial location, we can utilize images obtained in real time (these, too, in Gradient Echo) without electrocardiographic synchronization. Although the images lose somewhat in quality, this technique enables to obtain images in fractions of seconds on a single plane and to vary the scanning plane in an interactive manner, allowing to "chase" the anatomical detail required.

Classically, the study of the morphology is based on "black blood" sequences (Spin Echo, SE) that generate static images with an excellent spatial resolution (1-1.5 mm on the plane) (Fig. 7.1a-f), while the "white blood" techniques (Gradient Echo, Fast Cine Gradient Echo, cine Spoiled Gradient Echo, and the most up to date ultrafast sequences, such as Steady-State Free Precession (SSFP) pulse sequences) are used for obtaining reconstructions of the cardiac cycle (20-30 phases) and are thereby suitable for evaluating cardiac function. Conversely, this distinction remains true only in part when referring to modern equipment since some sequences, such as SSFP, provide anatomical information of great detail (Fig. 7.2) and present a high contrast between the circulating blood and the myocardial wall.

According to the complexity of performances demanded to the MRI exam, the operator can conduct the study in the most appropriate manner by choosing among several options and sequences offered by the hardware of the equipment available: the traditional Spin Echo sequences (TR 400-1000 ms, TE > 20 ms and such to allow the de-phasing of spins and consequent erasing of blood flow) can be obtained in free breathing while the Fast Spin Echo "black blood" sequences (with flow suppression by double inversion pulse) and the Triple Inversion Recovery Fast Spin Echo can be obtained in breath-hold (18-22 seconds per each breath-hold). Nowadays, the SE in free breathing are only used occasionally owing to their mediocre quality, the inevitable interferences of breathing, and a long acquisition time (3-5 minutes); yet they are appreciated for their greater weight in T1 due to the shorter TR (350-600 msec) that may be important whenever we wish to characterize the composition of an abnormal tissue or the presence of fatty infiltrations of the myocardial tissue. T2-weighted sequences (TE is typically 50 to 90 ms) have an increased image contrast, which may be helpful for tissue characterization. Moreover, the signal dynamics of these sequences are well known to those performing imaging with MR, and therefore the sequences are extremely precious in cases of uncertainty. These sequences are also the only feasible solution in case of arrhythmias that make breath-held sequences unsuitable.

The most suitable sequences for the study of organs in continuous motion are the Fast SE images (breath held), even if they are extremely sensitive to breathing artifacts and require more collaboration on behalf of the patient. The Fast SE "black blood" can either have a long TR (more than 1 sec) which would allow to acquire the signal every other beat, or have a shorter TR (less than 1 sec) which would allow to acquire the signal at every R-R interval. The latter has a stronger weight in T1, a better SNR ratio and is less prone to breath motion or flow artefacts (Fig. 7.1a-f). All Fast SE T1 sequences can be used with the fat suppression option, which is very helpful whenever there is suspicion of ARVC or of cardiac lipoma.

Triple Inversion Recovery sequences are more suitable when we need to characterize abnormal tissue (see Chapter on cardiac masses). In fact, differently from what happens for the study of other organs, the use of images in T2 (with TR>2000) both in breath-hold and synchronized with breathing

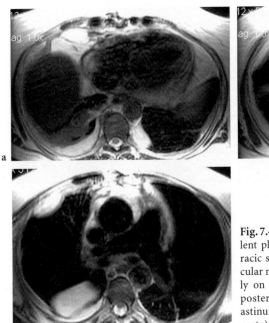

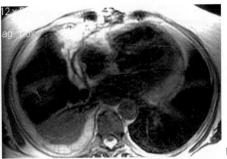

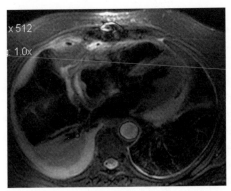

Fig. 7.4 a-c. Images in T2 in a patient with purulent pleural-pericardial-mediastinitis after thoracic surgical intervention. In evidence corpuscular matter at the level of the pleura (prevalently on the right), the pericardium (prevalently posterior), and the superior-anterior mediastinum (prevalently anterior to the ascending aorta)

and with ECG, produces very mediocre results because of the extreme sensitivity of the images caused by motion and haematic flow (Fig. 7.4a). Conversely, triple IR images are generally of excellent quality (Fig. 7.5 and Fig. 7.6a, b).

Generally speaking, T2 images are useful in the characterization of pericardial effusions or collections of fluid, while the triple IR images can be utilized for suppressing fatty tissue and are thereby the natural evolution and complement of sequences in the classical SE with FAT suppression, because of their

Fig. 7.5. Image in IR obtained along an axial plane. The same patient as in Figure 7.4 with pleural-pericardial-medistinitis. In this case the corpuscular matter appears hypointense, while the more fluid component appears hyperintense

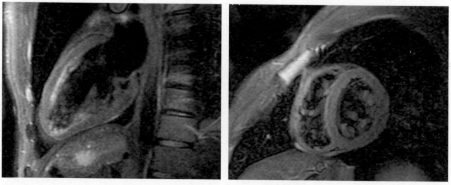

a b

Fig. 7.6 a, b. Images in IR performed in the intent of saturating the signal from the adipose tissue, which appears homogeneously hypointense. Image on the long vertical axis (**a**), and on the short axis (**b**)

higher acquisition speed (12-16 vs 18-22 sec) and excellent spatial resolution. The worst defect in triple IR sequences is the presence of a high signal from blood flowing at lower circulation velocity (as that close to the ventricular wall).

Thus a standard morphological study should foresee images in Fast SE "black blood" (8 mm thick, interslice gap 0 or 1 mm) in axial or para-axial planes (15-20 slices); images in para-axial view in Fast SE "black blood" with fat saturation and/or in triple IR of the left and right ventricle (12-20 slices) whenever there is a suspicion of fatty infiltrations, or a tissue characterization is required. Furthermore, a morphological study of the heart calls for cine-GRE, SPGR, or ultrafast sequences (SSFP) that provide images on the vertical and horizontal long axis for the study of the diameters and thickness of the cardiac chambers (Fig. 7.7a-d). Once the images are obtained, the operator decides to perform other planes to visualize a morphological detail or an anatomical relation. With the modern equipment available today it is rare that a cardiac study be restricted to the morphological aspect alone, while it is practically the rule to perform a deeper cognitive investigation also including the evaluation of function.

7.1.5 Techniques for measuring wall thickness and cardiac diameters

Similarly to Echocardiography, the measurement of thickness and cardiac diameters is performed in end-diastole and therefore in the end-diastolic frame obtained in the cine images. For this purpose, images on the horizontal axis of the heart (Fig. 7.2a) or on the short axis are generally utilized [3].

To date, there are no systematic polycentric studies that indicate the measuring technique in detail, which instead can only be inferred by similar measurements made during Echocardiography. In the case of the atria, end-sys-

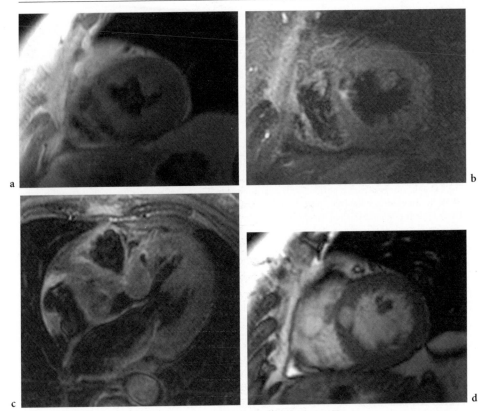

a

b

c

d

Fig. 7.7 a-d. Images from a patient with a diverticulum at the inter-ventricular septum. (**a**) Image in SE T1, (**b**) and (**c**) images in triple IR, (**d**) diastolic image obtained with the dynamic sequence (FIESTA)

tolic frames obtained on the horizontal long axis and eventually on the vertical long axis are used (Fig. 7.2b). It must, however, be underlined that since MRI is capable of highly accurate volumetric measurements, it is preferable to evaluate the volumes of the cavities and the weight of ventricular mass (see Chapter on cardiac function). Images in static "black blood" are not suitable for dimensional evaluations as they do not meet the photographic requirement of the end-diastolic or end-systolic phase.

7.1.6 Advantages and limitations

With no doubt the possibility of obtaining images on any plane, with a wide field of view and great contrast between different chest structures, greatly facilitates the diagnostic process in defining the picture of the disease. Moreover, the patient must be somewhat compliant and in stable clinical

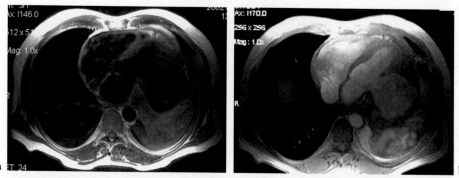

Fig. 7.8 a, b. Images from a patient with postinfarction heart rupture. Images in SE (**a**) and in cine SPGR (**b**). In evidence the large pseudo-aneurysmatic formation that occupies the left hemi-thorax. There is clear evidence of the passage between the true ventricular cavity and the pseudo-aneurysm

condition. For these reasons, MRI remains a third level test for morphological studies, but its use is gaining ground within the scenery of cardiac imaging, and is assuming the dignity of a technique of reference to turn to when a definition of the diagnostic problems is required at the highest level possible (Fig. 7.8).

References

1. Cerqueira MD, Weissman NJ, Dilsizian V et al (2002) Standardized myocardial segmentation and nomenclature for tomographic imaging of the heart: a statement for healthcare professionals from the Cardiac Imaging Committee of the Council on Clinical Cardiology of the American Heart Association. Circulation 105:539-542
2. Edwards WD, Tajik AJ, Seward JB (1981) Standardized nomenclature and anatomic basis for regional tomographic analysis of the heart. Mayo Clin Proc 56:479-497
3. Higgins CB, De Roos A (2003) Cardiovascular MRI and MRA. Lippincott Williams & Wilkins Philadelphia

7.2 Study of heart function

Anna Maria Sironi, Massimo Lombardi, Alessia Pepe, Daniele De Marchi

7.2.1 Main issues

One of the fundamental targets of cardiac imaging is to evaluate cardiac function in an accurate and reproducible manner, in order to provide the proper tools for the diagnostic-prognostic management of a vast array of heart-specific and multi-systemic disorders characterized by an altered cardiac function.

The study of cardiac function concerns practically all cardiological patients; in order to have an idea – even if partial – on the magnitude of the phenomenon, one need only consider the epidemiological data according to which 2% of the population under 65 years of age and 10% of the population over 65 is affected by heart failure [1].

The complex follow-up of a patient with heart failure or with the probability of developing heart failure not only requires that a methodology be accurate, but also highly reproducible. Accuracy and reproducibility are also indispensable requirements in the study of populations in the setting of pharmacological trials.

7.2.2 MRI: a complementary response to Echocardiography

An emblematic example of the effects of the technological evolution on cardiovascular MRI is the study of ventricular function. In the eighties, obtaining motion images of the heart was an uncertain objective and of little diagnostic significance, whereas today quick dynamic images with high spatial and temporal resolution have become a reality, making MRI, over the past 5 years, the method of reference for clinical and research purposes.

From the practical point of view Echocardiography fulfills the clinician's expectations in the vast majority of cases. Diffusion, availability, exam cost and the image quality of modern echocardiographic equipments is such that this technique remains the key examination in assessing cardiac function.

However, MRI is nowadays a sophisticated alternative when Echocardiography, which is still largely dependent on the operator and on the patient's acoustic window, gives suboptimal results. The quantification of cardiac function by MRI is not limited by geometrical assumptions, which are progressively weakened by the degree of cardiac remodeling [2]. The procedures quantifying ventricular volumes must match an excellent definition of the subendocardial borders, which often cannot be obtained through Echocardiography. Such limits are amplified when functional quantification is evaluated for the right ventricular chamber, the functionality of which is also an important diagnostic determinant in coronary heart disease [3], in congenital heart disease and in pulmonary disease. All the issues connected to a functional quantification of the ventricles in Echocardiography are stigmatized by the fact that in clinical practice the qualitative evaluation of cardiac function performed by expert operators, the quality still dominates over any effort of quantification [4].

The advantages of a functional evaluation by MRI, compared to other techniques, are represented by its non-invasiveness, the use of non-ionizing radiation, the independence from anatomical windows, and the non-administration of contrast mediums. In addition, MRI acquisition techniques can produce 3D reconstructions of the heart with ab initio digital images, oriented on any plane of space, and with high contrast between muscular structures and blood, hence providing, from these follow-ups, accurate and reproducible quantitative evaluations, independent from geometrical assumptions. MRI represents the complementary survey to Echocardiography, especially when one wants to pass from a qualitative to a quantitative evaluation.

7.2.3 Imaging strategies

The consolidated protocol for obtaining quantitative data on the cardiac ventricular chambers [5] starts with the acquisition of a coronal scout (Fig. 7.9a). Then, positioning the plane of the following acquisition at half of the cardiac profile, a sequence of dynamic images is obtained on the axial plane (Fig. 7.9b). On the end diastolic frame of this sequence of images the operator identifies the plane connecting the ventricular apex and the middle of the mitral valve in order to acquire the vertical long axis (2 chambers) (Fig. 7.9c). On the end diastolic frame of this sequence of images on the long axis the operator locates the plane connecting the heart apex and the middle of the mitral valve ring to obtain the long horizontal axis (4 chambers) (Fig. 7.9d). Following the long vertical view of planes parallel to the septum could erroneously lead to the acquisition of images on the long horizontal axis that do not necessarily pass through the center of the basal ring of the left ventricle or that could cut the tip of the apex, introducing problems of inaccuracy and reproducibility in quantitative evaluations. To obtain images on the short axis view of the left ventricle, the long horizontal plane is the preferred reference. The operator can identify the axis that connects the ventricular apex to the middle of the mitral valve on the end diastolic frame and position the planes to obtain the short axes with orthogonal orientation to this axis independent from the direction of the interventricular septum (Fig. 7.9.d). Alternatively, the short axis planes can be obtained starting from the long vertical axis, keeping the axis that connects the ventricular apex to the middle of the mitral valve as a reference (Fig. 7.9e). When acquiring the planes on the short axis we generally proceed from the atrio-ventricular groove to the apex to span the entire left and right ventricles.

It is also noteworthy to mention the technical variant for obtaining images on the long horizontal axis that utilizes a projection on the short axis at the medium ventricular level as a scout. In this case in order to obtain images on the long horizontal axis the operator positions the scanning plane on the vir-

Fig. 7.9 a-f. (a) Coronal scout; (b) end-diastolic image in axial projection; (c) end-diastolic image on long vertical axis; (d) end-diastolic image on long horizontal axis; (e) end-diastolic image on long vertical axis that is used in alternative for obtaining images on the short axis; (f) end-diastolic image on short axis at medium ventricular level that is used in alternative for obtaining images on the long horizontal axis

→

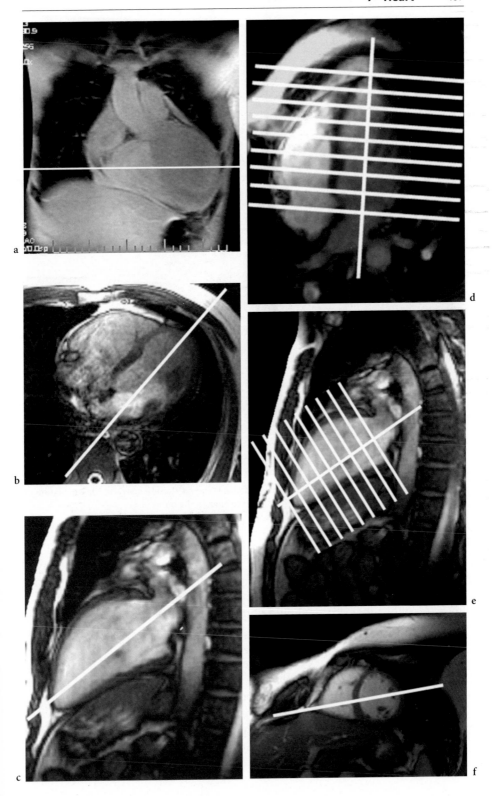

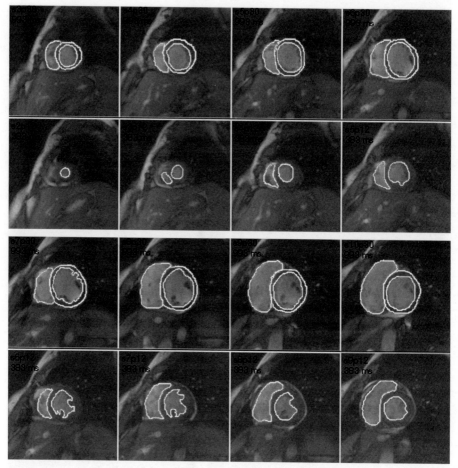

Fig. 7.10. Series of images on the short axis of the heart in end-diastole used for the calculation of the ventricular volumes (from left to right, from the apex to the base)

tual line that connects the anterior angle of the free wall of the right ventricle and the center of the left ventricular cavity (Fig. 7.9f).

If possible, the operator should obtain the dynamic sequences on the long vertical axis, on the long horizontal, and on the short axis in breath-hold (preferably in mild expiratory apnea).

To optimize the accuracy of measurements, a slice thickness of 8-10 mm and a distance of 0-2 mm between planes is generally used in a scanner of 1.5 Tesla. This way, the two ventricles are covered over their entire extension with 10-12 planes on the short axis (Fig. 7.10).

With collaborative patients, an expert operator can perform a study of ventricular function in about 10-15 minutes.

7.2.4 Sequences used for evaluation of cardiac function

The sequences in Spoiled Gradient Echo (SPGR) in free breathing (typical parameters being: TE 8.5 msec, TR 30 msec, FA 20°), with ECG gating has opened the way to the study of cardiac function, yet the time required to obtain such sequences makes them obsolete and limits their use exclusively to non-collaborative or arrhythmic patients. Modern scanners are equipped with fast sequences such as the SPGR itself – but with a different setting of acquisition parameters (TE 4.3 msec, TR 7.9 msec, FA 15°, 8-12 lines per segment) (Fig. 7.11a, b), and ultrafast sequences (steady-state free precessing, SSFP) (TE 2.1 msec, TR 4.9 msec, FA 45°, 12-16 lines per segment) (Fig. 7.11c, d) to be performed in breath-held acquisition.

Both the fast SPGRE and the ultrafast sequences (SSFP) allow to achieve 30 or more cardiac phases per heart beat (going under 11 phases leads to inadequate information on cardiac dynamics!).

The SPGR generates images of the muscular structures and blood with an adequate contrast, but optimal contrast is obtained with SSFP, which has the advantage of further reducing the acquisition time (8-20 seconds for the SPGR, 8-12 seconds for the SSFP). In addition to these sequences, there are even faster ones of echo planar derivation that are able to generate a cardiac cycle in 4-8 seconds per slice (24-30 lines per segment). As all SSFP images, they are very sensitive to flow artifacts and result noisy along the long axes of the heart (Fig. 7.9b), however the images on the short axis are almost always of excellent quality.

In order to obtain good quality images, it is extremely important to optimize in all breath-held sequences the lines per segment (Fig. 7.11g, h), i.e. the quantity of K-space to fill for each cardiac cycle: with a long R-R the number of lines per segment can be increased to reduce acquisition time; conversely with a short R-R, the number of lines per segment should be reduced. For what concerns the tolerance threshold of R-R variability, the tighter this parameter is (compatibly with the patient's conditions), the better the quality of the images.

7.2.5 Evaluation of the cardiac function with MR and postprocessing

The images obtainable in MRI are generally of high quality, and considerably facilitate the experienced eye when evaluating regional myocardial contractility and the global functional level of the ventricles. However, utilizing MRI as a "superecho" is a temptation that clashes with the reality of an expensive, lengthy exam that in these terms, hardly competes with Echocardiography. Except for cases of patients with a bad acoustic window, the qualitative evaluation alone depreciates the added value of obtaining functional quantitative

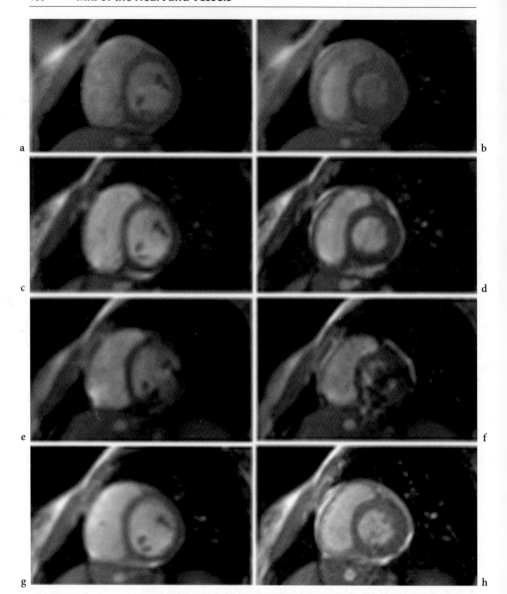

Fig. 7.11 a-h. (a, b) Images in SPGR (end-diastole and end-systole); (c, d) images obtained with FIESTA (end-diastole and end-systole) that produce a better contrast between structures than the images above; (e, f) images obtained by FIESTA Echo Train (end-diastole and end-systole) with a shorter acquisition time at the expense of a worse SNR and the presence of flow artifacts; (g, h) images obtained by FIESTA Echo Train (end-diastole and end-systole), after optimization of the sequence with a reduction of the amount of signal sampled per heartbeat (lines per segment) and reducing the R-R variability tolerance (arrhythmia rejection)

parameters in an operator independent manner, offered by such a refined technique. For this purpose transferring the images to a work-station with an adequate postprocessing program is unavoidable. The analysis of the images

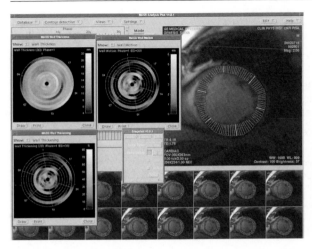

Fig. 7.12. Semi-automatic evaluation of ventricular function in a patient with dilatative cardiac disease. The bull's eye view gives an immediate picture of regional function

is based on the manual or semiautomatic recognition of the endocardial and epicardial edges of each ventricle, at least in end-diastolic and end-systolic phases in each slice. The papillary muscles and the endocardial trabeculae should be included in the calculation of the mass, except for when one wishes to evaluate regional function. It is important to exclude the atria that emerge from the basal images during systole. The mass is given by the volume of the myocardium multiplied by its specific weight of 1.05 g/cm³. The end-diastolic and end-systolic ventricular volumes are equal to the sum of the endocardial surfaces multiplied by the distance between the center of each slice (Fig. 7.12): their evaluation is independent from geometrical assumptions [6]. The stroke volume is given by the difference of end-diastolic and end-systolic volumes. The ejection fraction is given by the ratio between the stroke volume and the end-diastolic volume. The cardiac output is given by the product of the stroke volume multiplied by the heart rate. In presence of valvular disease however, the cardiac output determined as above is obviously higher than the real anterograde flow. In such situations it is advised to add to the measurements of the volumes performed as indicated above, the measurements of flow in the ascending aorta measured with PC contrast images [7] (see Chapter 2). The aortic flow measured on a complete cardiac cycle represents the stroke volume of the left ventricle. Likewise, the flow in the pulmonary artery measured over a complete cardiac cycle represents the stroke volume of the right ventricle. It is thereby possible to easily quantify the real anterograde flow and the regurgitation volume precisely, and compare such data with those obtained by the ventricular planimetry. The manual or semi-automatic identification of the sub-endocardial and sub-epicardial edges allows the regional functional evaluation in a very precise manner. The measurement of the diastolic and systolic segmental thickness, of wall thickening, and derivable parameters (Fig. 7.12) reduces the intrinsic bias of qualitative evaluations.

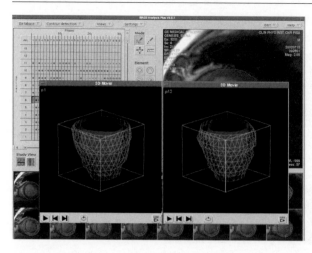

Fig. 7.13. 3D reconstruction of the left ventricle from short-axis images (same patient of previous figure, affected by dilatative cardiac disease)

For an experienced operator, postprocessing time is on average 20 minutes, depending on the quality of the images. The postprocessing systems available today allow an efficient and elegant representation of the regional function, facilitating the clinical work (Figs. 7.12, 7.13).

7.2.6 MRI quantification of left and right ventricular dimensions: accuracy and reproducibility

Cardiac Magnetic Resonance Imaging has shown to be an accurate and reproducible tool for the estimation of both Left Ventricular (LV) and Right Ventricular (RV) measurements, and is being increasingly recognized as the gold standard for non-invasive evaluation of cardiac function. MRI is completely non-invasive and its availability is widely increasing. It allows the acquisition of sequential 2D slices or 3D volumes in any desired plane with high spatial and temporal resolution. One major advantage is the high accuracy and reproducibility for volumetric assessment of both the left and right ventricle [8]. Previous studies found substantial differences for the determination of global LV function by comparing early MRI techniques with Echocardiography, Left Ventriculography and Radionuclide Ventriculography [9]. More recently, a better correlation with MRI has been found when adopting the most advanced echocardiographic techniques [10]. However, Cardiovascular Magnetic Resonance (CMR) has shown a better inter-study reproducibility in the assessment of Left Ventricular (LV) parameters. The inter- and intra-observer variability of the evaluation of the cardiac function, LV mass and ventricular volumes is very low compared to the other imaging techniques, since it is around 5% in normal subjects as in patients with altered cardiac function [11-14]. Therefore, breath-held CMR is a fast comprehensive technique for the assessment of cardiac volumes, function, and mass in cardiac patients because of its accuracy but also its high reproducibility. This allows to reduce considerably the number of patients required to prove the hypothesis in research studies, which suggests a potential for important research cost savings [15].

Lorenz *et al.* [11] published the first normal range of values for cardiac MRI LV mass and volumes, utilizing a conventional cine Gradient Echo sequence performed with free breathing. A different normal range for turbo Gradient Echo (turbo GRE) in breath holding was developed by Marcus *et al.* [12]. But the most frequently used technique now, and likely in the future, is the Steady-State Free Precession pulse sequence (SSFP), because of improved delineation of the endocardial borders and faster acquisition time. The comparisons between the two techniques (turbo GRE and SSFP) showed systematic differences: SSFP yields larger end-diastolic volumes (EDVs) and end-systolic volumes (ESVs) and smaller LV mass measurements than turbo GRE. The difference between these two pulse sequences may be due to the difference in endocardial border definition. Slow flow of blood at the endocardial border results in a poor signal, reduced contrast between blood and myocardium, and therefore potential overestimation of wall thickness in the turbo GRE pulse sequences. Hence the normal ranges for the different pulse sequences are not interchangeable. Furthermore, differences related to the age of the patient must also be considered [13] (Tables 7.1, 7.2).

Table 7.1. Mean values ± SD of left and right ventricle dimensions based on acquisition with cine GRE and SSFP*

	GRE		SSFP	
	Male	Female	Male	Female
LV-EDV (ml)	152.6±34.3	123.0±19.7	168.5±33.4	134.9±19.3
LV-ESV (ml)	52.7±13.8	40.6±9.2	60.8±16.0	48.9±10.7
LV-SV (ml)	99.9±23.0	82.5±13.5	107.7±20.7	86.0±12.3
LV-EF %	65.5±4.1	67.1±4.6	64.2±4.6	64.0± 4.9
LV-Mass (g)	159.7±25.7	106.7±12.6	133.2±23.9	90.2±12.0
LV EDV/BSA (ml/m^2)	74.4±14.6	70.9±11.7	82.3±14.7	77.7±10.8
LV Mass/BSA (g/m^2)	77.8±9.1	61.5±7.5	64.7±9.3	52.0± 7.4
RV-EDV (ml)	160.4±32.6	117.4±23.2	176.5±33.0	130.6±23.7
RV-ESV (ml)	67.8±14.8	44.5±9.3	79.3±16.2	52.3±9.9
RV-SV (ml)	92.7±22.1	72.9±16.9	97.8±18.7	78.3±16.9
RV-EF %	57.6±5.4	61.8±5.3	55.1±3.7	59.8±5.0
RV EDV/BSA (ml/m^2)	78.4±14.0	67.5±12.7	86.2±14.1	75.2±13.8

* LV-EDV, RV-EDV and LV mass have been indexed to BSA.

EDV = End Diastolic Volume, ESV = End Systolic Volume, SV = Stroke Volume, EF = Ejection Fraction, BSA = Body Surface Area (modified by Alfakih et al. [12])

Table 7.2. Mean values ± SD for left ventricular dimensions based on by acquisition cine GRE and SSFP.

	GRE		SSFP	
	Male	Female	Male	Female
Age ranging between 20 and 39 years				
EDV (ml)	161.8±27.7	126.0±22.2	178.6±30.1	137.0±20.7
EDV/BSA (ml/m²)	79.3±13.7	76.1±13.2	87.6±15.3	82.6±11.5
ESV (ml)	57.2 ±11.2	42.7±10.0	64.5±16.0	50.2±11.2
SV (ml)	104.6±18.8	83.4±15.1	114.2±16.4	86.7±11.7
EF %	64.7±3.6	66.2±4.9	64.3±4.2	63.6±4.5
Mass (g)	166.9±23.4	110.9±10.3	138.9±24.5	92.9±12.2
Mass/BSA (g/m²)	81.4±8.5	67.0±5.9	67.8±10.7	56.2±7.7
Age ranging between 40 and 65 years				
EDV (ml)	145.5±37.8	120.6±17.9	160.8±34.6	133.3±18.7
EDV/BSA (ml/m²)	70.6 ±14.6	66.9±8.9	78.3±13.2	73.9±8.9
ESV (ml)	49.3±14.8	39.0±8.5	57.9±15.9	47.8±10.5
SV (ml)	96.2±25.6	81.8±12.5	102.8±22.8	85.5±13.0
EF %	66.2±4.4	67.8±4.3	64.1±5.0	64.3±5.3
Mass (g)	154.2±26.7	103.4±13.5	128.8 ±23.2	88.1±11.7
Mass/BSA (g/m²)	75.1± 8.8	57.3±5.6	62.4±7.6	48.8±5.4

EDV = End Diastolic Volume, ESV = End Systolic Volume, SV = Stroke Volume, EF = Ejection Fraction, BSA = Body Surface Area (modified by Alfakih et al [12])

7.2.7 Evaluation of diastolic function

The evaluation of diastolic function represents a relevant clinical and methodological problem. About one third of patients with heart failure have exclusively, or prevalently, a compromised diastolic function in presence of a conserved – or at least severely impaired – systolic function. The consequences in terms of morbidity and healthcare costs are comparable to those brought by systolic compromising. Risk factors are hypertension, age, diabetes, myocardial hypertrophy, and ischemic heart disease [16, 17]. Some myocardial diseases appear exclusively as a diastolic compromission (as endomyocardial fibrosis).

Catheterism (pressure-volume curves) is considered the technique of reference, but obviously cannot be used on a large scale or repeatedly on a single patient. At present, the most used imaging technique remains, with good results, Echocardiography and in particular the study of the transmitral flow by the Doppler technique.

MRI is emerging as the alternative choice, also in consideration of the fact that it is a very accurate and reproducible three-dimensional technique [17]. Several different approaches have been proposed to evaluate diastolic function: indexes derived from the time-volume curves, indexes derived from the transmitral flow as measured by the PC technique [19, 20], and 31P-MR spectroscopy measurements of the myocardial energy for the active energy-dependent process of myocardial relaxation [21].

Time-volume curves generating from GRE images provide accurate assessment of global left ventricular function without the need for geometrical assumptions; GRE and SSFP imaging yield highly reproducible measurements of ventricular volumes throughout the cardiac cycle. From the contours describing the endocardial and epicardial border of the myocardium we can measure ventricular volumes, from which the volume-versus-time curves of both ventricles can be plotted. The same principles derived from Echocardiography can be applied to these curves, although no systematic study on their accuracy has been published yet.

The maximal change of milliliters per second calculated during the rapid filling phase, gives the Peak Filling Rate (PFR). The time between end systole and the time point at which PFR occurs (Fig. 7.14) is identified as the time to PFR. PFR can be expressed relative to the end-diastolic volume (PFR/EDV) and to the stroke volume (PFR/SV).

The measurement of flow by PC sequence leads to findings similar to those commonly used in Echo-Doppler for trasmitral and pulmonary vein flows. In such cases it is mandatory to position the scan plan perpendicular to the local flow direction.

The most commonly used parameters are: early peak filling rate of E wave (defined as the max velocity detectable between the end of systole and the middle of diastole); the acceleration time (time to peak filling rate, defined as the time between the beginning of the diastole and the max velocity of filling in the middle of diastole); the peak of the A-wave (peak late filling rate, corresponding to the maximum velocity of flow measured between the middle

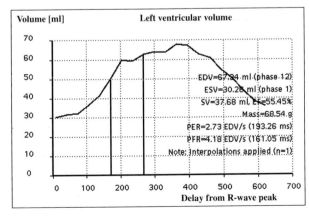

Fig. 7.14. Volume-time curve obtained from cine FIESTA images. The region between the two bars encloses the values used to calculate the peak filling rate

and the end of diastole); the E/A ratio. In the case of pulmonary vein flow, the systolic, diastolic, and reversal components [18] have been measured accurately by use of cine magnetic resonance with velocity encoding, showing close agreement with Doppler data [19, 20].

Furthermore, a good correlation has been demonstrated between velocity-based indexes and volumetric data [21]. Additionally, flow measurement by PC images is not restricted by poor acoustic windows and allows reproducible alignment with jets of any orientation, avoiding operator-dependent uncertainties in obtaining correct flow velocity profiles.

However, it must be underlined that ventricular filling patterns and flows reflect only indirectly diastolic myocardial function, as compared with patterns of myocardial wall motion. During diastole, the left ventricle rotates (*untwisting*), translates, and extends radially. Segmental contribution to this complex motion is different: untwisting is opposite in basal (counter-clockwise rotation when viewed from the apex) compared with apical segments (clockwise rotation), and radial displacement is highest in the endocardial layer compared with the epicardial layer.

Finally, 31P-MR spectroscopy has the ability of analyzing P-MR spectra and measuring the ratio of myocardial phosphocreatine and adenosine triphosphate levels (PCr/ATP) reflecting the energy status of tissue of the human heart in vivo. Myocardial relaxation is an active, energy-dependent process. Changes in 31P-MR spectra have been associated with disturbed diastolic function [21].

7.2.8 Evaluation of cardiac function by tagging images

Tagging consists in marking the myocardium with demagnetization axes (parallel lines or a grid of lines orthogonal to each another) that remain visible during the cardiac cycle (Fig. 7.15). It is one of the most fascinating innovations on the scenery of cardiac imaging in the last years. With tagging methods the magnetization of the heart (and surrounding structures) is locally perturbed in order to create MRI-visible markers (tags) within the heart wall that will move with the underlying myocardium. This, however, is only a minimal aspect compared to the computerized analysis of the behavior of such lines during the cardiac cycle. The mathematical analysis – which is still being optimized in its methodology, considering deformation, acceleration, deceleration

Fig. 7.16 a-f. Analysis of the images obtained by tagging, with the HARP technique. The Fourier analysis of the single image allows to avoid the recognition of the demagnetization lines, making the procedure operator independent: (**a, b**) the original images obtained with demagnetization lines with a different orientation (perpendicular to each other). (**c, d**) The results of the Fourier analysis on the original images; the spectral peaks are expressed as bright pixels. Only the sequences containing information on movement are retained, while all others are canceled. (**e, f**) The results of the aforementioned filter. The procedure is repeated for all images of the cardiac cycle and the tracing of the single pixel is performed over time

$\longrightarrow$

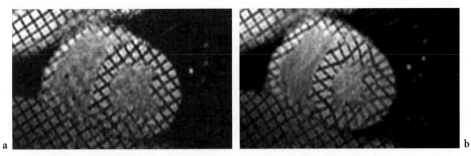

Fig. 7.15 a, b. End-diastolic (**a**) and end-systolic (**b**) images by means of tagging

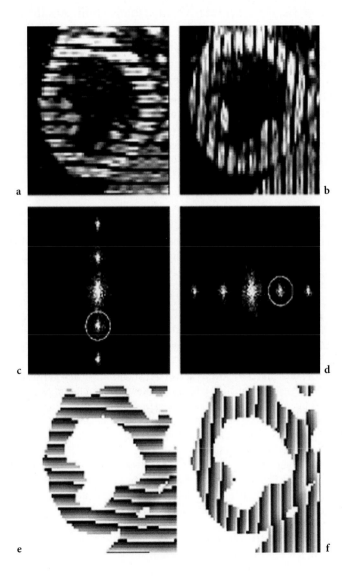

of such lines – can provide absolute quantitative information on regional myocardial contractility intended as systolic function, diastolic function, and wall strain [22]. It is noteworthy to underline that tagging represents the only possible non-invasive alternative for performing a sophisticated study of diastolic function, which at present can only be performed with intraventricular catheterism techniques available in few clinical research centers.

Before tagging becomes a routine technique with important clinical results, there are some open issues that must be solved in regards to the automatic locating systems for desaturation lines and to the standardization of the postprocessing approach.

One method of image analysis, recently put on the market, is HARP (Harmonic Analysis of Phase) [22], which actually eliminates the need for recognizing saturation lines and thereby greatly simplifies postprocessing (Fig. 7.16). Whatever the approach used, it is, however, fundamental to obtain images in which the desaturation lines remain clear during the entire cardiac cycle.

If the data provided by research centers so far is confirmed on a clinical scale, tagging could soon become a vital standard in the evaluation of systolic and diastolic functions – a technique without which we would not be able to perform advanced studies of cardiac function finalized for clinical purposes.

References

1. Ho KK, Pinsky JL, Kannel WB, Levy D (1993) The epidemiology of heart failure: The Framingham Study. J Am Coll Cardiol 22:6A-13A
2. Teichholz LE, Kreulen T, Herman MV, Gorlin R (1976) Problems in echocardiographic volume determination: Echocardiographic-angiographic correlation in presence or absence of asynergy. Am J Cardiol 37:7-11
3. Zehender M, Kasper W, Kauder E, Schonthaler M, Geibel A, Olschewski M, Just H (1993) Right ventricular infarction as an independent predictor of prognosis after acute inferior myocardial infarction. N Engl J Med 328:981-988
4. Amico AF, Lichtenberg GS, Reisner SA et al (1989) Superiority of visual versus computerized echocardiography estimation of radionuclide left ventricular ejection fraction. Am Heart J 118:1259-1265
5. Bellenger NG, Francis JM, Davies CL et al (2000) Establishment and performance of a magnetic resonance of cardiac function clinic. J Cardiovasc Magn Reson 2:15-22
6. Chuang ML, Hibberd MG, Salton CJ et al (2000) Importance of imaging method over imaging modality in non invasive determination of left ventricular volumes and ejection fraction: assessment by two- and three-dimensional echocardiography and magnetic resonance imaging. J Am Coll Cardiol 35:477-484
7. Mohiaddin RH, Longmore DB (1993) Functional aspects of cardiovascular nuclear magnetic resonance imaging: techniques and application. Circulation 88:264-281
8. Mogelvang J, Lindvig K, Sondergaard L, Saunamaki K, Henriksen O (1993) Reproducibility of cardiac volume measurements including left ventricular mass determined by MRI. Clin Physiol 13:587-597
9. Bellenger NG, Burgess MI, Ray SG, Lahiri A, Coats AJS, Cleland JGF, Pennel DJ (2000) Comparison of left ventricular ejection fraction and volumes in heart failure by echocar-

diography, radionuclide ventriculography and cardiovascular magnetic resonance: are they interchangeable? Eur Heart J 21:1387-1396

10. Morales MA, Positano V, Lombardi M, Rodriguez O, Passera M, Rovai D (2004) Semiautomatic detection of left ventricular contours in contrast-enhanced echocardiographic images: comparison with magnetic resonance imaging. J Am Soc Echocardiogr 17:876-882

11. Lorenz CH, Walker ES, Morgan VL, Graham TP, Klein SS (1999) Normal human right and left ventricular mass, systolic function and gender differences by cine magnetic resonance imaging. J Cardiovasc Magn Reson 1:7-21

12. Marcus JT, DeWaal LK, Gotte MJ, van der Geest RJ, Heethaar RM, Van Rossum AC (1999) MRI-derived left ventricular function parameters and mass in healthy young adults: relation with gender and body size. Int J Card Imaging 15:411-419

13. Alfakih K, Plein S, Thiele H, Jones T, Ridgway JP, Sivananthan MU (2003) Normal human left and right ventricular dimensions for MRI as assessed by turbo gradient echo and steady-state free precession imaging sequences. J Magn Reson Imaging 17:323-329

14. Pennel DJ (2002) Ventricular volume and mass by CMR. J Cardiovasc Magn Reson 4:4

15. Bellenger NG, Davies LC, Francis JM, Coats AJS, Pennel DJ (2000) Reduction in sample size for studies of remodelling in heart failure by the use of cardiovascular magnetic resonance. J Cardiovasc Magn Reson 2:271

16. Zile MR, Brutsaert DL (2002) New concepts in diastolic dysfunction and diastolic heart failure: Part I: diagnosis, prognosis, and measurements of diastolic function. Circulation 105:1387-1393.

17. Zile MR, Brutsaert DL (2002) New concepts in diastolic dysfunction and diastolic heart failure: Part II: causal mechanisms and treatment. Circulation 105:1503-1508

18. Paelinck BP, Lamb HJ, Bax JJ, Van der Wall EE, de Roos A (2002) Assessment of diastolic function by cardiovascular magnetic resonance. Am Heart J 144:198-205

19. Mohiaddin RH, Gatehouse PD, Henien M et al (1997) Cine MR Fourier velocimetry of blood flow through cardiac valves: comparison with Doppler echocardiography. J Magn Reson Imaging 7:657-663

20. Hartiala JJ, Mostbeck GH, Foster E et al (1993) Velocity-encoded cine MRI in the evaluation of left ventricular diastolic function. Measurement of mitral valve and pulmonary vein flow velocities and flow across the mitral valve. Am Heart J 125:1054-1066

21. Lamb HJ, Beyerbacht HP, van der Laarse A, Stoel BC, Doornbos J, van der Wall EE, de Roos A (1999) Diastolic dysfunction in hypertensive heart disease is associated with altered myocardial metabolism. Circulation 99:2261-2267

22. Osman NF, Kerwin WS, McVeigh E and Prince LJ (1999) Cardiac motion tracking using CINE harmonic phase (HARP), magnetic resonance imaging. Magnetic Resonance in Medicine 42:1048-1060

7.3 Study of myocardium

7.3.1 Stress MRI

ALESSANDRO PINGITORE, BRUNELLA FAVILLI, PETRA KEILBERG, GIOVANNI AQUARO, ELISABETTA STRATA

7.3.1.1 Introduction

The coronary artery system is anatomically divided into two districts: large conductive epicardial arteries and resistance arterioles. Excluding, for simplicity, the resistances dependant on cardiac mechanics and those linked to the rheological properties of the blood, we can state that great part of the coronary flow resistance is given by the muscular tone of the arterioles. The systems of conductance and resistance are in series, therefore the total resistance is given by the sum of the two. In normal conditions, the resistance determined by the large epicardial vessels is so modest that it can be neglected, but in the presence of a coronary stenosis, the narrowing provokes a substantial change in the relative distribution of the resistances and may condition regional myocardial flow [1]. As the other dynamic fluid conditions (perfusion pressure, rheology, etc.) remain unmodified; velocity of flow through the stenosis increases keeping flow constant, according to the Bernoulli's continuity law. The resistance to flow at level of the stenosis causes a drop in pressure and the formation of a trans-stenotic pressure gradient that increases proportionally with the severity of the stenosis – the severity depending on the fourth power of the radius of the residual lumen. The loss of pressure at level of the stenosis depends on the friction that blood meets passing through the stenosis (viscous losses) – a preponderant factor in conditions of low flow – and also depends on the turbulence, which is the main factor in high flow conditions. The relationship between trans-stenotic pressure gradient and flow is illustrated in Figure 7.17 [2]. It is evident that the pressure gradient rises exponentially with the increase in flow and that the more severe the stenosis is, the steeper is the curve for small flow variations. Arterial vasodilation is a mechanism that compensates, within certain limits, the increase of resistances occurring at the level of the epicardial coronaries. In the absence of stenosis, arterial vasodilation or coronary vasodilatatory reserve increase the coronary flow (up to fourfold the basal value) in response to the increased metabolic needs of the myocardium. In the presence of stenosis, the vasodilatatory reserve is used to keep coronary flow constant at basal conditions. Obviously, the ability of increasing flow in response to the myocardium's higher metabolic demand progressively reduces. When the stenosis is subocclusive (over 90%) the vasodilatatory reserve is unable to keep the flow constant any longer, even at basal conditions. The relation between stenosis and flow in basal conditions and of maximum vasodilation is illustrated in Figure 7.18 [3].

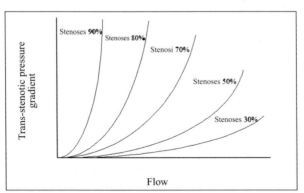

Fig. 7.17. Relationship between trans-stenotic pressure gradient and coronary flow (modified from Klocke FJ [2])

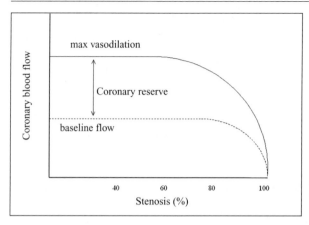

Fig. 7.18. Progressive reduction of coronary reserve in relation to the severity of the stenosis (modified from Klocke FJ [3])

Secondary myocardial ischemia is the result of a transient unbalance between oxygen demand and supply, which manifests either under stress when the mechanisms compensating the presence of a coronary stenosis are able to guarantee an adequate basal flow but cannot face demand increases (reduction of coronary reserve), or at rest when the stenosis is so severe that the basal coronary flow decreases despite the activation of all the compensation mechanisms (a quite rare event).

Myocardial ischemia determines a sequence of events, included in the so-called ischemic cascade (Fig. 7.19); this sequence has a precise temporal order [4]. Metabolic alterations are the first to ensue to the reduction in coronary flow. Alterations of the diastolic function (altered relaxation) then set in, followed by alterations of the systolic function (reduction of regional contractility). Subsequently, electrocardiographic changes occur, which ultimately announce the manifestation of precordial pain. These ischemic signs have been exploited by the imaging techniques for diagnostic purposes. Each technique has its own

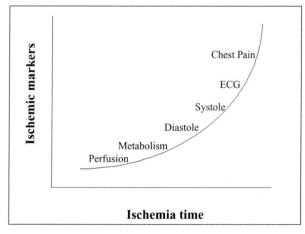

Fig. 7.19. Ischemic cascade. Myocardial ischemia triggers a series of chronologically ordered alterations (modified from Picano E [9])

diagnostic accuracy, intended in terms of sensitivity and specificity. Generally, perfusion and metabolic alterations can manifest in the presence of even mild coronary stenoses, while contractile dysfunction requires more severe stenoses. Hence, Positron Emission Tomography (PET) with 18-Fluorodeoxyglucose, which studies the cardiac metabolism, and perfusion scintigraphy are very sensitive but relatively less specific for the diagnosis of coronary disease as compared to Echocardiography and stress MRI, which base their diagnostic accuracy on the appearance of alterations in regional contractile function.

7.3.1.2 Semiotics of cardiac stress imaging

7.3.1.2.1 Induction of ischemia

The induction of myocardial ischemia by physical or pharmacological stress is a fundamental step in the diagnostic itinerary of a patient with suspected or known coronary disease. According to the current guidelines for stable angina [5], a physical or pharmachological diagnostic test associated to an imaging technique is identified as class I in the diagnostic classification of a patient with an intermediate risk of ischemia. The ischemic response to stress with the employment of an imaging technique allows a direct visualization of the area at risk and, therefore, the identification of the corresponding vascular territory. Furthermore, the characterization of the ischemic response according to temporal and spatial coordinates that include extension, severity, induction time of ischemia, and reversibility of the induced ischemia (Fig. 7.20) allows to make an accurate risk stratification of the patient, which will obviously determine the therapeutic strategy.

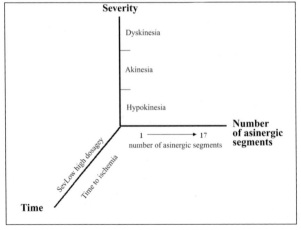

Fig. 7.20. Stratification of ischemic response according to spatial-temporal coordinates: time of ischemia, extension of asynergy, and severity of induced asynergy

7.3.1.2.2 Assessment of the ischemic area

Imaging techniques can directly visualize the ischemic area of the myocardium. Conventionally, the left ventricle is divided longitudinally (from the base to the apex) into four regions (proximal or basal, medium, distal, and real apex). According to the recommendations of the Scientific Societies, each region is then divided into segments. The proximal and the medium regions are divided into 6 segments each: anterior and inferior septum, anterior, antero-lateral, infero-lateral and inferior segments. The distal region is divided into 4 segments: interventricular septum, and the anterior, lateral and inferior walls. These segments plus the apical segment, which is the part of the myocardium beyond the cavity, add up to a total of 17 segments (Fig. 7.21) [6]. This subdivision reflects the distribution of the three large epicardial vessels: the anterior wall and the anterior septum are supplied by the left anterior descending coronary a., the inferior septum and the inferior segments are supplied by the right coronary a., and the antero-lateral and infero-lateral segments by the circumflex a. (Fig. 7.22). There can be, however, bordering myocardial segments that are supplied by different arteries according to the vascular dominance. The visualization of the area at risk and the knowledge of the corresponding vascular territory allows to identify indirectly the location of the coronary stenosis, or stenoses, responsible for the induced ischemia in patients with known or suspected coronary artery disease. Furthermore, this potentiality can be extremely useful in patients with previous myocardial

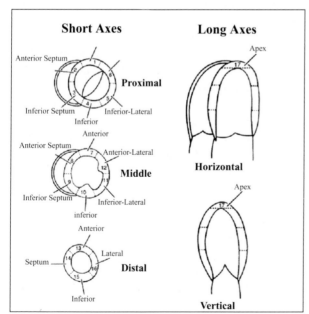

Fig. 7.21. Segmentation of the left ventricle (modified by Cerqueira et al [6])

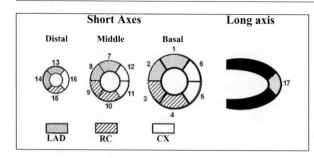

Fig. 7.22. Coronary vascular territories: LAD: Left anterior descending artery, RC: right coronary, CX: circumflex arteries (modified by Cerqueira et al [6])

infarction, in whom despite the presence of regional contractile dysfunction at rest, it is possible to discriminate between ischemia within the same vascular territory (homozonal) and ischemia in a different territory (heterozonal) – the latter being indicative of multivessel coronary disease.

7.3.1.2.3 Severity of contractile dysfunction

The severity of contractile dysfunction is directly correlated to the extent of the myocardial ischemia. Forrester et al. experimentally demonstrated increasing levels of contractile dysfunction in relation to the progressive reduction of coronary flow [7]. Moreover, experimental studies have demonstrated that the systolic thickening closely correlates to the subendocardial thickening during ischemia, as well as to the subendocardial flow and transmural perfusion, but has little to do with the systolic shortening and the flow of the subepicardium [8]. In clinical practice, the changes of regional contractile function are estimated on three levels of increasing severity: hypokinesia when there is a reduction of systolic thickening; akynesia when there is no systolic thickening, dyskinesia when systolic wall motion occurs outward towards the ventricular cavity (systolic bulging) in addition to a thinning of the wall. This condition can be described by a scoring system in which each degree of dysinergy is assigned a numerical value: 2 to hypokinetic segments, 3 to akinetic segments, and 4 to dyskinetic segments; 1 is assigned as reference value to normal segments. The score index of contractile function is obtained by summing these values and dividing them by the number of segments analyzed (Wall Motion Score Index). The higher the value of this index, the more severe the dysfunction and /or the extension of the contractile dysfunction [9].

7.3.1.2.4 Extension of the ischemic area

The extension of the area at risk can be quantified calculating the WMSI that represents an integrated index of extension and severity of the induced asyn-

ergy. The variation of the WMSI between basal and stress conditions correlates with the severity of the coronary disease and identifies those patients at
higher cardiac risk.

7.3.1.2.5 Time to ischemia

The time to ischemia corresponds to the period between the beginning of the
test (start of exercise or infusion of drug) and the onset of ischemia. The less
the time to ischemia, the greater the severity of heart disease and the risk for
cardiac ischemic events.

7.3.1.2.6 Reversibility of ischemia

Once ischemia has been induced and the images needed for diagnostic aims
have been obtained, the physical stress is interrupted or, in the case of pharmacological stress, the patient is administered a specific antidote. A slow or
incomplete recovery is a sign of the severity of the coronary disease.

7.3.1.3 Semiotics of cardiac stress with MRI

The possibility of stratifying the ischemic response according to time-space
coordinates depends on the kind of technique utilized. Techniques such as
Echocardiography that allow a continuous monitoring of the contractile
function can accurately evaluate "time to" and "reversibility of" ischemia.

To date, these two parameters have not been evaluated by MRI, where the
acquisition of the images suitable for evaluating the cardiac function usually
occurs only at stress peak or in the presence of angina. The definition of the
extension of the risk area and the severity of the contractile dysfunction are
parameters that can be accurately evaluated by MRI, since it is a technique
that permits a high spatial resolution and gives a good definition of endocardial contours of all the cardiac segments.

7.3.1.4 Pharmacological protocols

Because stress MRI with the use of physical effort is still limited to the few
research centers, generally pharmacological protocols are applied. The most
frequently used are those with dipyridamole and dobutamine. Table 7.3
reports evaluation studies for the accuracy in the diagnosis of myocardial
ischemia with stress MRI [10-17].

Table 7.3. Stress MRI. Publications on the diagnostic accuracy of inducible myocardial ischemia (Dobatro = Dobutamine + Atropine; Dob = Dobutamine; Dipy = Dipyridamole)

Authors	Protocol	Patients	Sensitivity	Specificity
Schalla S JACC 2001	Dobatro	22	97	97
Wahl A EHJ 2000	Dobatro	80	86	81
Hundley W Circulation 1999	Dobatro	153	83	83
Wahl A Circulation 2001	Dob	170	84	86
Nagel E Circulation 1999	Dob	208	86	85
Van Rugge F JACC 1993	Dob	45	81	100
Zhao S Magn Reson Imaging 1997	Dipy	60	80	75
Baer FM Int J Card Imaging 1993	Dipy	33	84	89

7.3.1.4.1 Dobutamine

Dobutamine is a sympatho-mimetic drug with a brief action time (half life 2 min) that basically acts on β-1 cardiac receptors and, to a lesser degree, on α1 and β1 receptors. Its main actions are: positive inotropic effect – well visible immediately after the administration of low doses – and positive chronotropic effect. The induction of ischemia mainly occurs due to the increase of oxygen consumption mediated by an increase of both contractility and cardiac rate. Other potential mechanisms are the regional changes of flow induced by β2-mediated coronary vasodilation and the α-mediated coronary vasospasm mechanism.

The commonly used protocol is drafted in Figure 7.23. The maximum dose is 40 microg/kg/min. The increase of the dose occurs every three minutes [18]. In the case the maximal expected heart rate is not reached, the protocol foresees the administration of atropin at the maximum dose of 1 mg distributed in 4 doses of 0.25 mg/min [19]. The antidote used for dobutamine/atropine belongs to the family of β-blockers (propranolol, atenolol, esmolol), which is not needed in all cases, if not strictly required, because of dobutamine's short time of action.

7.3.1.4.2 Dipyridamole

Dipyridamole provokes arteriolar vasodilation mediated by adenosynergic receptors A2. The mechanism of action does not directly involve the receptors but is mediated by endogenous adenosine, the metabolic degradation of which is reduced by dipyridamole. The increase of coronary flow is up to

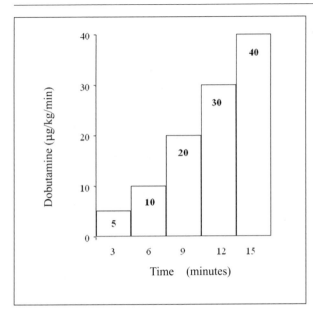

Fig. **7.23.** Dobutamine stress protocol: all dosages last 3 minutes. If the maximal frequency is not reached after the dose of 40 μg/kg/min, then atropine is added (1 mg divided into 4 administrations of 0.25 mg/min each)

eightfold the basal value. The mechanism of induction of myocardial ischemia is the so-called 'steal' phenomenon. There are two kinds of 'stealing': horizontal and vertical. In the vertical steal the mechanism is the loss of perfusion pressure downstream the stenosis, secondary to the increase of flow through the stenosis itself and to the conversion of kinetic energy to potential energy. Because the range of the coronary flow self regulation curve is located at pressure perfusion levels higher than those of the subepicardium, the steal reduces the flow at the level of the subendocardium. This hypoperfusion, occurring despite the increase of flow in the subepicardium, provokes a decrease in regional contractility.

The horizontal steal requires the presence of a collateral vascularization between two vascular districts. The steal occurs in the district supplied by the most stenotic vessel, where the vasodilatory reserve is lower than in the non-stenotic vascular district. The steal mechanism therefore depends on the reduction of vascular resistances of the so-called "donating-flow" district, following to the vasodilatation induced by dipyridamole. The standard protocol is shown in Figure 7.24 and foresees the administration of two doses of dipyridamole: the low dose (0.56 mg/kg in 4 minutes) followed by the high dose (0.28 mg/kg in 2 minutes), with a 4-minute time lapse in between [20]. Atropine can be administered in the case of a negative test, following the same procedure utilized for dobutamine [21]. The antidote is aminophillin, that is routinely administered because of dipyridamole's long action time (several hours).

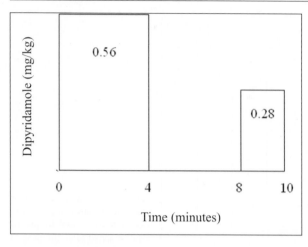

Fig. 7.24. Dipyridamole stress protocol: the first dosage lasts 4 minutes, then follows a 4 minute pause, and a second dose is administered in two minutes. After the second dose, in the case of test negativity, atropine is added (1 mg divided into 4 administrations of 0.25 mg/min each)

7.3.1.4.3 Adenosine

Adenosine differs from dipyridamole as it acts directly on the adenosynergic receptors and has a very short time of action (seconds). The induction mechanism is similar to that of dipyridamole. The administration of the antidote (aminofillin) is not necessary if not clinically required. Adenosine is prevalently used in studies of myocardial perfusion. Because it has a very short time of action, it is difficult to manage in the evaluation of contractile function or in combined studies of function and perfusion.

7.3.1.5 MRI and Echocardiography

Magnetic Resonance and Echocardiography are the two most accurate techniques for evaluating regional contractile function of the left ventricle in basal conditions and during stress. The main differences between the two techniques can be summarized as in Table 7.4. Today, Echocardiography is the most used method for evaluating contractile function during pharmacological or physical stress because of its high diagnostic accuracy, feasibility, versatility and low cost. The major limits of this technique are its non-optimal image quality in 5-10% of patients, its dependence on experience of the operator, and the non-optimal visualization of some myocardial segments. The introduction of a second harmonic has somewhat redimensioned these limits, as it better defines the contours of the endocardium. Reports on comparisons between the diagnostic accuracy for myocardial ischemia of the two techniques are few. The studies published so far demonstrate a higher accuracy for MRI compared to Echocardiography, independently from the drug used. There is also reason to believe that MRI with high doses of dobutamine is superior to Echocardiography in terms of sensitivity and specificity; the superiority is found in the better image definition, especially of the inferior

Table 7.4. Main differences between MRI and Echocardiography

	Echo	MRI
Feasibility	+++	++
Safety	+++	++
Diagnostic accuracy	++	+++
Costs	+	+++
Temporal resolution	+++	++
Spatial resolution	++	+++

and infero-lateral walls of the left ventricle where Echocardiography often fails [14]. Moreover, MRI allows a better analysis of regional contractility by means of its capacity of visualizing the same myocardial segment from different regions, a task, which is not performed easily with Echocardiography.

The measurement of systolic thickening, as a quantitative index of contractility, is more accurate by MRI than by Echocardiography because of its better definition of the endocardium. On the other hand, the complex motion of twisting and untwisting of the heart makes it difficult to measure the same portion of myocardium in systole and diastole on the short axis, and thus represents a limit of this approach. Image acquisition by tagging allows to follow the same portion of myocardium during the cardiac cycle and to facilitate the measurements of systolic thickening. The use of this approach has produced results similar to those obtained with the experimental method of reference involving intramyocardial ultrasound crystals [22]. This refined technique is purely quantitative, operator independent, and allows to evaluate the intramural myocardial contractile function, clearly distinguishing the subendocardial function from the subepicardial one. To underline the potentiality of this approach, one may simply consider that the measurement of the segmental circumferential shortening has permitted to document in basal conditions the presence of an intramyocardial contraction gradient with values of circumferential shortening of 25% for the subendocardium and of 18% for the subepicardium. Moreover, this parameter has resulted higher at level of the postero-lateral and infero-septal walls as compared to the antero-septal and antero-lateral walls – a difference that sees an increase during dobutamine [23]. Recently, the application of tagging to the dobutamine test has significantly increased its sensitivity for the diagnosis of coronary artery disease [24]. Tagging still remains, for the moment, a technique confined to few research laboratories but the growing interest it is attracting and the evidence of its effectiveness are such to predict it will become a clinical procedure in short time. From what has been stated so far, we can understand MRI's added value as compared to Echocardiography, which still remains the technique of reference and most used at a clinical level.

7.3.1.6 Feasibility and safety

Also feasibility and safety are fundamental aspects in studies of cardiac stress. If for Echocardiography the most important feasibility limit lies in the quality of the acoustic window, for MRI these limits lie in the complexity of its execution, difficult access to the equipment, and the sometimes sub-optimal electrocardiographic monitoring, especially during the phases of high heart rate.

Performing an exam in adherence to safety regulations recommends a continuous electrocardiographic and pressure monitoring of cardiac function. However, while for arterial pressure there are systems compatible with high magnetic fields, for ECG we must consider that the electrocardiographic signal can only allow to evaluate the heart rhythm, because of electromagnetic interference affecting the repolarization phase.

Communication between physician and patient is not always immediate; it is therefore good practice that nursing staff keep close contact with the patient as much as possible. In general, images are acquired basally at each increased dose of pharmacological stressor, at the end of the stress and always in the case of patient symptoms.

These important differences also influence the safety profile of these two techniques: although the safety profile has been well defined for the echocardiographical stress, it must still be defined for MRI – even if the two techniques appear to be quite similar.

7.3.1.7 MRI stress protocol

Images in cine are acquired using fast sequences that must be performed with breath holding. The most used sequences are the Spoiled Gradient Echo (SPGR) or the ultrafast (SSFP) type. The heart walls are visualized according to three longitudinal axes and three transversal ones; the latter traced at the level of the basal, medium, and distal regions of the left ventricle. Acquisition during stress is taken upon appearance of the typical symptomatology of the patient, or once the estimated maximum pharmacological dose – or the maximum dose tolerated by the patient – has been reached.

In order to maintain patient collaboration and avoid excessive hazards, it is advisable to keep image acquisition at peak stress, or in the case of pain, within the time span of a minute.

It is also advisable that the test be performed by medical personnel experienced in exams using drug-induced myocardial ischemia, because of the peculiarity of the environmental situation and the potential hazard to the patient. The medical and paramedic staff should be preventively trained on how to evacuate rapidly the patient from the magnet room if it were to become necessary. Because the time available for acquiring the images is stringent, the patient must be informed ahead of the test on the eventual clinical problems that might ensue (palpitations, precordial pain and other symptoms) and must be reassured on the personnel's ability for intervention.

In order to perform a comparative evaluation, the same sequence in cine along the same short axis or on the long axis of the left ventricle has to be repeated in basal conditions and during stress. Before administering the pharmacological stress, the operator will have to optimize the sequence that will be performed at the peak of stress or in presence of pain in order to be ready for acquisition. Lastly, two venous tubes – one for the pharmacological stressor, and the other for drugs to be administered in case of need – should be positioned on the two superior limbs.

7.3.1.8 Analyzing the images obtained during stress MR

Generally there is a qualitative evaluation (Fig. 7.25) that assigns a score to each segment, as previously seen. This implies that the reading of the images in cine-loop be read by skilled personnel to avoid loosing diagnostic accuracy. The WMSI is calculated in basal conditions and at peak stress. Such index integrates the information on the extension and severity of the induced contractile dysfunction.

The studies on diagnostic accuracy, performed on limited and selected groups of patients in ultraspecialized centers is not in our opinion sufficient to justify yet the routine use of stress MRI in place of stress Echocardiography. Rather, MRI is to be considered a third level technique to be restricted to those cases in which Echocardiography cannot be performed [13].

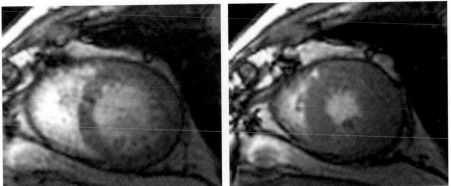

Fig. 7.25 a, b. End-diastolic (**a**), and end-systolic (**b**) images obtained at peak stress with dobutamine (40 µg/kg/min). As compared to the other walls, the intraventricular septum is hypokinetic (with a reduced thickening with respect to the other segments)

References

1. Epstein SE, Cannon III RO, Talbot TL (1985) Hemodynamic principles in the control of coronary blood flow. Am J Cardiol 56:4E-10E
2. Klocke FJ (1982) Clinical and experimental evaluation of the functional severity of coronary stenoses. Newsletter of the Council on Clinical Cardiology of the American Heart Association, Inc 7:1-9
3. Gould KL (1980) Dynamic coronary stenosis. Am J Cardiol 45:286-292
4. Heyndrickx CR, Baic H, Nelkins P et al (1978) Depression of regional blood flow and wall thickening after brief coronary occlusion. Am J Physiol 234:H653-H660
5. The European Society of Cardiology. Management of stable angina pectoris (1997) Recommendations of the task force of the European Society of Cardiology. Eur Heart J 18:394-413
6. Cerqueira MD, Weissman NJ, Dilsizian V et al (2002) Standardized myocardial segmentation and nomenclature for tomographic imaging of the heart: a statement for healthcare professionals from the cardiac imaging committee of the council on clinical cardiology of the American Heart Association. Circulation 105: 539-542
7. Forrester JS, Wyatt HL, da Luz PL et al (1976) Functional significance of regional ischemic contraction abnormalities. Circulation 54:64-70
8. Gallagher KP, Kumada T, Koziol JA et al (1980) Significance of regional wall thickening abnormalities relative to transmural myocardial perfusion in anesthetized dogs. Circulation 62:1266-1274
9. Picano E (1997) Stress Echocardiography. 3rd Edition Springer Verlag
10. Wahl A, Roethemeyer S, Paetsch I et al (2001) Simultaneous assessment of wall motion and perfusion during high-dose dobutamine-atropine stress MRI improves diagnosis of ischemia. Eur Heart J 184:P1058
11. Schalla S, Nagel E, Paetsch I et al (2001) Real-time magnetic resonance image acquisition during dobutamine stress for the detection of left ventricular wall motion abnormalities in patients with coronary artery disease J Am Coll Cardiol 391A:1108
12. Whal A, Roethemeyer S, Paetsch I et al (2001) Value of high-dose dobutamine stress MRI for follow-up after coronary revascularization procedures. Circulation II-769:3622
13. Hundley WG, Hamilton CA, Thomas MS et al (1999) Utility of fast cine magnetic resonance imaging and display for the detection of miocardial ischemia in patients not well suited for second harmonic stress echocardiography. Circulation 100:1697-1702
14. Nagel E, Lehmkuhl HB, Bocksch W et al (1999) Noninvasive diagnosis of ischemia-induced wall motion abnormalities with the use of high-dose dobutamine stress MRI: comparison with dobutamine stress echocardiography. Circulation. 99:763-770
15. van Rugge FP, van der Wall EE, de Roos A, Bruschke AV (1993) Dobutamine stress magnetic resonance imaging for detection coronary artery disease. J Am Coll Cardiol 22:431-439
16. Zhao S, Croisille P, Janier M et al (1997) Comparison between qualitative and quantitative wall motion analyses using dipyridamole stress breath-hold cine magnetic resonance imaging in patients with severe coronary artery stenosis. Magn Reson Imaging 15:891-898
17. Baer FM, Smolarz K, Theissen P et al (1993) Identification of hemodynamically significant coronary artery stenoses by dipyridamole-magnetic resonance imaging and 99mTc-methoxyisobutyl-isonitrile-SPECT. Int J Card Imaging 9:133-145
18. Mazeika PK, Nadazdin A, Oakley CM (1992) Dobutamine stress echocardiography for detection assessment of coronary artery disease. Am J Cardiol 69:1269-1273
19. Mcneill AJ, Fioretti PM, El-Said EM et al (1992) Enhanced sensitivity for detection of coronary artery disease by addition of atropine to dobutamine stress echocardiography. Am J Cardiol 70:41-46

20. Picano E, Lattanzi F, Masini M, Distante A, l'Abbate A (1986) High dose dipyridamole echocardiography test in effort angina pectoris. J Am Coll Cardiol 8:848-854
21. Picano E, Pingitore A, Conti U et al (1993) Enhanced sensitivity for detection of coronary artery disease by addition of atropine to dipyridamole echocardiography. Eur Heart J 14:1216-1222
22. Lima JCA, Jeremy R, Guier W et al (1993) Accurate systolic wall thickening by nuclear magnetic resonance imaging with tissue tagging: correlation with sonomicrometers in normal and ischemic myocardium. J Am Coll Cardiol 21:1741-1751
23. Power TP, Kramer CM, Shaffer AL et al (1997) Breath-hold dobutamine magnetic resonance myocardial tagging: normal left ventricular response. Am J Cardiol 80:1203-1207
24. Kuijpers D, Ho KY, van Dijkman PRM, Vliegenthart R, Oudkerk M (2003) Dobutamine cardiovascular magnetic resonance for the detection of myocardial ischemia with the use of myocardial tagging. Circulation 107:1592-1597

7.3.2 Myocardial perfusion

Massimo Lombardi, Piero Ghedin

7.3.2.1 Introduction

The use of MRI in the study of myocardial perfusion has experienced a great drive from the technological advancements seen in recent years and many studies that have confirmed the remarkable clinical potentialities of this methodological approach.

The most commonly used technique consists in injecting the contrast bolus into a peripheral vein and monitoring its "first pass" through the myocardium [1]. The equipment available today can acquire 3-5 images per heartbeat (Fig. 7.26), so that perfusion throughout the entire myocardium can

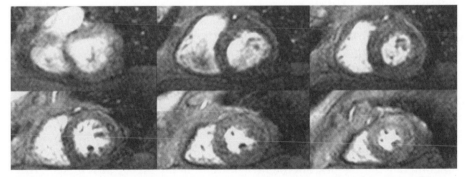

Fig. 7.26. Left Ventricle. Six sections on parallel planes on the short axis of the left ventricle. In this case all images were obtained during the same heartbeat during the first pass of paramagnetic contrast medium injected in a peripheral vein. The lack of homogeneity of signal from the myocardium, which is unavoidable, derives partially from technical issues and partially from the physiological pattern of myocardial perfusion

be studied with a single injection of contrast. Studies of comparison between MRI and SPECT or PET have evidenced a substantial competitiveness of MRI, confirming some of its advantages [2-4]. At present, MRI is in the phase of clinical validation by international multi-center studies. However, it is widely believed that MRI could already be proposed as a robust method for the study of perfusion in the diagnosis of inducible myocardial ischemia.

7.3.2.2 Pulse sequences

Virtually, all the different types of equipment for magnetic resonance differ one from the other, and consequently so do the sequences used – even if some of these share some common elements.

The requirements for studying myocardial perfusion with the first-pass technique are:

a) a temporal resolution that permits the acquisition of a number of images (at least three), synchronized with ECG, in less than a second, which means within a single heartbeat
b) the possibility of repeating image acquisition during each consecutive heartbeat, for about one minute in order to follow the first pass of a bolus of contrast agent through the myocardium
c) the preparation (nulling) of the myocardium that amplifies as much as possible the intramyocardial enhancement given by the arrival of the contrast bolus
d) an adequate spatial resolution.

At present the most utilized sequences are the fast and ultrafast Gradient Echo, FLASH or turbo-FLASH, (Fast Low Angle Shot) and Echo-planar derived sequences (EPI).

The fast Gradient Echo are T_1-weighted sequences. When used in combination with a Gd-based contrast agent, they produce signal enhancement in the myocardium. These sequences have a short time of echo (TE) (less than 4 msec) and a very fast repetition time (TR) (less than 8 msec) that can cancel out the effect of a local lack in homogeneity of the magnetic field, and thus cancel the effect of $T2^*$, allowing a rapid acquisition.

They typically present a preparatory 180° inversion pulse that inverts magnetization and provides strongly T_1-weighted images followed by a delay (TI, time of inversion). TI determines signal intensity and is generally chosen to eliminate the signal from the myocardium in the precontrast images. After the delay, radio frequency pulses are emitted inducing a small change of angle (flip angle usually 15°), which allows a fast image acquisition. The choice of a small FA is due to the fact that a reduced TR allows a short time to the complete recovery of longitudinal magnetization.

The Echo Planar Imaging (EPI) technique collects all the data of the lines composing the matrix of raw data (K-space) within a single RF pulse. Thanks to a rapidly switching magnetic field gradient following a single RF pulse, EPI sequences generate many Gradient Echoes (GRE), this allows to acquire the entire set of data needed to create the image in a single shot.

EPI has the advantage of being an extremely fast acquisition method (50-100 msec per acquisition) and intrinsically determines strongly $T2^*$-weighted images. It can be applied to Gradient Echo or Spin Echo techniques.

Compared to the other techniques, images obtained with EPI are characterized by a lower SNR than conventional imaging because of the short acquisition time. This problem can be overcome by increasing the number of excitations, which however reduces the technique's time resolution. A better SNR is given by the most recent multi-shot techniques that allow to split the acquisition of image data over several shots.

With these techniques the TE can be reduced (to less than 2 ms) and yield $T1$-weighted images, so as to avoid some of the inconveniences of $T2^*$-weighted techniques. Generally, a 180° inversion pulse is associated to the procedure, with the incorporation of dephasing gradients to eliminate the signal of the blood pool and of the myocardium. The results obtained so far indicate that such $T1$-weigted images have an excellent quality and contrast enhancement during the first passage of the contrast medium. Moreover, multi-shot techniques avoid the susceptibility artifact that often affects $T2^*$-weighted images and reduce distortions of the magnetic field caused by the presence of the contrast medium in the ventricular cavity.

7.3.2.3 The technique of execution

The operator generally acquires cardiac images on the short axis of the left ventricle (from 1-7 according to the performance of the equipment available) using as scout image the long horizontal axis or the long vertical axis of the heart. The standard approach considers three slices on the short axis of the ventricle. Considering the ideal line that connects the mitral valvular plane to the true apex of the left ventricle, the scanning planes are positioned at 25, 50, and 75% of such line starting from the apex down (Fig.7.27). In this manner the three scanning planes allow to study the perfusion of 16 of the 17 myocardial segments, leaving out only the true apex. This approach is simple and extremely accurate from a diagnostic point of view [5]. Usually, images are not acquired on the long axis, as it is more difficult to coordinate the acquisition of all the myocardial segments. In consideration of respiratory motion, which can make the following analysis of images difficult, it is preferable to acquire the images during the first pass in mild apnea (at least 20 seconds). The ideal acquisition includes precontrast images (5-6 beats for each plane), and at least 15-20 images for each

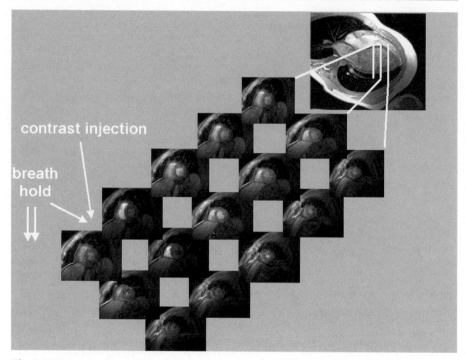

Fig. 7.27. Diagram of a study of myocardial perfusion by means of the first pass technique. In this case, there are three images per beat. The figure at the upper right corner shows the position of three scanning planes on the scout image (long horizontal axis of the left ventricle). These planes are used to obtain a sequence of images for consecutive beats during a preset number of cycles. The bolus of contrast agent is injected after the acquisition of part of the images (3-5 cardiac cycles) in order to have a reference value for precontrast signal intensity. Images during the first passage are acquired in breath-hold

plane during the passage of the contrast medium; the injection is performed with a speed of 3-5 ml per sec with an automatic injector, so that the entire injection does not last over 3 seconds.

Figure 7.27 shows a simplified representation of one of the techniques used in studies of myocardial perfusion. It is indispensable to have an optimal triggering to avoid the risk of losing temporal resolution right at the moment of the first passage. If the test foresees a basal injection of contrast medium and another injection during pharmacological stress (for e.g. adenosine 140 µ/kg min × 6 minutes; dipyridamole 0.84 mg/kg in 10 minutes, etc.) it is better to let at least 20 min time lapse between the two injections. When using pharmacological stressors, a venous tube should be positioned for each arm in order to have an immediate venous drug-free access in which the contrast agent or an eventual antidote can be injected.

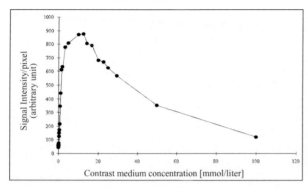

Fig. 7.28. Relationship between the concentration of Gd–based contrast medium and the signal obtained by means of turbo flash sequence with short TR (T1-weighted images). At lower concentrations of contrast agent, signal intensity follows a linear increase until an intensity plateau is reached; at higher concentrations susceptibility phenomena cause a fall in signal

The use of pharmacological stressors requires the use of a monitor for vital signs and trained personnel who can perform rapid maneuvers of intervention for evacuating the patient from the magnet room in case of need.

The contrast agent is used at the lowest dose foreseen by theory in order to maintain a linear relation between the concentration and the signal detected, which is lost at higher concentrations.

The doses suggested are 0.05-0.075 mmol/kg. At these doses, it is unlikely that saturation caused by prevalence of the $T2^*$ lead to a reduction in signal intensity (Fig. 7.28). Finally, the dose to be injected will also have to be optimized in consideration of whether there will be a qualitative or quantitative postprocessing of the images. The latter seems to be facilitated by higher dosages of contrast agent [6].

7.3.2.4 Image postprocessing

As a first approach, the study of the perfusion of an organ with the first pass technique evaluates the qualitative changes of the signal within a single region of tissue. The presence of signal change, or its absence, classifies the tissue as perfused or hypoperfused. One of the prerequisites for such a classification is the relationship of linearity between the concentration of the contrast agent and the extent of signal change, which implies a signal enhancement for positive agents, and a reduction for negative contrast agents. In reality the concept of an indirect contrast agent has much more complicated implications. It must be considered, for example, that the atoms of H in water, no matter what their compartment of origin (red blood cells, plasma, interstitium, or tissue cell), change compartment between blood and interstitium at a rate of about 40 times during their passage through a capillary [7]. All acquisition techniques must deal with this issue, which becomes relevant only when going from a qualitative to a semi-quantitative or quantitative evaluation (see Chapter 4).

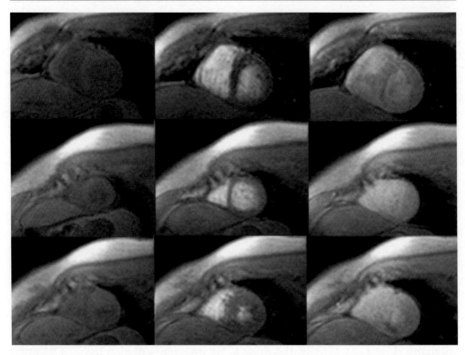

Fig. 7.29. Study of myocardial perfusion performed by means of three scanning planes on the short axis of the left ventricle. The images obtained in the myographic phase (right) evidence a defect of transmural perfusion at the level of the inferior wall in the distal segment of the left ventricle

Nowadays, in studies of myocardial perfusion, the preference goes toward the use of agents that are more efficient on T_1, for example the Gd-based contrast agents. This is due to the fact that susceptibility contrast agents present disadvantages, such as higher sensitivity to distortions and artifacts, and a lower degree of signal change as compared to that of agents acting on T_1. This latter statement is not, however, an absolute truth but only an indication, because the action on the surrounding protons depends very much on how the ions are "assembled" within the molecules forming the agent.

Once the image sequences have been acquired, they must then be evaluated so that the hypoperfused regions, if present, can be identified with certainty.

A very simple method of evaluation consists in having expert observers visualize the images in cine-loop (Fig. 7.29). This method of inspection does not require any particular postprocessing program, but implies an interpretation on behalf of the operator with inevitable intra- and inter- observer variability. This kind of analysis may be applied as a first approach and lacking dedicated postprocessing software, provided the operators are specifically trained for this task. Otherwise, the analysis can be performed by a dedi-

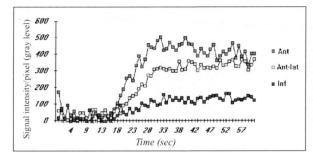

Fig. 7.30. Time-intensity curves in an animal model of induced severe myocardial ischemia at the level of the inferior wall. Contrast medium evidences the different dynamics (a slowed entrance of contrast medium, a lower peak intensity, etc.) of this region as compared to the other walls

cated postprocessing software, made relatively easy by the fact that the images are originally in digital form.

The basic concepts of the software that analyze perfusion images can be summarized as follows: the myocardial regions of interest are identified in each image (generally regions correspond to the segments of coronary distribution). The software is generally semi-automatic and allows identification of cardiac contours and of some reference points such as the connection between the free wall of the right ventricle and the left ventricle. Then the myocardial profile is segmented in a number of regions of interest (ROIs). Signal intensity inside each ROI is automatically measured. By repeating the procedure for each image, the time/intensity curves can be plotted, describing the first passage of the contrast medium through each segment of the myocardium (Fig. 7.30). These curves are then processed according to the general tracer theory in order to obtain semi-quantitative or quantitative measurements.

The parameters that can be obtained from the time/intensity curves are quite a few and have been utilized and compared by many authors. Such parameters are the max amplitude of the curve (peak intensity of the signal), time to reach peak intensity of the signal (time to peak), slope of the contrast-agent wash-in curve in the myocardium, area under the curve, Mean Transit Time (MTT); all have been demonstrated to be variously correlated to myocardial flow [8-12].

On the basis of these parameters, we can obtain parametric images that visually describe the phenomenon of perfusion, similarly to the way it happens in nuclear medicine (Fig. 7.31).

Which parameter is the most suitable for giving a better indication on the difference of perfusion in the various regions is still to be established.

For example, the parameter relative to the area under the time/intensity curve, that in other imaging techniques such as PET can allow an estimate of perfusion, is unsuitable in MRI because of the presence and permanence of the contrast agent in the interstitium for relatively long periods (even longer in the postischemic interstitium), or because of the recycling of contrast medium.

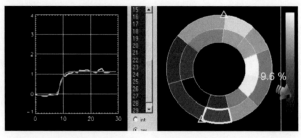

Fig. 7.31. On the left, a time-intensity curve obtained from a region of interest selected by the operator from the myocardial profile. Once the time-intensity curves have been obtained for each of the regions of interest, the program analyses the parameter selected (relative wash-in slope corrected by the wash-in slope from a region of interest inside the left ventricular cavity) on each curve and lastly creates a parametric image (image on the right), in which the level of gray encodes the level of the parameter

The slope of the curve evaluated in the period of signal enhancement (up-slope) seems to be more reliable compared to other parameters that are more influenced by local factors such as the multi-compartmental distribution of the contrast agent, the presence of artifacts, recycling, and the dispersion of the medium.

Generally, it is preferred to correct the up-slope of the segment being examined for the up-slope of a curve obtained in a region of interest inside the ventricular cavity [13]. This allows to compensate for the changes in compactness and velocity of the contrast agent bolus from one patient to another, and from one injection to another within the same patient (input function). A further improvement of the use of the corrected wash-in slope is the so-called index of perfusion reserve. This robust and recommended parameter is calculated dividing the value obtained during maximum vasodilatation (adenosine) by the value obtained in basal conditions.

Some authors have attempted to find an effective quantification of myocardial perfusion through MRI. Several approaches have been designed, but are based on mathematical-physical models and present a number of limitations. Among these, the fact of not including all variables involved, such as the relative uncertainties concerning the true determination of the contrast medium concentration in the haematic pool; the irregular relationship between agent concentration, intensity of the signal and myocardial perfusion level; and lastly, the role taken on by the amount of the contrast agent that ends up in the interstitium.

Several models have been proposed, ranging from the simplest mono-compartment (Kety's model) to the more complex multi-compartment ones [8-12, 14].

In conclusion, while semi-quantitative evaluation is well available and usable on a routine basis, the true quantification of regional myocardial perfusion by MRI still remains a troublesome objective of uncertain application; much hope is put on the use of contrast agents with monocompartimental kinetics, on condition that they keep a linear correlation between concentration and signal intensity, with the absence of hemodynamic effects of the contrast agent, etc. Figure 7.32 shows an example of myocardial perfusion studied with a mono-compartment contrast agent.

7.3.2.5 Clinical applications

At present, all works published underline the efficacy of this approach in the description of regional perfusion, both in basal conditions and during pharmacological stress [3, 5, 9, 15], using contrast mediums that had initially been developed for other organs such as the brain.

Despite the good results univocally obtained, the ultra-structural characteristics of the myocardium lead toward the use of a contrast agent with mono-compartmental distribution [16, 17]; the main pharmaceutical companies are developing this class of agents (Fig. 7.32) and the first results appear promising.

However, at present, contrast agents with extravascular distribution are the only ones proposable in the study of myocardial perfusion in patients with suspected myocardial ischemia, or in the evaluation of the state of perfusion after revascularization procedures [11-18]. Pilot studies hypothesize the use of the agents in the diagnosis of acute coronary syndrome to complement normal diagnostic tools [19]. If on one hand the study of myocardial perfusion by MRI appears a robust technique in an advanced stage of technological stabilization, on the other it is still early to tell what role it will have in the clinical setting, which already has many well-known and validated imaging procedures.

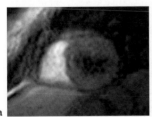
a

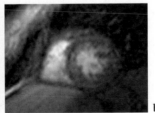
b

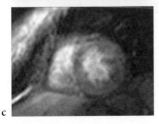
c

Fig. 7.32 (a-c). Images from a patient affected by ischemic heart disease during pharmacological stress with adenosine. The molecules of the Gd-based contrast agent used in this case have a structure that constrain them to the vascular district (blood pool). The quality of the images allows to identify the hypoperfused region easily at the level of the lateral wall. (a) Contrast medium in right ventricular cavity; (b) contrast medium in left ventricular cavity; (c) myographic phase

References

1. Atkinson DJ, Burnstein D, Edelman RR (1990) First pass cardiac perfusion evaluation with ultrafast MR Imaging. Radiology 174:757-762
2. Matheijssen NA, Louwerenburg HW, van Rugge FP et al (1996) Comparison of ultrafast dipyridamole magnetic resonance imaging with dipyridamole SestaMIBI SPECT for detection of perfusion abnormalities in patients with one-vessel coronary artery disease: assessment by quantitative model fitting. Magn Reson Med 35:221-288
3. Schwitter J, Nanz D, Kneifel S et al (2001) Assessment of myocardial perfusion in coronary artery disease by magnetic resonance: a comparison with positron emission tomography and coronary angiography. Circulation 103:2230-2235
4. Ibrahim T, Nekolla SG, Schreiber K et al (2002) Assessment of coronary flow reserve: comparison between contrast-enhanced magnetic resonance imaging and positron emission tomography J Am Coll Cardiol 39:864-870
5. Nagel E, Klein C, Paetsch I et al (2003) Magnetic resonance perfusion measurements for the noninvasive detection of coronary artery disease. Circulation 108:432-437
6. Giang TH, Nanz D, Coulden R, Friedrich M, Graves M, Al-Saadi N, Luscher TF, von Schulthess GK, Schwitter J (2004) Detection of coronary artery disease by magnetic resonance myocardial perfusion imaging with various contrast medium doses: first European multi-centre experience. Eur Heart J 25:1657-1665
7. Lombardi M, Jones RA, Westby J et al (1999) Use of the mean transit time of an intravascular contrast agent as an exchange-insensitive index of myocardial perfusion. J Magn Reson Imaging 9:402-408
8. Wilke N, Simm C, Zhang J et al (1993) Contrast-enhanced first pass myocardial perfusion imaging: correlation between myocardial blood flow in dogs at rest and during hyperemia. Magn Reson Med 29:485-497
9. Wilke N, Jerosch-Herold M, Wang Y et al (1997) Myocardial perfusion reserve: assessment with multisection, quantitative, first-pass MR imaging. Radiology 204:373-384
10. Wilke NM, Jerosch-Herold M, Zenovich A, Stillman AE (1999) Magnetic resonance first-pass myocardial perfusion imaging: clinical validation and future applications. J Magn Reson Imaging 10:676-685
11. Jerosch-Herold M, Wilke N, Stillman AE (1998) Magnetic resonance quantification of the myocardial perfusion reserve with a Fermi function model for constrained deconvolution. Med Phys 25:73-84
12. Jerosch-Herold M, Wilke N (1997) MR first pass imaging: quantitative assessment of transmural perfusion and collateral flow. Int J Card Imaging 13:205-218
13. Cullen JH, Horsfield MA, Reek CR, et al (1999) Myocardial perfusion reserve index in humans using first-pass contrast-enhanced magnetic resonance imaging. J Am Coll Cardiol 33:1386-1394
14. Santarelli MF, Landini L, Lombardi M et al (2000) A model-based method for myocardium flow estimation MAGMA. 11:87-88
15. Eichenberger AC, Schuiki E, Kochli VD et al. (1994) Ischemic heart disease: assessment with gadolinium-enhanced ultrafast MR imaging and dipyridamole stress. J Magn Reson Imaging 4:425-431
16. Wilke N, Kroll K, Merkle H et al. (1995) Regional myocardial blood volume and flow: first-pass MR imaging with polylysine-Gd-DTPA. J Magn Reson Imaging 5:227-237
17. Saeed M, Wendland MF, Higgins CB (2000) Blood pool MR contrast agents for cardiovascular imaging. J Magn Reson Imaging 12:890-898
18. Al-Saadi N, Nagel E, Gross M et al (2000) Improvement of myocardial perfusion reserve early after coronary intervention: assessment with cardiac magnetic resonance imaging. J Am Coll Cardiol 36:1557-1564

19. Kwong RY, Schussheim AE, Rekhraj S et al. (2003) Detecting acute coronary syndrome in the emergency department with cardiac magnetic resonance imaging. Circulation 4;107:531-537

7.3.3 Myocardial viability

ALESSANDRO PINGITORE, BRUNELLA FAVILLI, VINCENZO POSITANO, MASSIMO LOMBARDI

7.3.3.1 Introduction

The damage caused by long-term reduced myocardial perfusion can manifest in several ways through changes in metabolism and functional condition of the myocardium. The most classic examples are the stunned myocardium and the hibernating myocardium. The study of myocardial viability has several goals: to identify the presence and extension of viable tissue, to give a topographic description, and to characterize some physiopathological properties such as the presence of contractile reserve by means of an "ad hoc" stimulation [1, 2]. The reason for such a diagnostic effort is due to the fact that such tissue can recuperate a normal spontaneous contractility after coronary revascularization [3, 4] and its presence has important prognostic implications [5, 6].

In a stunned myocardium, a metabolic change causes an unbalance between the function and the energetic supply causing a contractile dysfunction, despite the presence of a normal myocardial blood flow (mismatch function-flow). Functional recovery often appears spontaneously days or months after the ischemic event. The stunned myocardium has been described in different clinical conditions among which: reperfused acute myocardial infarction; unstable angina; induced ischemia; after the use of cardioplegic solutions in the procedures of heart surgery; and after revascularization (surgical or percutaneous) [7-10].

In the hibernating myocardium, the contractile dysfunction is associated to a chronic reduction of myocardial flow (match function/flow), which remains in all cases higher than the critical threshold sufficient to guarantee cellular survival. Functional recovery occurs only after the re-establishment of normal conditions of myocardial flow. The hibernating myocardium has been named "smart heart" for its capacity to adapt to conditions of non-favorable flows, maintaining the anatomic and physiological integrity of the cells [11].

The two models of viable myocardium do not exclude each other and repeated ischemic episodes that provoke the stunning of the myocardium in the presence of reduced flow can lead to a hibernating myocardium.

Myocardial viability has an important prognostic impact and its identification is fundamental in the decision-making process. The assessment of the prognostic value has to take into account different parameters, such as the presence of global or regional dysfunction of the left ventricle, the time of evaluation compared to the acute event (acute or previous myocardial infarction), the extension of viable tissue, etc. [12-14]. At present, nuclear medicine and stress Echocardiography represent the most used methods for this purpose [15]. 201-Thallium is a marker of cellular viability that penetrates into the cells, replacing the potassium through the ATPase-dipendent sodium-potassium pump at the level of the cellular membrane. The defect of reversible captation within few hours from the injection of the marker is the scintigraphical sign of viability. Positron Emission Tomography (PET) can assess in quantitative terms, both the myocardial flow and cellular metabolism, permitting to obtain accurate information on the presence of metabolic viability and simultaneously to quantify the myocardial flow in the segments of hibernating and stunned myocardium. Today this technique represents the diagnostic gold standard for viability in virtue of the fact that the areas maintain a glucose metabolism quantitatively similar to that of normal areas.

The marker for stress Echocardiography is the contractile reserve documented by positive inotropic stimuli (dobutamine).

In general, there is a certain grade of consequentiality between the impairment of perfusion, of metabolism, and of function, but frequently these alterations are associated in different ways within the same myocardial segment [16, 17]. Particularly, the presence of the contractile reserve can indicate relatively severe myocardial damage with a high probability of functional recovery, while the presence of reserve metabolism with the absence of contractile reserve can indicate more severe cellular damage.

At present, myocardial viability, evaluated in terms of both perfusion and function, is considered a dichotomous variable, i.e. absent or present. Hence, a myocardial segment is viable if it has contractile reserve or a perfusion above an established limit or if it recovers contractile function after revascularization.

MRI has adopted the entire semiological background of myocardial viability built with classical methods, and has enriched it with new elements that have the potential of defining new diagnostic therapeutic and prognostic algorithms.

7.3.3.2 Evaluation of myocardial viability with MRI techniques

7.3.3.2.1 End-diastolic wall thickness

Wall thinning is a morphological sign of transmural necrosis [18]. Indeed, autoptic studies have demonstrated that transmural myocardial necrosis is commonly associated to a wall thickness of less than 6 mm [19]. This becomes evident after 4 months from an acute event as the conclusion of the fibrous repairing of the necrotic area. In the extended anterior myocardial infarction, thinning can ensue early and thus occur before the completion of the scarring process as an expansion of the infarction area [20]. Several clinical studies with Echocardiography have demonstrated that thinned myocardial segments with an increased backscattering have a low probability of recovering their contractile function after revascularization and are to be considered necrotic [21, 22]. Moreover, in patients with postischemic dilatative cardiomyopathy, a diastolic thickness below 6 mm is associated to a low probability of functional recovery after revascularization (negative predictive value of 93%).

MRI techniques for the study of end-diastolic wall thickness.
The evaluation of myocardial thickness and regional and global wall kinetics of the left ventricle requires the use of cine sequences (SPGR, SSFP, etc.). The acquisition planes are those according to the axis of the heart (long horizontal axis, long vertical axis and planes on the short axis), and the temporal resolution must take into account the heart rate. It is advisable to have at least 20 phases for a temporal resolution not over 50 msec. Obtaining a higher number of cycle reconstruction phases (for example 30) would facilitate the evaluation of the diastolic thickness. The clear and natural contrast between blood and myocardial tissue, in particular that obtained with the most up to date sequences, allows an accurate definition of the endocardium and of the subepicardium, and hence a more accurate and reproducible quantitative measurement of the diastolic and systolic thickness compared to Echocardiography [23]. In patients with previous myocardial infarction, a criterion of myocardial necrosis has been identified in a diastolic thickness below 5.5 mm [24]. Metabolism is taken as the gold standard of reference and is evaluated as the uptake of 18-fluorodeoxyglucose (FDG) at PET scanning; the segments with diastolic thickness below 5.5 mm have a metabolic activity significantly lower than that of the segments with preserved thickness. The sensitivity and specificity of the end-diastolic thickness for the diagnosis of myocardial viability resulted to be respectively 72 and 89%. The correlation between metabolic activity and diastolic thickness in akinetic segments resulted scattered but significant (r=.48), and 44% of the segments resulted viable at PET [24]. The negative predictive value of diastolic thickness in relation to the recovery of function after revascularization resulted 90% [25]. The wide variability between diastolic wall thickness and metabolic activity can be explained by the fact that myocardial segments, even of reduced thickness and asyngergic, can maintain viable the subepicardial layer, which is more resistant to ischemia. This would explain the relative independence of the uptake of FDG from wall thickness [26]. It is likely that in patients with postischemic dilatative cardiomyopathy the relation between diastolic thickness and myocardial viability can be influenced by geometrical alterations of the non-functioning left ventricle, which are dependant on the ventricular remodeling and by the tethering of the necrotic areas over the viable myocardial areas, potentially capable of modifying the diastolic thickness independently from the transmural extension of the necrosis.

7.3.3.2.2 *Contractile reserve*

Echocardiography has had the merit of developing and refining, in time, the evaluation of regional contractile reserve during stress. At first, Echo-stress (physical exercise, dipyridamole, dobutamine) was introduced for the evaluation of myocardial ischemia, the diagnosis of which was based on the worsening of contractile function. Later on it was employed for evaluating myocardial viability, the diagnosis of which was based instead on the evidence of contractile reserve, and thus on the improvement of contractile function of a baseline asynergic segment that becomes normokinetic from hypokinetic, or becomes hypo or normokinetic from akinetic.

The same stressors are used for inducing myocardial ischemia (physical stress, dipyridamole and dobutamine) with the proper adaptations of the case. Among these stressors, the most used is dobutamine, exploited for its inotropic effect at the dose of 5-10 µg/kg/min. Many studies have documented the diagnostic accuracy and the prognostic impact of viability as assessed by dobutamine [12-15].

The same pharmacological protocols can be applied to MRI by cine sequences to assess patients with recent [27] or chronic myocardial infarction [24] or with postischemic left ventricular dysfunction [18]. The comparison between MRI-dobutamine and scintigraphy both with 201-thallium and 99m-Tc sestamibi has evidenced that the first technique is less sensitive but more specific than the two nuclear techniques with respect to the recovery of contractile function after revascularization, the sensitivity and specificity being: 50 and 81% for MRI, 76 and 44% for 201-thallium at rest, 68 and 51% for 201-thallium rest-redistribution, and 66 and 49% for 99m-Tc sestamibi at rest [18]. Considering PET as the gold standard, sensitivity and specificity of dobutamine MRI for the diagnosis of myocardial viability have resulted to be 81 and 95% respectively with an 86% agreement [24].

It is presumed that the discrepancy between the presence of metabolic activity and the absence of inotropic reserve depends on the transmural extension of the necrosis which obstacles functional recovery, and by the simultaneous presence of residual metabolically active tissue on the outer layers of the cardiac wall [28]. Hence, the same dysfunctioning myocardial segments can result viable or necrotic according to the evaluation criterion used: necrotic if judged in relation to functional recovery, or viable if judged in relation to the presence of metabolic activity or to the status of regional perfusion.

The epicardial layer normally participates in a minor fashion to the thickening of the transmural wall [29]. Some studies have, however, discovered the importance of the subepicardium in the recovery of contractile function in dysfunctioning segments in patients with recent acute myocardial infarction. MRI could offer, as an additional advantage, the possibility of studying intramural contractility that differentiates the function of the endocardium from that of the epicardium.

The analysis of images obtained by tagging in fact allows to make a quantitative evaluation of cardiac mechanics in both systole and diastole. The normal myocardium has a physiological gradient of transmural contraction that is higher in the endocardium than in the epicardium [30], and persists also during the infusion of dobutamine [31]. In subjects with acute myocardial infarction, the increase in contractility (expressed in terms of percentage of systolic thickening) of the subepicardium is predictive of recovery – whether it be spontaneous or after reperfusions – of the segmental and global left ventricle function [32, 33]. The clinical and prognostic significance of the residual metabolic activity of the epicardial layer is still under investigation.

MR techniques for the study of contractile reserve.
The techniques are the same as for stress MRI, introduced in Paragraph 7.3.1. The typical approach is to use low dosages of dobutamine (5-10 µg/kg/min up to 5 min) to induce the improvement of regional function in those segments with baseline impaired contractility. To this purpose, dynamic images with SPGR or preferably SSFP sequences are acquired either at baseline or during infusion of dobutamine.

7.3.3.2.3 Evaluating viability with contrast agents

MRI has the intrinsic advantage of allowing the contrast between tissues according to their different relaxivity (T1 and T2) characteristics and their proton density. Since necrotic tissues present different histochemical differences from non–necrotic tissue, the two can easily be discriminated and a necrotic region can be identified throughout its entire extension [34, 39]. Acute myocardial infarction can be viewed from its first stages by using SE T1-weighed, T2-weighed, or SE IR sequences. Variations can be detected quite early (60-240 min after a coronary occlusion) and can persist for weeks after the event. The types of variation that can be detected depends on the technique employed, but all basically involve an increase in signal intensity, which can be amplified by the administration of a contrast medium (Fig. 7.33) [40]. Although the interpretation of these variations is not univocal, the alteration of the signal foresees the presence of oedema, compartmentalization of aqueous content, concentration and nature of the lipid component, presence of macromolecular structures, temperature, and presence of granulation tissue [33-39]. A different approach to the study of necrotic tissue foresees the sequential acquisition of images repeated over time, so that the operator can follow the dynamics of the contrast agent over a several-minute period and/or obtain images aimed at studying the first pass of a bolus of contrast agent (see perfusion – Paragraph 7.3.2). Myocardial flow has variable physiopathological characteristics according to the ischemic insult and to the

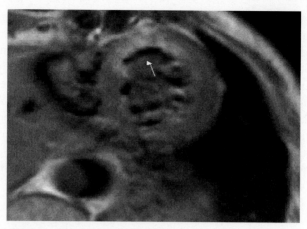

Fig. 7.33. SE T1 image on the short axis of the left ventricle after administration of the contrast medium (0.1 mmol/kg Gd-DTPA-BMA, gadodiamide) in a patient with recent myocardial infarction (1 week). The subendocardial infarcted region of the anterior wall appears hyperintense compared to the normal myocardial tissue (from Trends in Contrast Media, H.S. Thomsen, R.N. Muller, R.F. Mattrey Eds, Springer-Verlag Berlin-Heidelberg (1999), Heart, M. Lombardi and A. L'Abbate, pp. 223-231)

anatomic/functional status of epicardial vessels. Thus, this information goes beyond the simple geographical location of the necrotic tissue.

In recent years there has been the diffusion of a new MRI acquisition technique that facilitates the characterization of the infarcted myocardium and the diagnosis of myocardial viability. The late acquisition of images after the administration of contrast medium (delayed contrast enhancement – DE) allows to distinguish clearly the necrotic tissue from the surrounding viable tissue. This technique yields a high Contrast-to-Noise Ratio (CNR), beyond that of other sequences.

The sequence used for delayed enhancement is an Inversion Recovery Gradient Echo (IR-GRE), in which the initial 180° inversion pulse greatly increases the T1 weight of images. The acquisition is performed in diastole, whereby it is necessary to define carefully the inversion delay time (TI)-defined as the time elapsing between the application of the 180° prepulse and the center of K-space [41]. In this phase the magnetization of the normal myocardium is close to zero. Hence the viable myocardium is hypointense while the necrotic myocardium appears strongly hyperintense. If the acquisition sequence is properly optimized (especially for what concerns the TI that ranges between 150 and 600 msec at 1.5 T), the increase in signal intensity of the necrotic area is so marked (>500% compared to baseline) that it produces a clear distinction between necrotic and viable tissue (Fig. 7.34) [42].

Histological studies have documented that the tissue in which the contrast medium collects closely corresponds to the necrotic tissue. However, it has to be underlined that the planimetric measurement of hyperintense areas changes in relation to the delay between injection of contrast agent and acquisition of the signal, and after 20 minutes such measure matchs that of the infarcted area

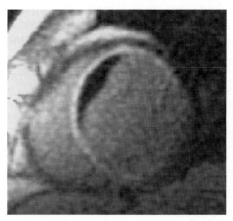

Fig. 7.34. Image on the short axis of the left ventricle obtained by IR-GRE – delayed enhancement – after administration of the contrast medium (0.2 mmol/kg Gd-DTPA-BMA, gadodiamide) in a patient with a recent extended anterior infarction. Anterior, anterior-septal and inferior-septal segments appear hyperintense and thinned compared to normal segments. The image evidences the presence of a highly hypointense structure inside the left ventricular cavity and adherent to the inter-ventricular septum, corresponding to thrombotic material

[43]. The mechanism of accumulation of the contrast medium in the necrotic region is not completely understood. Several mechanisms have been proposed: accumulation of contrast in the interstitial space, which becomes extremely large in the necrotic tissue; slow wash-out of the contrast medium from the necrotic tissue; binding with proteins from the necrotic tissue; etc. It is best to acquire the images both on the short and long axis so that all the cardiac segments can be visualized, including the true apex that cannot be detected in the images on the short axis; moreover, there should be two different observation points of the same myocardial segment. The parameters of the sequence are optimized for each single patient, in particular for what concerns TI. Typical values of acquisition parameters are TI 150-300 msc, matrix 256×160, slice thickness 8 mm, no slice gap, FA 20°, TR 9.1, TE 4.1, bandwidth 20.8, 2 NEX. Acquisition is performed 15-20 minutes after administration of the contrast medium at the dose of 0.2-0.3 mmol/kg.

7.3.3.3 Acute myocardial infarction

The extent of the necrotic tissue can be overestimated when using traditional static sequences (SE T1, SE T2) because of the presence of variable degrees of interstitial oedema. Obviously, the correlation between hyperintense areas and infarcted areas increases with the progressive absorbing of the interstitial oedema [44]. The use of a contrast medium surely improves the CNR, however one must consider all the pharmacokinetic changes induced by the structural alterations that have occurred in the necrotic tissue (see Chapter 4).

There are two contrast-medium enhancement patterns for viability in acute myocardial infarction [45]. The first pattern is characterized by an early phase of increase in signal intensity in the infarcted area; this increase is similar to that obtained in the non-infarcted area. In the minutes following, the signal intensity becomes more marked in the infarcted territory, while it progressively decreases in the non-infarcted area (Fig. 7.33). The second pattern

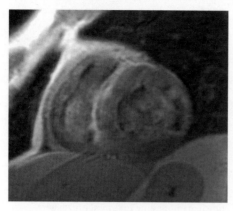

Fig. 7.35. Image on the short axis of the left ventricle obtained by SE T1 after administration of the contrast medium (0.2 mmol/kg Gd-DTPA-BMA, gadodiamide) in a patient with recent acute myocardial infarction (96 hrs). At the level of the inferior-lateral wall the image evidences a thin hyperintense external area surrounding a hypointense area corresponding to the necrotic-hemorrhagic tissue with no enhancement of the signal corresponding to the gross micro vascular damage. With coronary angiography a large marginal branch resulted to be occluded

is characterized in the early phase by the absence of an increase in signal in the layers at the center of the infarcted area. This hypointense area is surrounded by a hyperintense halo, in which there is a further increase of signal in the later phase (Figs. 7.35, 7.36).

These two patterns describe different degrees of alteration of coronary flow, and thus of myocardial damage. In particular the second pattern is more frequently associated to conditions of severe flow reduction (TIMI 0 or 1) and a severe impairment of regional contractile function. In addition, this pattern is associated to the absence of contractile reserve to dobutamine [27], and to a negative prognosis [46] as to functional recovery. The in-homogeneity of flow, as described in the second pattern, has been demonstrated experimentally and is associated to a greater reduction of subendocardial flow, which can be referred to as the no-reflow phenomenon characterized by a severe myocardial ischemic damage including cellular necrosis, microvascular lesions and hemorrhage [47, 48]. An interesting complement can be achieved by combining the information gathered from the perfusion study as with the first pass technique (see myocardial perfusion Paragraph 7.3.2) (Fig. 7.37) with those that can be derived from delayed images.

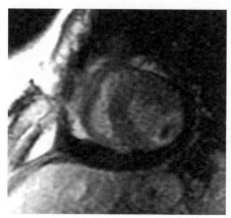

Fig. 7.36. Image on the short axis of the left ventricle obtained by IR-GRE after administration of contrast medium (0.2 mmol/kg Gd-DTPA-BMA, gadodiamide) in a patient with acute myocardial infarction. The image evidences a hyperintense area surrounding a hypointense area corresponding to the necrotic hemorrhagic tissue and a pericardial hemorrhagic effusion (cardiac rupture!)

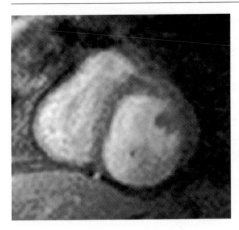

Fig. 7.37. The image of perfusion, during the first pass of the contrast bolus injected i.v., shows a vast hypointense area corresponding to transmural hypoperfusion at the level of the inferior wall in a patient with previous myocardial infarction in the same region

This combined approach allows to define three patterns of enhanced signal hyperintensity in patients with acute myocardial infarction, who have been efficiently reperfused: 1) signal hypointensity at the first pass (*early*) without late hyperintensity (*hypo*), 2) early and late hyperintensity (*hyper*); 3) early hypointensity and late hyperintensity (*comb*). The hypersegments evidence a better recovery of contractile function after a week, while the *hypo* do not improve, and the *comb* have an intermediate improvement [49].

This means that the late hyperintensity, as in the *hyper*, is indicative of the presence of viable tissue mixed to necrotic tissue in patients with acute myocardial infarction. Therefore, the time elapsed after the ischemic event is fundamental as the same pattern of late hyperintensity identifies a partially viable tissue in patients with acute myocardial infarction, and necrotic tissue in patients with previous myocardial infarction. The area of late hyperintensity can diminish within a few days from heart attack [50], probably due to the reabsorption of the interstitial oedema and to the scarring reaction of the necrotic tissue. The myocardial segments that present reduction of the hyperintense area have a greater chance of recuperating contractile function [51].

Lastly, it should be considered that the chance of function recovery is, however, function of the transmural extension of the hyperintense area in IR-GRE images, resulting highly probable in the segments that show an extension below 25%, intermediate in segments with extension between 25 and 75%, and practically null where segments exceed 75% [51]. These experimental data are confirmed also in human beings, in which the segments with hyperintensity located in the subendocardial area have a higher contractile reserve at dobutamine test than the akinetic segments with transmural necrosis [27]. However, it has been shown that in terms of functional recovery the presence of contractile reserve, as shown by dobutamine MRI, seems to have an higher predictive value than the measurement of transmural extension of the hyperintense area in IR-GRE images [52].

7.3.3.4 Chronic myocardial infarction

As for acute myocardial infarction, morphological and functional information on the infarcted tissue can also be obtained for patients with chronic myocardial infarction. The relaxation properties of the necrotic tissue are distinguishable from those of normal tissue, and in theory could be characterized with SE or GRE, T1- and T2-weighted images [53, 54]. In reality, an imaging approach that distinguishes necrotic from viable tissue exclusively on the basis of magnetic characteristics is less feasible than the technologies available today allow, which foresee the administration of a contrast agent and the use of "ad hoc" sequences. The cardiology packages today have optimized IR-GRE sequences for amplifying the signal from necrotic areas after the administration of the contrast medium. The hyperintensity detected with this technique is a direct signal of myocardial necrosis in patients with chronic myocardial infarction and closely correlates with the area of histologically determined necrosis [50]. The presence, location, and transmural extension are accurately determined with this method in patients with Q and non-Q myocardial infarction [55]. It has been demonstrated that segments that appear non viable at 201-thallium scintigraphy have a much higher signal intensity than the viable segments. By correlating regional kinetics to the presence of hyperintensity detectable by IR-GRE, it has been demonstrated that 58% of hypokinetic segments that show hyperintensity at DE are viable with 201-thallium, compared to 91% of the hypokinetic segments without hyperintensity. Conversely, in akinetic or dyskinetic myocardial segments, 83% of segments without hyperintensity and only 17% of those with hyperintensity were viable with 201-thallium [56]. The relation between transmural extension of the hyperintensity and the severity of the asynergy is not strictly linear. Indeed, it has been demonstrated that there is a marked reduction of systolic thickening in the presence of a transmural myocardial necrosis involving over 20% of the wall thickness, while there is no appreciable difference of systolic thickening for transmural necroses between 20 and 100% [57]. Hence, in conclusion, the severity of the defect of contraction is not a predictor of transmural extension of the necrosis.

In ischemic necrosis, the progression of a hyperintense area proceeds from the subendocardium to the subepicardium, thus mimicking the progression of the wave of necrotic injury. This particular location and progression of late hyperintensity is specific for postischemic myocardial fibrosis and differs from the other forms of myocardial fibrosis, such as marked hypertrophy, myocarditis, and non-ischemic dilatative cardiomyopathy in which late hyperintensity, if present, is distributed in a disorganized fashion inside the myocardium.

Although PET is considered today the most sensitive technique for assessing myocardial viability, when it comes to locating very small regions of myocardial infarction confined within the subendocardial layer, MRI shows better performance [58, 59]. Compared with this technique, sensitivity and specificity of late hyperintensity for MRI result to be respectively 0.86 and

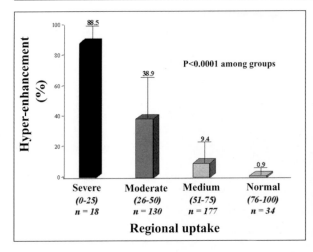

Fig. 7.38. Relationship between regional uptake of 99m-Tc sestamibi at G-SPECT and transmural extension of signal hyperintensity at DE. The lesser the uptake, the larger the transmural extension of the signal hyperintensity (personal data)

0.94. Similar results can be obtained comparing the results with 99m-Tc sestamibi with SPECT (Figs. 7.38-7.40) [60].

Transmural extension of hyperenhancement and the recovery of contractile function after coronary revascularization closely relate [61]. The chance of recovery decreases progressively with the transmural extension of late hyperintensity, since the average value is 10±7% in the segments that recover and

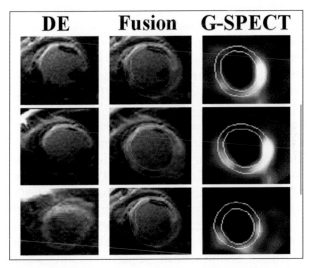

Fig. 7.39. Images in three planes on the short axis of the left ventricle (top to bottom: proximal to distal plane) of a patient with extended previous anterior myocardial infarction. The column on the left shows MRI DE images. In the central column, the fusion of the MRI DE images with the corresponding G-SPECT images. In the right column the corresponding G-SPECT images. In the DE images, hyperintensity signal is located at the level of the anterior, anterior-septal, and inferior-septal walls. The transmural extension of the hyperintensity at the level of the proximal inferior-septal segment (top) is 27% with a corresponding uptake value for 99m-Tc sestamibi of 62% (G-SPECT). The transmural extension of hyperintensity at the level of the middle anterior-septal wall (central panels) is 97% with a corresponding 99m-Tc sestamibi uptake value of 21% (G-SPECT)

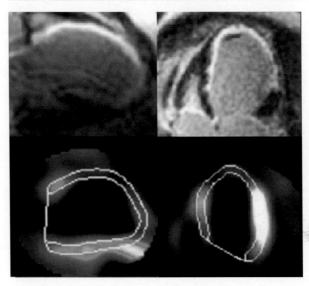

Fig. 7.40. Images on the vertical long axis (left) and on the horizontal long axis (right) of the left ventricle in a patient with extended previous anterior myocardial infarction. The hyperintensity signal in MRI DE images involves in all the apical segments with a 99m-Tc sestamibi uptake of 14%. the transmural extension

47±14% in the segments that do not recover contractile function. These data are in agreement with the histological evidence on intraoperator bioptic specimens obtained from dysfunctioning myocardial segments. The myocardial areas with preserved viability have a loss of myocardial tissue significantly lower than the necrotic areas [62]. The myocardial segments with no contractile reserve should, therefore, be considered necrotic in relation to the evaluation criteria of myocardial viability based on the contractile recovery after revascularization [63]. This non-visible viability, and hence non-identified in terms of contractile reserve, could contribute to preserving the shape and size of the left ventricle, and thus preventing the postinfarction remodeling of the ventricle and the development of heart failure [64]. The functional recovery represents only one scenario of myocardial viability – the visible one. Conversely, there are intermediate forms of myocardial viability in which the isles of viable myocardium, stunned and hibernating, are mixed with isles of necrotic and normal tissue. For these intermediate forms of myocardial viability that do not appear as functional recovery, the potential scenario is still unknown. The severity of cell impairment and transmural extension of myocardial necrosis are two fundamental elements of myocardial viability and its potential. Transmural extension of myocardial necrosis can be quantified through MRI and could be important asset in understanding other physiopathological, clinical, and prognostic scenarios of myocardial viability that go beyond the current one based on the capability of functional recovery.

7.3.3.5 Conclusions

The characterization of myocardial viability with MRI can be done following a multi-parametric approach that integrates information on morphology,

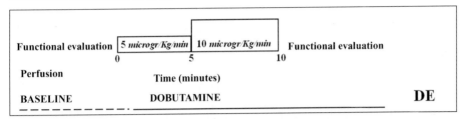

Fig. 7.41. Combined protocol for the study of myocardial viability. Cine MRI with low-dose dobut-amine (5-10 microgr/kg in 5+5 min) for the assessment of the functional reserve, study of basal myocardial perfusion with the first pass technique and finally images in IR-GRE for the evaluation of viability

function and perfusion. A protocol for the study of myocardial viability is proposed in Figure 7.41. The operator starts off by assessing baseline contractile function. This is followed by a study on perfusion in baseline condition. The contractile reserve is then evaluated during infusion of dobutamine. Finally, the operator acquires late images after the administration of the contrast agent. By following such a procedure, the evaluation of viability, defined in terms of contractile reserve, can be integrated with the information on perfusion and cellular viability.

References

1. Pierard LA, De Landsheere CM, Berthe C et al (1990). Identification of viable myocardium by echocardiography during dobutamine infusion in patients with myocardial infarction after thrombolytic therapy: comparison with positron emission tomography. J Am Coll Cardiol 15:1021-1031
2. Picano E, Marzullo P, Gigli G et al (1992) Identification of viable myocardium by dypiri-damole induced improvement in regional left ventricular function assessed by echocardiography in myocardial infarction and comparison with thallium function scintigraphy at rest. Am J Cardiol 70:703-710
3. Gheorghiade M, Cody RJ, Francis GS et al (1998) Current medical therapy for advanced heart failure. Am Heart J 135:231-248
4. Braunwald E, Rutherford JD (1986) Reversible ischemic left ventricular dysfunction: evidence for the "hibernating" myocardium. J Am Coll Cardiol 8:1467-1470
5. Eitzman D, Al-Aouar Z, Kanter HL et al (1992) Clinical outcome of patients with advanced coronary artery disease after viability studies with positron emission tomography. J Am Coll Cardiol 20:559-565
6. Lee KS, Marwick TH, Cook SA et al (1994) Prognosis of patients with left ventricular dysfunction, with and without viable myocardium after myocardial infarction. Relative efficacy of medical therapy and revascularization. Circulation 90:2687-2694
7. Nixon JV, Brown CN, Smitherman TC (1982) Identification of transient and persistent segmental wall motion abnormalities in patients with unstable angina by two-dimensional echocardiography. Circulation 65:1497-1503
8. Kloner RA, Allen J, Cox TA, Zheng Y, Ruiz CE (1991) Stunned left ventricular myocardium after exercise treadmill testing in coronary artery disease. Am J Cardiol 68:329-334
9. Breisblatt WM, Stein KL, Wolfe CJ et al (1990) Acute myocardial dysfunction and recovery: a common occurrence after coronary by-pass surgery. J Am Coll Cardiol 15:1261-1269

10. Touchstone DA, Beller GA, Nygaard TW, Tedesco C, Kaul S (1989) Effects of successful intravenous reperfusion therapy on regional myocardial function and geometry in humans: a tomographic assessment using two-dimensional echocardiography. J Am Coll Cardiol 13:1506-1513

11. Rahimtoola SH (1985) A perspective on the three large multivessel randomised clinical trials of coronary bypass surgery for chronic stable angina. Circulation 72 (Suppl V):V123-V135

12. Sicari R, Picano E, Landi P. et al (1997) The prognostic value of dobutamine-atropine stress echocardiography early after acute myocadilal infarction. J Am Coll Cardiol 29:254-260

13. Picano E, Sicari R, Landi P et al (1998) Prognostic value of myocardial viability in medically treated patients with global left ventricular dysfunction early after an acute uncomplicated myocardial infarction: a dobutamine stress echocardiography study. Circulation 98:1078-1084

14. Meluzin J, Cerny J, Frelich M et al (1998) Prognostic value of the amount of dysfunctional but viable myocardium in revascularized patients with coronary artery disease and left ventricular dysfunction. J Al Coll Cardiol 32:912-920

15. Bax JJ, Cornel JH, Visser FC et al (1996) Prediction of recovery of myocardial dysfunction after revascularization. Comparison of fluorine-18 fluorodeoxyglucose/thallium-201 SPECT, thallium-201 stress-reinjection SPECT and dobutamine echocardiography. J Am Coll Cardiol 28:558-564

16. Zamorano J, Delgado J, Almeria C et al (2002) Reason for Discrepancies in Identifying Myocardial Viability by Thallium-201 Redistribution, Magnetic Resonance Imaging, and Dobutamine Echocardiography. Am J Cardiol 90:455-459

17. Gunning MA, Anagnostopoulos C, Knight CJ et al (1998) Comparison of 201 TL, 99mTc-Tetrofosmin, and dobutamine magnetic resonance imaging for identifying hibernating myocardium. Circulation 98:1869-1874

18. Roberts CS, Maclean D, Maroko P, Kloner RA (1984) Early and late remodeling of the left ventricle after acute myocardial infarction. Am J Cardiol 54:407-410

19. Dubnow MH, Burchell HB, Titus JL (1965) Post infarction ventricular aneurysm. A clinico-morphologic and electocardiographic study of 80 cases. Am Heart J 70:753-760

20. Pirolo JS, Hutchins GM, Moore GW (1986) Infarct expansion: pathologic analysis of 204 patients witha a single myocardial infarct. J Am Coll Cardiol 7:349-354

21. Faletra F, Crivellaro W, Pirelli S et al (1995) Value of transthoracic two-dimensional echocardiography in predicting viability in patients with healed Q-wave anterior wall myocardial infarction. Am J Cardiol 76:1002-1006

22. Cwaig MJ, Cxaig E, Nagueh SF et al (2000) End-diastolic wall thickness as a predictor of recovery of function in myocardial hibernation: relation to rest-redistribution TL-201 tomography and dobutamine stress echocardiography. J Am Coll Cardiol 35:1152-1161

23. van Rugge FP, van der Wall EE, Spanjersberg SJ et al (1994) Magnetic resonance imaging during dobutamine stress for detection and localization of coronary artery disease. Quantitative wall motion analysis using a modification of centerline method. Circulation 90:127-138

24. Baer FM, Voth E, Schneider CA et al (1995) Comparison of low dose dobutamine gradient echo magnetic resonance imaging and positron emission tomography with 18F fluo-rodeoxyglucose in patients with chronic coronary artery disease: a functional and morpho-logical approach to the detection of residual myocardial viability. Circulation 91:1006-1015

25. Baer FM, Theissen P, Schneider CA et al (1998) Dobutamine magnetic resonance imaging predicts contractile recovery of chronically dysfunctional myocardium after successful revascularization. J Am Coll Cardiol 31:1040-1048

26. Perrone Filardi P, Bacharach SL, Dilsizian V et al (1992) Metabolic evidence of viable myocardium in regions with reduced wall thickness and absent wall thickening in patients with chornic ischemic left ventricular dysfunction. J Am Coll Cardiol 20:161-168

27. Dendale P, Franken PR, Block P, Pratikakis Y, De Roos A (1998) Contrast enhanced and functional magnetic resonance imaging for the detection of viable myocardium after infarction. Am Heart J 135:875-880

28. Dakik HA, Howell JF, Lawrie GM et al (1997) Assessment of myocardial viability with 99mTc-sestamibi tomography before coronary by-pass graft surgery: correlation with histopathology and postoperative improvement in cardiac function. Circulation 96:2892-2898

29. Gascho JA, Copenhaver GL, Heitjan DL (1990) Systolic thickening increases from subepicardium to subendocardium. Cardiovascular Research 24:777-780

30. Clark N, Reicheck N, Bergey P et al (1991) Circumferential myocardial shortening in the normal human left ventricle. Assessment by magnetic resonance imaging using spatial modulation of magnetization. Circulation 84:67-74

31. Power T, Kramer CM, Shaffer AL et al (1997) Breath-hold dobutamine magnetic resonance myocardial tagging: normal left ventricular response. Am J Cardiol 80:1203-1207

32. Geskin G, Kramer CM, Rogers WJ et al (1998) Quantitative assessment of myocardial viability after infarction by dobutamine magnetic resonance tagging. Circulation 98:217-223

33. Bogaert J, Maes A, Van de Werf F et al (1999) Functional recovery of subepicardial myocardial tissue in transmural myocardial infarction after successful reperfusion: an important contribution to the improvement of regional and global left ventricular function. Circulation 99:36-43

34. Williams ES, Kaplan JI, Thatcher F Zimmerman G, Knoebel SB (1980) Prolongation of proton spin lattice relaxation times in regionally ischemic tissue from dog hearts. J Nucl Med 21:449-453

35. van Rugge FP, van der Wall EE, van Dijkman PR et al (1992) Usefulness of ultrafast magnetic resonance imaging in healed myocardial infarction. Am J Cardiol 70:1233-1237

36. McNamara MT, Higgins CB, Schechtmann N et al (1985) Detection and characterization of acute myocardial infarction in man with the use of gated magnetic resonance. Circulation 71:717-724

37. Pflugfelder PW, Wisenberg G, Prato FS, Carrol SE (1986) Serial imaging of canine myocardial infarction by in vivo nuclear magnetic resonance. J Am Coll Cardiol 7:843-849

38. Tscholakoff D, Higgins CB, McNamara MT, Derugin N (1986) Early-phase myocardial infarction by MR imaging. Radiology 159:667-672

39. Wesbey G, Higgins CB, Lanzer P Botvinick E, Lipton MJ (1984) Imaging and characterisation of acute myocardial infarction in vivo by gated nuclear magnetic resonance. Circulation 69:125-130

40. McNamara MT, Tscholakoff D, Revel D et al (1986) Differentiation of reversible and irreversible myocardial injury by MR imaging with and without gadolinium-DTPA. Radiology 158:765-769

41. Simonetti OP, Kim RJ, Fieno DS et al (2001) An improved MR imaging technique for the visualization of myocardial infarction. Radiology 218:215-223

42. Fieno DS, Kim RJ, Chen EL et al (2000) Contrast-enhanced magnetic resonance imaging of myocardium at risk: distinction between reversible and irreversible injury throughout infarct healing. J Am Coll Cardiol 36:1985-1991

43. Oshinski JN, Yang Z, Jones JR, Mata JF, French BA (2001) Imaging time after Gd-DTPA injection is critical in using delayed enhancement to determine infarct size accurately with magnetic resonance imaging. Circulation 104:2838-2842

44. Choi SI, Jiang CZ, Lim KH et al (2000) Application of breath-hold T2 weighted, first pass perfusion and gadolinium-enhanced T1-weighted MR imaging for assessment of myocardial viability in a pig model. J Magn Reson Imaging 11:476-480

45. Lima JAC, Judd RM, Bazille A et al (1995) Regional heterogeneity of human myocardial infarcts demonstrated by contrast-enhanced MRI: potential mechanisms. Circulation 92:1117-1125

46. Wu KC, Zerhouni EA, Judd RM et al (1998) Prognostic significance of microvascular obstruction by magnetic resonance imaging in patients with acute myocardail infarction. Circulation 97:765-772

47. Judd RM, Lugo-Olivieri CH, Arai M et al (1995) Physiological basis of myocardial contrast enhancement in fast magnetic resonance images of 2-day-odl reperfused canine infarcts. Circulation 92:1902-1910

48. Kloner RA, Ganote CE, Jennings RB (1974) The "no-reflow" phenomenon after temporary coronary occlusion in the dog. J Clin Invest 54:1496-1508

49. Rogers WJ, Kramer CM, Geskin G et al (1999) Early contrast-enhanced MRI predicts late functional recovery after reperfused myocardial infarction. Circulation 99:744-750

50. Kim RJ, Fieno DS, Parrish TB, (1999) Relationship of MRI delayed contrast enhancement to irreversible injury, infarct age, and contractile function. Circulation 100:1992-2002

51. Hillebrand HB, Kim RJ, Parker MA, Fieno DS, Judd RM (2000) Early assessment of myocardial salvage by contrast enhanced magnetic resonance imaging. Circulation 102:1678-1683

52. Wellnhofer E, Olariu A, Klein C, Grafe M, Wahl A, Fleck E, Nagel E (2004) Magnetic resonance low-dose dobutamine test is superior to SCAR quantification for the prediction of functional recovery. Circulation 109:2172-2184

53. Hsu JCM, Johnson A, Smith WM et al (1994) Magnetic Resonance imaging of chronic myocardial infarcts in formalin-fixed human autopsy hearts. Circulation 89:2133-2140

54. Bouchard A, Reeves RC, Cranney G et al (1989) Assessment of myocardial infarct size by means of T2-weighted 1H nuclear magnetic resonance imaging. Am Heart J 117:281-289

55. Wu E, Judd RM, Vargas JD et al (2001) Visualization of presence, location, and transmural extent of healed Q-wave and non-Q-wave myocardial infarction. Lancet 357:21-28

56. Ramani K, Judd RM, Holly TA et al (1998) Contrast magnetic resonance imaging in the assessment of myocardial viability in patients with stable coronary artery disease and left ventricular dysfunction. Circulation 98:2687-2694

57. Lieberman AN, Weiss JL, Jugdutt BI et al (1981) Two-dimensional echocardiography and infarct size: relationship of regional wall motion and thickening to the extent of myocardial infarction in the dog. Circulation 63:739-746

58. Klein C, Nekolla SG, Bengel FM et al (2002) Assessment of myocardial viability with contrast enhanced magnetic resonance imaging: comparison with positorn emission tomography. Circulation 105:162-167

59. Kuhl HP, Beek AM, van der Weerdt AP et al (2003) Myocardial viability in chronic ischemic heart disease: comparison of contrast-enhanced magnetic resonance imaging with (18) F-fluorodeoxyglucose positron emission tomography. J Am Coll Cardiol 41:1341-1348

60. Giorgetti A, Pingitore A, Lombardi M et al (2002) Quantitative evaluation of trasmural extent of myocardial necrosis by means of contrast-enhanced magnetic resonance: comparison with nitrate 99mTC-tetrofosmin G_SPECT scintigraphy. J Nucl Med 46:4:92

61. Kim RJ, Wu E, Rafael A et al (2000) The use of contrast enhanced magnetic resonance imaging to identify reversible myocardial dysfunction. N Engl J Med 343:1445-1453

62. Nagueh SF, Mikati I, Weilbaecher D et al (1999) Relation of the contractile reserve of hibernating myocardium to myocardial structure in humans. Circulation 100:490-496

63. Sciagrà R, Pellegri M, Pupi A et al (2000) Prognostic implications of Tc-99m Sestamibi viability imaging and subsequent therapeutic strategy in patients with chronic coronary artery disease and left ventricular dysfunction. J Am Coll Cardiol 36:739-745

64. Kaul S (1995) There may be more to myocardial viability than meets the eye. Circulation 92:2790-2793

65. Samady H, Elefteriades JA, Abbott BG et al (1999) Failure to improve left ventricular function after coronary revascularization for ischemic cardiomyopathy is not associated with worse outcome. Circulation 100:1298-1304

7.3.4 Cardiomyopathies

Massimo Lombardi, Claudia Raineri, Alessia Pepe

7.3.4.1 Introduction

Cardiac MRI has found fertile ground in the field of cardiomyopathies thanks to its intrinsic possibilities of morphological, functional and, above all, tissue characterization. If Arrhythmogenic Right Ventricular Cardiomyopathy (ARVC) was one of the first pathologies to benefit from the potential of MRI, now other forms of cardiomyopathy dominate the cardiovascular MRI labs, with an ever-growing production of scientific works and clinical applications.

7.3.4.2 Arrhythmogenic right ventricular cardiomyopathy (ARVC)

7.3.4.2.1 Overview

Arrhythmogenic Right Ventricular Cardiomyopathy (ARVC) represents one of the most frequent diagnostic suspicions motivating the referral of young patients to cardiological MRI exams.

This disease discovered in the seventies, was described as a disease of the cardiac muscle with unknown etiology, characterized by structural and functional alterations of the right ventricle consequent to progressive myocardial atrophy with a fatty or fibrous replacement of the right ventricle myocardium [1]. Further macroscopic and histological alterations have been found throughout the last decade through a careful revision of clinical and instrumental data. In particular, a relatively frequent involvement of the left ventricle has been documented [2].

In consideration of such findings, its definition has been changed in the recent classification of cardiac diseases, which was recently reviewed by the World Health Organization task force. Indeed, ARVC has been defined as a true form of cardiomyopathy, characterized by a progressive fibro-fatty replacement of the myocardium of the right ventricle, which likely involves the intraventricular septum [3].

7.3.4.2.2 Epidemiology

The prevalence and incidence of the disease are not known but surely ARVC is among the most frequent causes of sudden death among children and young adults, mainly males; the age at which the diagnosis is made is generally between 20 and 50 years.

In 30-50% of cases ARVC has a familiar incidence [4]. The inheritance is autosomic dominant with incomplete penetration, also if there is a description of a recessive variant associated to non-epidermolytic palmoplantar keratoderma and wooly hair on the island of Naxos [4, 5]. Genetic linkage studies performed so far on many families have allowed to identify several chromosomal loci: 14q12-q22; 14q23-q24; 2q32; 3p23; 1q42-q43; 10p12-p14; 10q22.3 and 17q21, the last of which is the recessive variant [5-13]. The heterogeneity of the genetic findings could explain, at least in part, the heterogeneity of this disease. However, which genes included in these regions are actually involved and which are the real consequences from a biochemical and cellular point of view are still unknown. At present, only hypotheses can be made. For what concerns the 3p23 region, three genes are suspected; these encode for a *raf* serine-threonine protein kinase, for a DNA-binding protein, and for a protein thyroxine-phosphatase [6]. As for the region 1q42-q43, a possible gene responsible for arrythmogenic ARVC could be the one encoding for the cardiac ryanodine receptor gene [7], since a mutation of this gene has been found in some cases of familiar incidence.

7.3.4.2.3 Etiopathogenisis

The etiopathogenisis of the disease is still unknown. Three mechanisms have been proposed as an explanation of the fibro-adipose substitution of the myocardium: a) genetically determined myocardial dystrophy, b) inflammation associated with myocardial necrosis (myocarditis), c) programmed cell death (apoptosis).

According to the theory of dystrophy, the progressive loss of myocardium would be secondary to some genetically determined metabolic or ultra structural defect.

The inflammatory hypothesis is linked to the frequent histological findings of inflammatory infiltrations [1, 14]. Many infective and toxic agents have been investigated, along with several immunological mechanisms. In this context, fibro-adipose replacement would be the expression of a healing process in a picture of myocarditis. This theory does not conflict with the familiarity of the disease, as experimental studies have documented a genetic predisposition to viral infections that can trigger an immune response [15]; moreover, there are many reports of experimental myocarditis caused by the Coxsackie virus, with a selective involvement of the right ventricle; these cases in terminal stages seem to lead to the development of ventricular aneurysms similar to those observed in ARVC [16]. Finally, bioptic studies have demonstrated the presence of entero-viral RNA homologous to that of type B Coxsackievirus in 37% of patients with ARVC [17].

Recently, it has been proposed that cell death in ARVC may correspond to a mechanism of programmed cell death (apoptosis) [18]. According to this hypothesis, the progressive loss of myocardium would be the result of poussées of apotosis. Because myocardial cells are permanent, the empty spaces would be filled with adipocytes and collagen-synthesizing fibroblasts.

The presence of apoptotic cells, easily distinguishable from the necrotic cells, has been documented in autoptic studies [19] and on endomyocardial biopsies [20]. Recently, it has also been demonstrated that apoptosis can be set off not only by a programmed cellular mechanism but also by viral infections, which suggests a possible interaction between flogosis and apoptosis in the pathogenesis of progressive myocardial damage typical of ARVC [21].

7.3.4.2.4 Histopathological findings

The characteristic histological finding of the disease is myocardial atrophy of the free wall of the right ventricle, regional or diffuse, with fibro-adipose replacement that mainly involves the external two-thirds of the myocardial wall (Fig. 7.42) [22]. Residual myocytes, in various stages of degeneration, are located mostly at the level of the subendocardial trabecula, with only few sparse myocytes in the fibro-adipose tissue.

The dispersion of healthy myocytes, in the context of fibro-adipose replacement, accounts for the delay in transmission of the intraventricular pulse and the persistence of diastolic depolarization (late potentials), and even of the establishment of re-entry circuits that trigger ventricular arrhythmias [23].

If it is true that fibro-adipose tissue in the myocardium is one of the important histopathological characteristics of the disease, it must be however remembered that finding fatty tissue in the right ventricular myocardium does not necessarily mean ARVC; indeed, significant degrees of intramyocardial fatty infiltration are common normal findings, especially if the subject is of older age and the area involved is the antero-apical portion of the right ventricle (Fig. 7.43). Also a subendocardial fibrosis of variable degree is a common finding, just as the presence of fibro-muscular bundles penetrating epicardial fat [25].

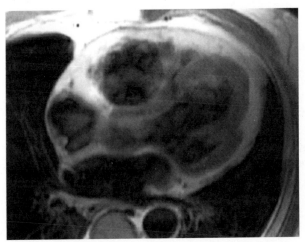

Fig. 7.42. Image on axial plane in FSE "black blood" of a patient with adipose infiltration of the free wall of the left ventricle at the level of the right ventricle outflow tract. The presence of fatty tissue determines a hyperintensity signal, which involves the entire thickness of the ventricular wall

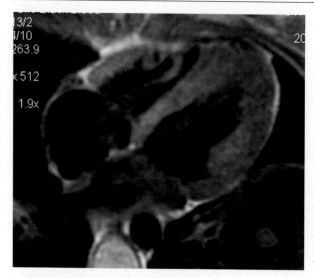

Fig. 7.43. Image on the long horizontal axis of the heart in FSE "black blood" of a patient with non-specific fatty infiltration of the free wall of the right ventricle. Occasional finding

7.3.4.2.5 Morphological findings

There are two variants of ARVC: a fatty form, exclusively involving the right ventricle without thinning of the free wall, and a fibro-adipose form characterized by the thinning of the free wall of the right ventricle and by the presence of aneurysms, often with involvement of the left ventricle [26].

The right ventricle can present several degrees of segmental or global dilatation with alterations of free wall kinetics. The most typical cases present thinning of the free wall of the right ventricle, and even aneurysmatic areas, which are more frequent in systole but that can also persist in diastole, and are most frequently located at the level of the infundibulus, of the apex, and of the basal part of the inferior wall (the triangle of dysplasia!) (Fig. 7.44).

In the cases involving the left ventricle, there usually is a dilatation of the ventricular chamber and asynergic areas, mainly at the apex and at the level of the postero-inferior wall.

7.3.4.2.6 Clinical manifestations

The clinical picture of patients with ARVC is extremely heterogeneous and ranges from completely asymptomatic forms to clinical heart failure [27]. Clinical manifestations are generally correlated to the onset of ventricular arrhythmias that can vary from isolated extrasystolic beat to sustained or non-sustained ventricular tachycardia, ventricular fibrillation; rarely, atrial fibrillation and atrial flutter might occur. Ventricular arrhythmias are always left bundle branch block-like and usually ensue to physical effort. The most frequent symptoms are palpitation and syncope; sometimes also dyspnea and angina-like chest pain occur. In some cases the first sign of the disease is sudden death.

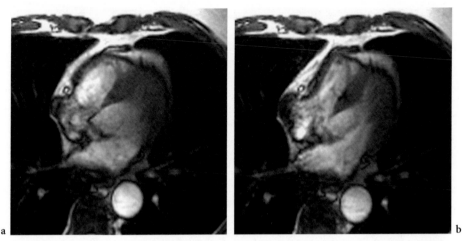

Fig. 7.44 a, b. Images on the long axis of the heart in cine FIESTA of a patient with ARVC. (a) The image in end-diastole evidences a segmental bulging of the free wall of the right ventricle at the middle-distal level; (b) the image of the same segment in systole shows a clear aneurysmatic behavior

7.3.4.2.7 Diagnosis

Given the extreme morphological and functional heterogeneity of the disease, the diagnostic path is very complex and generally leads to a diagnosis of probability, and only rarely to a diagnosis of certainty. In the anamnesis, the elements to search for are family history for ARVC or sudden death, a personal history of palpitation, lipothymia, and syncope. The first diagnostic step is obviously the electrocardiographic characterization. Often a prolonged QRS is found at ECG (>110 msec) with complete or incomplete right/left bundle branch block; there may also be a negative T-wave in the right precordial leads and sometimes an epsilon wave in V1. In most proclaimed cases, high resolution ECG shows the presence of late potentials. Ventricular arrhythmias are common (premature ventricular beats, sustained and non sustained tachycardia with left bundle branch block morphology) at dynamic Holter ECG and during the physical stress test. Lastly, Echocardiography and MRI, allow to identify morphological and functional alterations of the heart.

7.3.4.2.8 Differential diagnosis

Differential diagnosis of ARVC foresees multiple pathological situations often with common denominators from an electrophysiological and clinical point of view, even if in reality some of these are not accompanied by evident morphological or histological alterations.

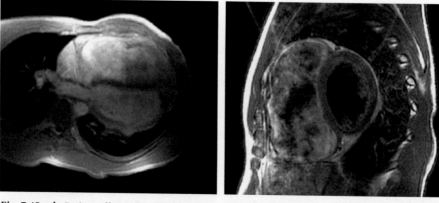

Fig. 7.45 a, b. Patient affected by Uhl's disease and atrial fibrillation. (**a**) Image of the heart in cine SPGR on the long horizontal axis showing a large dilatation of the right ventricle; (**b**) same case in an image of the heart obtained on the short axis by SE "black blood". The quality of the images is reduced by the concomitant atrial fibrillation and the numerous artifacts inside the cavity caused by the slow blood flow

The wide array of pathologies includes:

a) ventricular tachycardia originating from the *outflow tract* of the right ventricle, characterized by non-specific structural alterations at the level of the outflow tract and variable electrophysiological properties

b) benign ventricular extra-systolic activity with left bundle block morphology. The morphology of QRS suggests an infundibular origin of the arrhythmia; morphologic findings and function of right ventricle are normal

c) Brugada's syndrome: genetic disease characterized by ST elevation in V1-V3 and complete or incomplete right bundle branch block. The clinical picture is characterized by malignant ventricular arrhythmias; often sudden death is the first sign of the disease. Differently from ARVC, the syndrome is not accompanied by any histological, morphological, or functional alterations of the myocardium

d) Uhl's anomaly: the disease is characterized by a partial or complete substitution of right ventricular myocardium by fibrous tissue, which translates into a clinical picture of right ventricular failure. It may remain asymptomatic for many years and lead to sudden death (Fig. 7.45).

7.3.4.2.9 Diagnosis of ARVC with MRI

In recent years MRI has regularly been used for the morpho-functional study of the right ventricle whenever there was a suspicion of ARVC. In reality, if on one hand the potentiality of the method in that direction has always been clear, on the other the inadequacy of the equipment available has often appeared as the most limiting factor for a correct diagnosis. Obtaining good quality images of the heart requires an extremely efficient synchronization with the ECG; but sometimes not even this is enough, due to the presence of arrhythmias (typically ventricular extra-systolic activity, BBS type); therefore, pretreatment of the patient (e.g. propafenon 150 mg ter i.d. in the 7-10 preceding days) is often recommended.

The objectives of MRI in subjects with suspected ARVC can be synthesized in three points:

a) morphological information, with particular concern for the volumetric dimensions of the right ventricle
b) evaluation of the global and, especially, regional function of the free wall of the right ventricle and segmental function of left ventricle
c) presence of fatty infiltration in the myocardium.

Morphological findings.
The sizing of the right ventricle covers a fundamental role in the diagnostic procedure for ARVC. Because the right ventricle has a decisively irregular morphology, it is unsuitable for linear measurements. Moreover, there are no systematic data available to provide clear references as to the different segments of the right ventricle. There are, however, reference values for right ventricular volumes (see Paragraph 7.2.6). MRI is the only technique that allows volumetric measurements of the right ventricle without the aid of geometrical assumptions.

MRI also gives the possibility of measuring the thickness of the free wall of the right ventricle. Because this wall is very thin, it is necessary to rely on the highest acquisition matrix possible, the most closely compatible to the acquisition time. For this measurement it is suggested to use end-diastolic images obtained with cine-MRI techniques. In detail, the measure of the free-wall thickness is taken at its different segments (normal value 4-6 mm) [28]. When drawing up the final evaluation, the operator should consider that there are different physiological or para-physiological conditions, such as considerable physical activity, that can lead to significant variations of this parameter.

Assessment of function.
MRI offers the possibility of evaluating both the global function, expressed as right ventricle Ejection Fraction (EF), and the regional function of the free wall with the demonstration of asynergic areas.

The typical finding in ARVC is systo-diastolic bulging, frequently located in correspondence to the so-called triangle of dysplasia. Usually the localization of the asynergic areas correspond to the localization of the areas with the most extended fatty infiltration, and thus with reduced mechanical resistance. The presence of asynergic regions does not imply diagnosis of ARVC, as it can also be appreciated in other pathologies such as congenital or inflammatory diseases. Conversely, its absence does not allow to exclude the diagnosis, since the diastolic bulging requires a significantly extended fibro-adipose infiltration in order to develop.

Analysis of MRI signal.
MRI can provide characteristics on the wall signal since the hydrogen atoms of the different tissues show slight differences in frequency of precession (chemical shift) in virtue of different molecular bonds. The method is used for differentiating the signal coming from hydrogen atoms in the fatty tissue from the signal of the other tissues, and sometimes for cancelling it out (fat suppression) or saturating it.

The images generally used are those in T_1-weighted Spin Echo in free breathing or preferably the FSE "black blood" in breath-hold. In both images, the fatty tissue shows a high signal intensity that contrasts with the hypointense myocardial tissue. The proof of adipose infiltration can also come from images with signal suppression from the adipose tissue. This procedure is perhaps more efficient in free-breathing images, which indeed allow a shorter T_1 than those in breath-hold but requires long acquisition times and especially have a lower image quality. Other extremely useful images are those obtained by fat suppression or by Inversion Recovery (Short Time Inversion Recovery – STIR). This sequence, which foresees the use of an extremely short inversion time, efficiently cancels-out fatty tissue. Its main limitation lays in the fact that with very short inversion times, there are more artifacts linked to the slowed flow in proximity of the left ventricle free wall that can compromise the quality of images. If the suppression/saturation of the fatty tissue can result very efficient in some patients (hyperintense areas that become largely hypointense), in other patients it is impossible to separate the signal emitted by fat from that emitted by the surrounding myocardium, as the differences of precession frequencies within the single subject can be very limited.

Moreover, finding fatty infiltrations areas in the context of the free wall of the right ventricle or at the apex is not pathognomonic of ARVC. In fact, it is known that a certain degree of fat infiltration in the right ventricle myocardium can represent, for a number of subjects, a finding with no pathological value, especially for those subjects in older age or patients with a marked increase in subepicardial fat (obese) [22, 24].

MRI strategy.
Given the prevalence of alterations in the dysplasia triangle (which has the inferior margin of the heart as its base and the right ventricular outflow tract

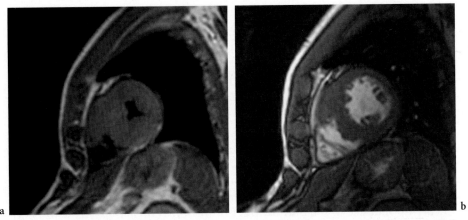

Fig. 7.47 a, b. Patient with hypertrophic cardiac disease involving the interventricular septum and the free wall of the right ventricle. (a) Image on the short axis of the heart in Fast SE "black blood". (b) Image on the short axis of the heart in cine FIESTA

death, recurrent syncope events, the presence of non-sustained ventricular tachycardia with Holter-ECG, the altered pressure response during the ergono- metric test, and marked wall hypertrophy (thickness >30 mm) [52]. In patients with HCM, sudden death is linked to the onset of ventricular tachycardia or ventricular fibrillation [53]. The anatomic substrate for such arrhythmias is likely to be represented by structural alterations of the myocardium, which is characteristic of the disease, and seems to be associated to the presence of areas of disorganized myofibril distribution and marked fibrosis [44, 45].

Many autoptic studies have demonstrated that in patients with HCM, fibrous areas are frequently found also in absence of significant coronary lesions [43, 44, 54, 55].

The diagnosis of HCM is based on the echocardiographic finding of a hypertrophic left ventricle (wall thickness >2SD in the normality range adjusted to age and weight) in absence of other cardiac or systematic pathologies that can justify a hypertophy of such magnitude [3, 56].

The echocardiographic exam documents the presence and regional distri- bution of wall hypertrophy in patients with HCM, in addition to the presence, in a lesser number of patients, of a dynamic gradient in the outflow tract of the left ventricle accompanied by an anomalous systolic shift of the anterior mitral limb against the intraventricular septum.

7.3.4.3.1 MRI in HCM

Many studies on MR have demonstrated great accuracy of the method in the morphological and functional assessment of patients with HCM and in the screening of family members.

Cine images (SPGR, SSFP, etc.), allow to give a precise measure of wall tickening, end-diastolic and end-systolic volumes of the left ventricle and thus of the ejection fraction. Thickness and ventricular diameters are generally measured in the end-diastole images in the horizontal, vertical long-axis and short axis projections of the left ventricle.

Compared to Echocardiography, MRI has been demonstrated to be superior in the evaluation of cardiac mass and in identifying hypertrophy at the level of the apex and of the right ventricle [57-59] and represents the technique of choice for monitoring and quantifying the postsurgical changes after surgical myectomy or through catheter selective alcohol-mediated necrosis of the interventricular septum [60, 61] (Fig. 7.48).

The use of cine sequences allows to verify if there is an obstructive pattern in correspondence to the outflow tract of the left ventricle [62] as with Echo-Doppler. In the regions of turbulent blood flow, blood is hypointense. A new approach to the dynamic gradient has recently been proposed for measuring the actual area of the outflow tract of the left ventricle using regional mappings of turbulent flow during systole in images on short axis of the left ventricle [61]. This method, if proved to be valid, would allow to overcome the problem of pressure recovery that usually leads to an overestimation of the gradient and of inter-observer variability, which represent two important limits to Echocardiography in the evaluation of the obstructive forms in HCM.

Tagging has been proposed for evaluating diastolic dysfunction in patients with HCM [63]. In fact the technique allows to analyze the rotational movement of the heart, characteristic of the iso-volumetric relaxation and radial distension of the walls during the filling phase. Preliminary studies on patients with left ventricular hypertrophy by pressure overload have docu-

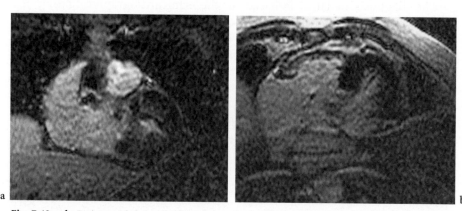

a   b

Fig. 7.48 a, b. Patient with hypertrophic obstructive cardiomyopathy treated with selective septal alcoholization. The images obtained in 3D IR-FGR DE show a hyperintense area at the level of the interventricular septum. (a) Image on the short axis of the heart; (b) image on the long horizontal axis of the heart

mented an increase of systolic torque motion, in addition to a prolonging of the rotational movement of the apical structures and a reduction in radial distension of the myocardium at the level of the basal septum [64, 65]. This technique is however still in an experimental stage that must be verified for its feasibility in a clinical setting.

Compared to other imaging techniques, MRI offers a further advantage in the study of HCM as to the possibility of providing a tissue characterization of the myocardium with great prognostic relevance.

In recent years the development of MRI sequences (IR-Fast Gradient Echo – delayed enhancement) with the use of extra cellular contrast agents has allowed to identify fibro-necrotic areas in patients with pregressed myocardial infarction [66, 67]. In these MR images the necrotic areas appear hyperintense (see Paragraph 7.3.3) [67-69]. The mechanism of accumulation of the contrast agent in the site of pregressed necrosis is still unclear. Among the different hypotheses, the most probable implies an alteration of the pharmaco-dynamics of the contrast agent in the diseased interstitium.

Recently, it has been reported that images in delayed enhancement can be used to identify the eventual presence of fibrous areas also in patients with HCM [70]. Previous papers indicate that the hyperenhanced areas are found in most patients (>80%) and typically only in correspondence to the hypertrophic regions, most often at the level of the third medium of the ventricular wall with multi-focal distribution (Fig. 7.49). There are no correlations between the fibrous areas and the territory of distribution of the epicardial coronary arteries. The fibrous process typically involves the conjunction area between the intraventricular septum and the free wall of the right ventricle.

The extension of the areas of fibrosis correlates to the degree of wall hypertrophy and inversely to systolic thickening

The presence of fibrous areas alone is not indicative of an unfavorable prognosis, but an extended fibrous area is [70].

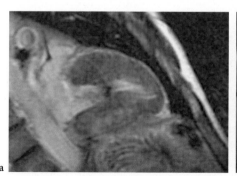 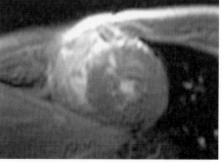

a   b

Fig. 7.49 a, b. Patient with hypertrophic cardiomyopathy: Images obtained with 2D IR-FGR DE: (a) image on the long vertical axis of the heart showing hyperintense area at the level of the inferior wall; (b) image on the short axis shows hyperintensity area at the level of the anterior-septal wall

In a recent study the data on delayed enhancement and the clinical risk factors for sudden death seem to correlate [71]. The areas of delayed enhancement would result significantly more extended in patients who develop heart failure (28.5% vs 8.7%) and in patients presenting one or two risk factors of sudden death (15,7% vs 8.6%).

There are two patterns of enhancement: diffused and regional. Patients with diffused hyperenhancement seem to present two or more risk factors for sudden death (87% vs 33%) more often than patients with regional patterns of hyperenhancement. These results are in agreement with autoptic studies that show the correlation between a higher degree of myocardial fibrosis and sudden death [54, 72-73]. It must be underlined that, to date, there are no systematic histological correlations between the areas of delayed enhancement and autopsy findings in patients with HCM.

The interpretation according to which the areas of delayed enhancement corresponds to areas of fibrous replacement is at present purely speculative. Other kinds of fibrosis that increase the distribution volume of the contrast agent, such as interstitial fibrosis, could be at the base of increased signal intensity. Surely, the fibrous areas that are evidenced in patients with HCM present different characteristics from those found in patients with pregressed necrosis. Probably, in patients with HCM, such regions are the results of a series of pathological processes that determine the formation of different fibrous types (fibrous replacement or absence of myocytes) may be attributed to myofibril disarray and the consequent spreading of the interstitial space.

Despite the limitations, MRI studies performed so far seem to suggest a close correlation between fibrous areas and an unfavorable remodeling of the left ventricle, in addition to the presence of several risk factors for sudden death [71].

The use of MRI in the study of HCM, in addition to providing precise morphological and functional indications, allows an accurate tissue characterization of the myocardium, which might provide additional information for the prognostic stratification of patients and in particular for the identification of that smaller group of patients with HCM who are at high risk of sudden death.

7.3.4.4 Non-compaction of the myocardium

Non-compaction of the myocardium is a rare congenital disease caused by an interruption or by an uncompleted compacting process of the myocardial trabeculas during embriogenesis. It can be isolated to the left ventricle, or involve both ventricles [73], and sometimes has a familial tendency [74, 75].

According to a recent classification by WHO, the non-compacted myocardium falls into the group of non-classified cardiomyopathies [4].

The diagnosis, which is often unknown, is based on precise echocardiographic criteria [78]:

a) absence of coexisting congenital defects
b) increased myocardial wall thickness formed by a thin compacted epicardial layer and a more extended non-compacted endocardial layer. The endocardial layer is basically formed by trabeculas and blind-end recesses connected with the ventricle cavity. The two layers can be better differentiated by measuring the thickness of the epicardium and the endocardium on the parasternal short axis projection at the end of systole. The ratio of non-compacted area to compacted area must >2
c) the segments most frequently involved are the apex (>80%) and the medium portion of the inferior and lateral wall
d) the spaces between trabeculas of the myocardium are in direct continuity with the ventricular cavity and, differently do not communicate with the coronary circulation.

The description of the location of the segments involved requires that the left ventricle be divided into nine segments [75, 77]: an apical segment, 4 medium segments, and 4 basal segments (inferior, lateral, anterior, and septal).

At present there are no established echocardiographic criteria for the diagnosis of non-compacted right ventricle due to the natural wealth of trabecula of the right apex and to the difficulty of differentiating normal variants from diseased patterns.

The morbidity and mortality of patients affected by non-compacted myocardium is high among both young and adult subjects. The clinical picture includes heart failure, thromboembolic events, and sudden cardiac death [76].

The physiopathological substrate of arrhythmias and heart failure in these patients is still source of discussion. According to some authors myocardial ischemia could play a crucial role [79]. In patients with non-compaction of the ventricle, the flow of the great epicardial coronary vessels is normal [75, 80]. However, in correspondence to the non-compact regions there is clear evidence of subendocardial fibrosis. Therefore, the most probable hypothesis would seem to be that the fibrous areas in these segments are the consequence of a process of subendocardial ischemia [81-84].

In a small group of patients, PET has evidenced a reduction of myocardial perfusion both at basal conditions and after pharmacological stress with dipyridamole limited to the non-compacted areas [85], perhaps correlated to a reduced development of the microvasculature, eventually linked to wall hypertrophy [85].

According to other authors, myocardial perfusion in patients with a non-compaction of the ventricle [78] would result normal at baseline conditions and reduced during pharmacological stress; moreover, it would not involve the areas of the myocardium alone but also segments of morphologically normal myocardium. Hence, findings would be pointing to a hypothesis of alteration of microvasculature.

7.3.4.4.1 MRI in the study of non-compaction of the myocardium

In virtue of the high spatial resolution and the possibility of tissue characterization, MRI is spreading as a technique of great diagnostic relevance in patients with ventricular non-compaction [86]. Spin Echo sequences allow an accurate morphological definition of the myocardial wall and of the ventricular cavities. In cine sequences (SPGR, SSFP, etc.) compaction and non-compaction appear more clearly distinguishable (Fig. 7.50). Moreover, delayed images acquired after the administration of contrast agent allow to identify

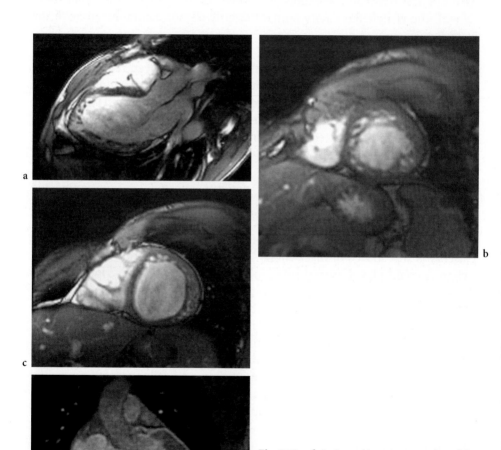

Fig. 7.50 a-d. Patient with non-compaction of the left ventricle. Images obtained by cine FIESTA. (**a**) Long vertical axis of the heart. The image evidences many blind-end recesses in continuity with the ventricular cavity and the presence of a thin subepicardial region. The same findings can be appreciated in images on the short axis obtained at several levels of the left ventricle (**b-d**)

the presence of fibrous areas in correspondence to the subendocardium. The study of myocardial perfusion with the first pass technique (see Chapter 7) has evidenced in a recent case reported in literature a reduction of perfusion in correspondence to non-compacted regions [87].

7.3.4.5 Hemochromatosis

Hemochromatosis is a relatively frequent pathology, characterized by intracellular deposit of hemosiderin and ferritin. The organs most often involved are liver, heart, and the central nervous system. The disease is distinguished into its two forms, primitive and secondary. Primitive hemochromatosis is a genetic disease with recessive autosomic transmission, among the most frequent worldwide as to prevalence [87]. Secondary hemochromatosis in most cases develops after an exaggerated iron uptake due to a chronic transfusional therapy or due to chronic hyperhemolysis. In view of higher life expectancy among these patients, iron overload caused by this condition is becoming a growing concern.

Independently from the underlying pathology, iron overload yields relatively uniform signs, with cardiac dysfunction being the first cause of death among patients with hemochromatosis [89].

The difficulty of picturing hemosiderotic cardiomyopathy properly under a physiopathological profile lies in the variety of concomitant mechanisms. There is no doubt that iron overload at the level of cardiac myocytes determines a diastolic and systolic dysfunction, in either an alternating, progressive, or simultaneous manner, following a restrictive, and dilatative pattern. This makes the diagnostic pathway and follow-up of hemochromatosic cardiomyopathy difficult, imposing the use of a technique that allows an accurate morpho-functional evaluation and a reliable tissue characterization.

Echocardiography is able to evaluate, to a satisfying degree, the preserved wall thicknesses, changes of volume and left ventricular function; however the limits of the technique are amplified when trying to quantify functionality of the right ventricle chamber, which is another important prognostic determinant of hemochromatosic cardiomyopathy [90, 91].

7.3.4.5.1 MRI in the study of hemochromatosis

The quantitative data on either right or left cardiac function obtained by MRI represent the gold standard of modern non-invasive cardiology with significantly low values of intra-and inter- operator variability [28, 92].

A frequent finding among patients with hemochromatosis is a variable degree of mitral insufficiency, as this appears to have a somewhat prognostic value. The standard approach requires its quantitative evaluation, which can easily be achieved with MRI using cine Gradient Echo or phase velocity encoding sequences [93].

MRI has the peculiarity of allowing the myocardial tissue characterization of such patients, identifying iron deposits as specific markers for disease. It has to be considered that values of serum ferritin [94] and the iron deposits at the hepatic level are not reliable predictors of iron upload in the myocardium. This accumulation does not lead to significant alterations of echogenicity and, therefore, cannot be detected. The deposit is prevalently subepicardial, patchy, and affecting the left ventricle, which is the reason why endomyocardial biopsy has a low diagnostic sensitivity [88]. Conversely, iron is a strongly paramagnetic substance that introduces some local inhomogeneities into the magnetic field, and its deposits cause a shortening in T1-, T2- and T2* [94]. To date, the GRE T2* technique seems to provide a quick and reproducible evaluation of iron accumulation at the level of the myocardium (Fig. 7.51).

In patients with Thalassemia major β, the indices of left ventricular dysfunction seem to correlate with the evaluation of intra cardiac iron deposit measured by assessing the values of T2* [95]. Normal T2* reference values at the level of the myocardium have been measured at 52±16 ms (single echo technique) [96] and at 33.3±7.8 ms (multi-echo technique) [97]. T2* values <20 ms would always associate to a reduced left ventricular function. However, a validation of T2* through pathological findings still has not been made, while further studies are needed to provide some data on how to evaluate the effects of fibrosis and desaturation in the evaluation of T2* [96-98].

Recent studies have documented the possibility of identifying through MRI areas of fibrosis in patients with pregressed myocardial infarction and patients with hypertrophic cardiomyopathy. This method, however, has not been validated for hemochromatosis [98].

Remaining within the field of tissue characterization, T1-weighted sequences, after the administration of Gd-based contrast agents [99], or T2-weighted, have shown to be valid in identifying the accumulation of liquid deposits such as oedemas or deposits from myocardial-pericardial inflammatory processes that often concur in determining hemosiderotic cardiomyopathy.

MRI can hence be considered a valid non-invasive tool for managing hemosiderotic cardiomyopathy in terms of diagnosis and prognosis. Moreover, considering the potential reversibility of cardiac morbidity in hemochromatosis [100-102] by, for example, chelating therapy or bone marrow transplant, therapeutic monitoring is an objective of great respect in which MRI can be qualified as the ideal tool.

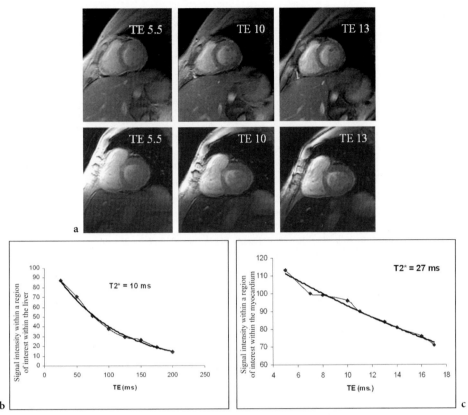

Fig. 7.51 a-c. (a) T2*-weighted images with single echo technique. Short axis of the heart obtained with increasing values of TE. Top: images obtained from a healthy volunteer. Bottom: images obtained with the same technique in a patient with thalassemia major. There is an evident signal hypointensity at level of the liver caused by a deposit of Fe++. (b) The graph illustrates the relationship between signal intensity, measured at the level of a region of interest positioned in the liver, and the increasing values of TE. These values provide data used to calculate T2* of the tissue. The T2* of this patient with thalassemia major is reduced (normal range 37±7 msec), the graph (c) illustrates the relationship between the intensity of the signal measured at the level of a region positioned in the mid-ventricular septum of the patient with thalassemia major and increasing TE values. The derived value of the myocardium's T2* results normal (normal ranges 52±16 msec)

7.3.4.6 Endomyocardial fibrosis

Endomyocardial fibrosis is a rare form of secondary cardiomyopathy. At present, two forms have been found: Loeffler's disease, typical of temperate climates, and another occurring in tropical and subtropical areas. Loeffler's endocarditis is a rapidly progressive disease that arises in about 75% of patients with hypereosinofilia [103]. It can either be idiopathic or secondary

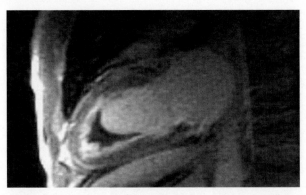

Fig. 7.52. Patient with endomyocardiofibrosis. The image on the long vertical axis of the heart obtained by IR-GRE delayed enhancement after contrast agent administration evidences an obliteration of the distal part of the left ventricular cavity on behalf of highly hypointense thrombotic material. The endocardium appears diffusely hyperintense due to the uptake of contrast medium, which confirms important fibrous phenomena at this level

to one of several pathologies (autoimmune, infectious, parasitic, allergic syndromes, or neoplastic). The tropical form, compared to the former, has a slower clinical evolution and is not associated with hypereosinofilia.

Although, the two have separate pathogenetic processes, both are characterized by a rigid thickening of the subendocardium, which is more often thicker at the level the apex of one or both ventricles, of the papillary muscles and of the valvular systems; often there are voluminous thrombotic endocavitary masses [104-106] (Fig. 7.52).

The clinical picture is that of a restrictive cardiomyopathy with evolution toward heart failure by diastolic dysfunction [107].

The echocardiographic exam frequently detects the presence of hyperechogenic material that obliterates the apex of one or both ventricles, and the further thickening and adherence to the posterior wall of the cordal system of the atrio-ventricular valves; often non-negligible mitral and/or tricuspidal insufficiency is detectable [104-108].

7.3.4.6.1 MRI in endomyocardial fibrosis

MRI allows an accurate evaluation of the site and extension of the subendocardial fibrosis, also providing the possibility of analyzing the tissue's characteristics [105, 109-112]. The employment of the different T1- and T2-weighted sequences, and the employment of contrast agents allows a precise definition of the endoluminal thrombotic masses.

Areas of subendocardial fibrosis can be identified by means of the IR-GRE (delayed enhancement) images acquired late after the administration of the contrast medium.

Cine sequences allow to measure the ventricular volumes and ejection fraction quite accurately, and also evaluate the diastolic function, the most compromised functional characteristic in these patients.

References

1. Basso C, Thiene G, Corrado D et al (1996) Arrhythmogenic right ventricular cardiomyopathy. Displasia, dystrophy, or myocarditis? Circulation 94:983-991
2. Pinamonti B, Sinagra G, Salvi A et al (1992) Left ventricular involvement in right ventricular dysplasia. Am Heart J 123:711-724
3. Richardson P, McKenna W, Bristow M et al (1996) Report of the 1995 World Health Organization/International Society and Federation of Cardiology Task Force on the definition and classification of cardiomyopathies. Circulation 93:841-842
4. Nava A, Thiene G, Canciani B et al (1988) Familial occurrence of right ventricular dysplasia: a study involving nine families. J Am Coll Cardiol 12:1222-1228
5. Aman Coonar S, Protonotarius N, Tsatsopoulou A et al (1998) Gene for arrhythmogenic right ventricular cardiomyopathy with diffuse nonepidermolytic palmoplantar keratoderma and wooly hair (Naxos disease) maps to 17q21. Circulation 97:2049-2058
6. Ahmad F, Li D, Karibe A et al (1998) Localization of a gene responsible for arrhythmogenic right ventricular dysplasia to chromosome 3p23. Circulation 98:2791-2795
7. Bauce B, Nava A, Ramazzo A et al (2000) Familial effort polymorphic ventricular arrhythmias in arrhythmogenic right ventricular cardiomyopathy map to chromosome 1q42-43. Am J Cardiol 85:573-579
8. Severini GM, Krajinovic M, Pinamonti B et al (1996) A new locus for arrhythmogenic right ventricular displasia on the long arm of chromosome 14. Genomics 31:193-200
9. Rampazzo A, Nava A, Miorin M et al (1997) DAVD4, a new locus for arrhythmogenic right ventricular cardiomyopathy, maps to chromosome 2 long arm. Genomics 45: 259-263
10. Tiso N, Stephan DA, Nava A et al (2001) Identification of mutations in the cardiac ryanodine receptor gene in families affected with arrhythmogenic right ventricular cardiomyopathy type 2. Hum Mal Genet 10:189-194
11. Li D, Gonzales O, Bachinski LL et al (2000) Human protein tyrosine phosphatase-like gene: expression profile, genomic structure and mutation analysis in families with DAVD. Gene 256:237-243
12. Li D, Ahmad F, Gardner MJ et al (2000) The locus of a novel gene responsible for arrhythmogenic right ventricular dysplasia characterized by early onset and high penetrance maps to chromosome 10p12-p14. Am J Hum Genet 66:148-156
13. Melberg A, Oldfors A, Blomstrom-Lundqvist C et al (1999) Autosomal dominant myofibrillar myopathy with arrhythmogenic right ventricular cardiomyopathy linked to chromosome 10q. Ann Neurol 46:684-692
14. Thiene C, Corrado D, Nava A et al (1991) Right ventricular cardiomyopathy: is there evidence of an inflammatory aetiology? Eur Heart J 12:22-25
15. Kodama M, Matsumoto Y, Fujwara M (1992) In vivo lymphocyte-mediated transfer of experimental autoimmune myocarditis. Circulation 85:1918-1926
16. Matsumori A, Kawai C (1980) Coxsackie virus B3 perimyocarditis in BALB/c mice: experimental model of chronic perimyocarditis in the right ventricle. J Pathol 131:97-106
17. Grumbach IM, Heim A, Vonhof S et al (1998) Coxsackievirus genome in myocardium of patients with arrhythmogenic right ventricular dysplasia/cardiomyopathy. Cardiology 89:241-245

18. James TN (1994) Normal and abnormal consequences of apoptosis in the human heart. From postnatal morphogenesis to paroxysmal arrhythmias. Circulation 90:556-573

19. Mallat Z, Tedgui A, Fontaliran F et al (1996) Evidence of apoptosis in arrhythmogenic right ventricular dysplasia. N Engl J Med 335:1190-1196

20. Valente M, Calabrese F, Thiene G et al (1996) In vivo evidence of apoptosis in arrhythmogenic right ventricular dysplasia. N Engl J Med 335:1190-1196

21. Colston JT, Chandrasekar B, Freeman GL (1998) Expression of apoptosis-related proteins in experimental coxsackie virus myocarditis. Cardiovasc Res 38:158-168

22. Fontaliran F, Fontaine G, Fillette F et al (1991) Frontières nosologiques de la dysplasie arythmogène. Variations quantitatives du tissu adipeux ventriculaire droit normal. Arch Mal Cœur 84:33-38

23. Fontaine G, Guiraudon G, Frank R, Tonet JL et al (1984) Arrhythmogenic right ventricular dysplasia: a clinical model for the study of chronic ventricular tachicardia. Jpn Circ 515-538

24. Thiene G, Basso C, Calabrese F et al (2000) Pathology and pathogenesis of arrhythmogenic right ventricular cardiomyopathy. Hertz 25:210-215

25. Burke AP, Farb A, Tashko G et al (1998) Arrhythmogenic right ventricular cardiomyopathy and fatty replacement of the right ventricular myocardium. Are they different diseases? Circulation 97:1571-1580

26. Corrado D, Basso C, Thiene G et al (1997) Spectrum of clinicopathologic manifestations of arrhythmogenic right ventricular cardiomyopathy/dysplasia: a multicenter study. J Am Coll Cardiol 30:1512-1520

27. Fontaine G, Fontaliran F, Frank R et al (1998) Arrhythmogenic right ventricular cardiomyopathies. Clinical forms and main differential diagnoses. Circulation 97:1532-1535

28. Lorenz Ch, Walker ES, Morgan VL et al (1999) Normal human right and left ventricular mass, systolic function and gender differences by cine magnetic resonance imaging. J Cardiovasc Magn Reson 1:7-21

29. McKenna WJ, Thiene G, Nava A et al (1994) Diagnosis of arrhythmogenic right ventricula dysplasi/cardiomyopathy. Br Heart J 71:215-218

30. Maron BJ (2003) Sudden death in young athletes. N Eng J Med 11;349(11):1064-1075

31. Thiene G, Nava A, Corrado D et al (1988) Right ventricula cardiomyopathy and sudden death in young people. N Engl J Med 318:129-133

32. Zeppilli P, La Rosa Gangi M, Santini C et al (1988) Right heart in athletics. Echocardiography 1988: proceedings of the 6th international congress on echocardiography, Rome, 1988. Excerpta Medica eds Amsterdam

33. Zeppilli P (1995) Cardiologia dello sport. CESI, Roma

34. Frank S, Braunwald E (1968) Idiopathic hypertrophic subaortic stenosis: clinical analysis of 126 patients with emphasis on the natural history. Circulation 37:59-788

35. Maron BJ, Bonow RO, Cannon Ro III et al (1987) Hypertrophic cardiomyopathy; interrelations of clinical manifestations, pathophysiology and theraphy. N Engl J Med 316:780-9, 844-852

36. Spirito P, Seidman CE, McKenna WJ, Maron BJ (1997) The management of hypertrophic cardiomyopathy. N Engl J Med 336:775-785

37. Marian AJ, Roberts R (2001) The molecular genetic basis for hypertrophic cardiomyopathy. J Moll Cell Cardiol 33:655-670

38. Klues HG, Schiffers A, Marron BJ (1995) Phenotypic spectrum and patterns of left ventricular hypertrophy in hypertrophic cardiomyopathy: morphologic observations and significance as assessed by two dimensional echocardiography in 600 patients. J Am Coll Cardiol 26:1699-1708

39. Maron BJ, Ferrans VJ, Henry WL, Clarke CE, Redwood DR (1974) Differences in distribution of myocardial abnormalities in patients with obstructive and nonobstructive asym-

metric septal hypertrophy (ASH). Light and electron microscopic findings. Circulation 50:436-446

40. Maron BJ, Roberts WC (1981) Hypertrophic cardiomyopathy and cardiac muscle cell disorganization revisited: relation between the two and significance. Am Heart J 102:95-110

41. Maron BJ, Wolfson JK, Roberts WC (1992) Relation between extent of cardiac muscle cell disorganization and left ventricular wall thickness in hypertrophic cardiomyopathy. Am J Cardiol 70:785-790

42. Maron BJ, Anan TJ, Roberts WC (1981) Quantitative analysis of the distribution of cardiac muscle cell disorganization in the left ventricular wall of patients with hypertrophic cardiomyopathy. Circulation 63:882-894

43. Unverferth D, Baker PB, Pearce LI, Lautman J et al (1987) Regional myocyte hypertrophy and increased interstitial myocardial fibrosis in hypertrophic cardiomyopathy. Am J Cardiol 59:932-936

44. Maron BJ, Wolfson JK, Epstein SE, Roberts WC (1986) Intramural ("small vessel") coronary artery disease in hypertrophic cardiomyopathy. J Am Coll Cardiol 8:545-557

45. Schwartzkoff B, Mundhenke M, Strauer BE (1998) Alterations of the architecture of subendocardial arterioles in patients with hypertrophic cardiomiopathy and impaired coronary vasodilatator reserve: a possibile cause for myocardic ischemia. J Am Coll Cardiol 31:1089-1096

46. Cannan CR, Reeder GS, Bailey KR et al (1995) Natural history of hypertrophic cardiomyopathy; a population-based study, 1976 through 1990. Circulation 92:2488-2495

47. Maron BJ, Casey SA, Poliac LC et al (1999) Clinical course of hypertrophic cardiomyopathy in a regional United States cohort. JAMA 281:650-655

48. Spirito P, Bellone P, Harris KM et al (2000) Magnitude of left ventricular hypertrophy predicts the risk of sudden death in hypertrophic cardiomyopathy. N Engl J Med 342:1778-1785

49. Spirito P, Chiarella F, Carratino L et al (1989) Clinical course and prognosis of hypertrophic cardiomyopathy in an outpatient population. N Engl J Med 320:749-755

50. Kofflard MJ, Waldestein DJ, Vos J et al (1993) Prognosis in hypertrophic cardiomyopathy: a retrospective study. Am J Cardiol 72:939-943

51. Cecchi F, Olivotto I, Montereggi A et al (1995) Hypertrophic cardiomyopathy in Tuscany: clinical course and outcome in an unselected regional population. J Am Coll Cardio 26:1529-1536

52. Elliott PM, Poloniecki J, Dickie S et al (2000) Sudden death in hypertrophic cardiomyopathy: identification of high risk patients. J Am Coll Cardiol 36:2212-2218

53. Maron BJ, Shen WK, Link MS et al (2000) Efficacy of implantable cardioverter-defibrillators for the prevention of sudden death in patients with hypertrophic cardiomyopathy. N Engl J Med 342:365-373

54. Basso C, Thiene G, Corrado D et al (2000) Hypertrophic cardiomyopathy and sudden death in the young: pathologic evidence of myocardial ischemia. Hum Pathol 31:988-998

55. Maron BJ, Epstein SE, Roberts WC (1979) Hypertrophic cardiomyopathy and transmural myocardial infarction without significant atherosclerosis of the extramural coronary disease. Am J Cardiol 43:1086-1102

56. McKenna WJ, Spirito P, Desnos M, Dubourg O, Komajada M (1997) Experience from clinical genetics in hypertrophic cardiomyopathy: proposal for new diagnostic criteria in adult members of affected families. Heart 77:130-132

57. Bottini PB, Carr AA, Prisant LM et al (1995) Magnetic resonance imaging compared to echocardiography to assess left ventricular mass in the hypertensive patient. Am J Hypertens 8:221-228

58. Posma JL, Blanksma PK, Van der Wall et al (1996) Assessment of quantitative hypertrophy scores in hypertrophic cardiomyopathy: magnetic resonance imaging versus echocardiography. Am Heart J 132:1020-1027

59. Pons Llado G, Carreras F, Borras X et al (1997) Comparison of morphologic assessment of hypertrophic cardiomyopathy by magnetic resonance versus echocardiographic imaging. Am J Cardiol 79:1651-1656

60. Franke A, Schondube FA, Kuhl HP et al (1998) Quantitative assessment of the operative results after extended myectomy and surgical reconstruction of the subvalvular mitral apparatus in hypertrophic obstructive cardiomyopathy using three dimensional transesofageal echocardiography. J am Coll Cardiol 31:1641-1649

61. Schultz-Menger J, Strohm O, Waigand J et al (2000) The value of magnetic resonance imaging of the left ventricular outflowtract in patients with hypertrophic obstructive cardiomyopathy after septal artery embolization. Circulation 101:1764-1766

62. White RD, Obuchowski NA, Gunawardena S et al (1996) Left ventricular outflow tract obstruction in hypertrophic cardiomyopathy: presurgical and post surgical evaluation by computed tomography magnetic resonance imaging. Am J Cardiol Imaging 10:1-13

63. Stuber M, Scheidegger M, Fischer S et al (1999) Alterations in local myocardial motion pattern in patients suffering from pressure overload due to aortic stenosis. Circulation 100:361-368

64. Maier SE, Fischer SE, McKinnon GC et al (1992) Evaluation of left ventricular segmental wall motion in hypertrophic cardiomyopathy with myocardic tagging. Circulation 90:1919-1928

65. Kramer CM, Reichek N, Ferrari VA et al (1994) Regional heterogeneity of function in hypertrophic cardiomyopathy. Circulation 90:186-194

66. Wu E, Judd RM, Vargas JD, Klocke FJ, Bonow Ro, Kim RJ (2001) Visualization of presence, location and transmural extent of healed Q-wave and non Q-wave myocardial infarction. Lancet 357:21-28

67. Kim RJ, Fieno DS, Parrisch TB et al (1999) Relationship of MRI delayed contrast enhancement to irreversible injury, infart age and contractile function. Circulation 100:1992-2002

68. Choi KM, Kim RJ, Gubernikoff G et al (2001) Transmural extent of acute myocardial infarction predicts long-term improvement in contractile function. Circulation 104:1101-1107

69. Kim RJ, Wu E, Rafael A et al (2000) The use of contrast-enhanced magnetic resonance imaging to identify reversible myocardial dysfunction. N Engl J Med 343:1445-1453

70. Choudhury L, Mahrholdot H, Wagner A et al (2002) Myocardial scarring in asymptomatic or middly symptomatic patients with hypertrophic cardiomyopathy. J Am Coll Cardiol 40:2156-2164

71. Moon JCC, Mckenna WJ, McCrohon JA et al (2003) Toward clinical assessment in hypertrophic cardiomyopathy with gadolinium cardiovascular magnetic resonance. J Am Coll Cardiol 41:1561-1567

72. Tanaka M, Fujiwura H, Onodera T et al (1986) Quantitative analysis of myocardial fibrosis in normal, hypertensive hearts and hypertrophic cardiomyopathy. Br Heart J 55:575-581

73. Varnava AM, Elliott PM, Mahon N, Davies MJ, McKenna WJ (2001) Relation between myocyte disarray and outcome in hypertrophic cardiomyopathy. Am J Cardiol 88:275-279

74. Sedemera D, Pexieder T, Vuillemin M, Thompson RP, Anderson RH (2000) Developmental pattering of the myocardium. Anat Rec 258:319-337

75. Chin TK, Perloff JK, Williams RG, Jue K, Mohrmann R (1990) Isolated noncompaction of left ventricular myocardium. A study of eight cases. Circulation 82:507-513

76. Oechslin EN, Attenhofer Jost CH, Rojas JR, Kaufmann PA, Jenni R (2000) Long-term follow-up of 34 adults with isolated left ventricular noncompaction: a distinct cardiomyopathy with poor prognosis. J Am Coll Cardiol 36:493-500

77. Ichida F, Hamamichi Y, Miyawaki T et al (1999) Clinical features of isolated noncompaction of the ventricular myocardium. J Am Coll Cardiol 34:233-240

78. Jenni R, Oechslin E, Scheider J, Attenhofer Jost C, Kaufmann P (2001) Echocardiographic

and pathoanatomical characteristics of isolated left ventricula noncompaction: a step towards classification as a distinct cardiomyopathy. Heart 86:666-671

79. Jenni R, Wyss CA, Oechslin EN, Kaufmann PA (2002) Isolated ventricular noncompaction is associated with coronary microcirculatory dysfunction. J Am Coll Cardiol 39:450-454

80. Bleyl SB, Mumford BR, Brown-Harrison MC et al (1997) Xq28-linked noncompaction of the left ventricular myocardium: prenatal diagnosis and pathologic analysis of affected individuals. Am J Med Gent 72:257-265

81. Hook S, Ratliff NB, Rosenkranz E, Sterba R (1996) Isolated noncompaction of the ventricular myocardium. Pediatr Cardiol 17:1733-1734

82. Dusek J, Ostadal B, Duskova M (1975) Postnatal persistence of spongy myocardium with embryonic blood supply. Arch Pathol 99:312-317

83. Hopkins WE, Waggoner AD, Gussak H (1994) Quantitative ultrasonic tissue characterization of myocardium in cyanotic adults with an unrepaired congenital heart defect. Am J Cardiol 74:930-934

84. Akiba T, Becker A (1994) Disease of the left ventricle in pulmonary atresia with intact ventricular septum. The limiting factor for long-lasting successful surgical intervention? J Thorac Cardiovascular Surg 108:1-8

85. Junga G, Kneifel S, Von Smeka A, Steiner H, Bauersfeld U (1999) Myocardial ischaemia in children with isolated ventricular noncompaction. Eur Heart J 20:910-916

86. Daimon Y, Watanabe S, Takeda S, Hijikata Y, Komuro I (2002) Two-layered appearance of noncompaction of the ventricular myocardium on magnetic resonance. Circ J 66:619-621

87. Borges AC, Kivelitz D, Baumann G (2003) Isolated left ventricular non-compaction: cardiomyopathy with homogeneous transmural and heterogeneous segmental perfusion. Heart 89:e21

88. Powell LW, George DK, Mc Donnell SM et al (1998) Diagnosis of hemochromatosis. An Intern Me 129:925-931

89. Olson LJ, Edwards WD, McCall JT, Ilstrup DM, Gersh BJ (1987) Cardiac iron deposition in idiopathic hemochromatosis: Histologic and analytic assessment of 14 hearts from autopsy. J A. Coll Cardiol 10:1239-1243

90. Koren A, Garty I, Antonelli D, Katzuni E (1987) Right ventricular cardiac dysfunction in b-thalassemia major. Am J Dis Child 141:93-96

91. Aessopos A, Stamatelos G, Skoumas V et al (1995) Pulmonary hypertension and right heart failure in patients with b-thalassemia intermedia. Chest 107:50-53

92. Pennel DJ (2002) Ventricular volume and mass by CMR. J Cardiovasc Magn Reson 4:507-513

93. Fujita N, Chazouilleres AF, Hartiala JJ et al (1994) Quantification of mitral regurgitation by velocity encoded cine nuclear magnetic resonance imaging. JACC 23:951-958

94. Kaltwasser J, Werner E (1989) Assessment of iron burden. Bailliere's Clin Hematol 2:195-207

95. Waxman S, Eustace S, Hartnell GG (1994) Myocardial involvement in primary hemochromatosis demonstrated by magnetic resonance imaging. Am Heart J 128:1047-1049

96. Anderson LJ, Holden S, Davis B et al (2001) Cardiovascular T2 star (T2*) magnetic resonance for early diagnosis of myocardial iron overload. EHJ 22:2171-2179

97. Westwood M, Anderson LJ, Firmin DN, Gatehouse PD, Charrier CC, Wonke B, Pennel JD (2003) A single breath-hold multiecho T2* cardiovascular magnetic resonance technique for diagnosis of myocardial overload. J Magn Reson Imaging 18:33-39

98. Aso H, Takeda K, Ito T et al (1998) Assessment of myocardial fibrosis in cardiomyopathic hamsters with gadolinium DPTA-enhanced magnetic resonance imaging. Invest Radiol 32:22-32

99. Friedrich MG, Srom O, Schults-Menger J et al (1998) Contrast-media enhanced magnetic

resonance imaging visualizes myocardial changes in the course of viral myocarditis. Circ 97:1802-1809

100. Rivers J et al (1987) Reversible cardiac dysfunction in hemochromatosis. Am Heart J 113:216-217
101. Mariotti E, Angelucci E, Agostini A et al (1998) Evaluation of cardiac status in iron-loaded thalassemia patients following bone marrow transplantation: improvement in cardiac function during reduction in body iron burden. Br J Haematol 103:916-921
102. Davis BA, Porter JB (2000) Long-term outcome of continuous 24-hour deferoxamine infusion via inwelling intravenous catheters in high risk b-thalassemia. Blood 95:1229-1236
103. Parrillo JE (1990) Heart disease and the eosinophil. N Engl J Med 323:1560-1561
104. Weller PF, Bulbley GJ (1994) The idiopathic hypereosinophilic syndrome. Blood 83:2759-2779
105. Puvaneswary M, Joshua F, Ratnarajah S (2001) Idiopathic hypereosinophilic syndrome: magnetic resonance imaging finding in endomyocardial fibrosis. Australasian Radiology 45:524-527
106. Katritsis D, Wilmshurst PT, Wendon JA et al (1991) Primary restrictive cardiomyopathy: clinical and pathologic characteristics. J Am Coll Cardiol 18:1230-1235
107. Schneider U, Jenni R, Turina J et al (1998) Long term follow up of patients with endomyocardial fibrosis: effects of surgery. Heart 79:362
108. Chil JS, Perloff JK (1988) The restrictive cardiomyopathies. Cardiol Clinics 6:289-316
109. D'Silva SA, Kohli A, Dalvi BV, Kale PA (1992) MRI in right ventricular endomyocardial fibrosis. Am Heart J 123:1390-1392
110. Pitt M, Davies MK, Brady AJ (1996) Hypereosinophilic syndrome: endomyocardial fibrosis. Heart 76:377-378
111. Chandra M, Pettigrew RI, Eley JW, Oshinski JN, Guyton RA (1996) Cine-MRI aided endomyocardetomy in idiopathic hypereosinophilic syndrome. Ann Thorac Surg 62:1856-1858
112. Bishop G, Bergin J, Kramer C (2001) Hypereosinophilic syndrome and restrictive cardiomyopathy due to apical thrombi. Circulation 104:e3-e4

7.4 Valvular disease

MASSIMO LOMBARDI

7.4.1 Introduction

MRI has a marginal role in valvular disease compared to Echocardiography and Doppler, which have demonstrated a very high efficiency, and often substitute cardiac catheterization.

The limited use of MRI in valvular disease must not induce one to believe that the technological aspects of MRI are inadequate for the issues involving these pathologies, rather it must be underlined that today scanners allow a very efficient and refined evaluation of valvular defects.

Visualization of the valves requires only a few minutes and the information on the presence of morphological deformations or functional alterations is substantially equal to that obtainable by Echocardiography. The advantages of MRI over Echocardiography are the possibility of obtaining very good quality images without spatial limitations – except for when there are arrhythmias with a disorganized cardiac rhythm. For example, the planimetric evaluation of a stenotic valve, or the measurement of the dimensions of the valvular ring is a relatively simple procedure and the quality of the images is such to leave few doubts on the feasibility of the measurements [1-4].

7.4.2 Indications for MRI in valve disease

There are indications on the use of MRI in cases of endocarditis in the bicuspid aortic valve, in the inflammatory processes involving mitral vascular leaflets, etc. [4-7] (Figs. 7.53, 7.54); however, there are basically two situations in which MRI offers the best advantages over other methods: the quantification of regurgitation that can accompany some forms of valvular disease and, when required, the evaluation of the origin and coursing of coronaries.

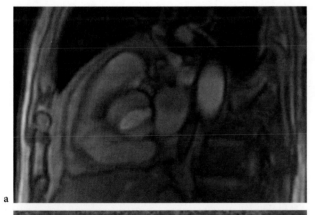

a

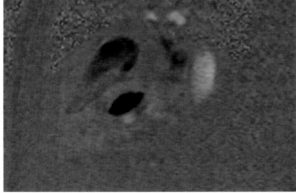

b

Fig. 7.53 a, b. Aortic bicuspid valve. (a) Morphologic image in Fast GRE that evidences the abnormal systolic opening of the bicuspid valve with typical ellipsoidal appearance. (b) The corresponding image in PC for the calculation of valvular flow.

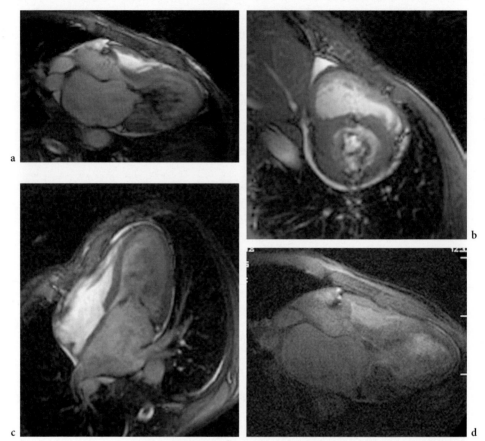

Fig. 7.54 a-d. Bacterial endocarditis on mitral valve. (a) Image in Fast cine-SPGR on the long vertical axis of the heart. The anterior-medial leaflet of the mitral appears thickened at its distal half. The
high turbulence of the transmitral flow can be appreciated as a loss of signal. (b) Image in Fast cine-
SPGR on the short axis of the heart, 1 cm approx below the plane of the mitral valve; the image evidences the irregularity of the valvular leaflets. (c) Image in Fast cine SPGR on the long horizontal
axis of the heart evidencing the thickening of the mitral valve leaflets at their distal parts. (d) Image
in cine SPIRAL GRE that allows a plane spatial resolution of about 0.8 mm; in evidence a thickening of the edge of the anterior-medial mitral leaflets

The quantification of regurgitation can be obtained by means of two different techniques: Fast cine images (SPGR or SSFP) (historically SPGR was
the first to be introduced) and PC images. The first method uses images on
"white blood" where the turbulent flow, as that of reflux, induces a local loss
of signal (loss of phase coherence) that contrasts with the hyperintensity of
the flowing blood (Figs. 7.55, 7.56). The mapping of regurgitant flow visualized
in this manner is performed on parallel slices in order to visualize the entire
turbulence in 3D and provides absolute measurements (in ml per heart beat)
that correlate well with the calculations performed with catheterization. The

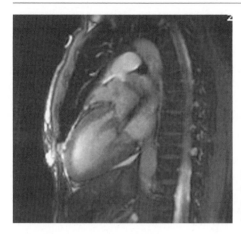

Fig. 7.55. Image in Fast cine SPGR on the long vertical axis of the heart showing the jet of mitral regurgitation that can be appreciated as a loss of signal in the left atrium

simultaneous planimetric measuring of the entire ventricular cavity allows to calculate the regurgitant fraction quite precisely.

Furthermore, phase contrast images represent a very elegant and fast way for evaluating valve disease. This technique provides images in cine Gradient Echo and, simultaneously on the same plane, provides parametric images in which the level of gray is in function of the direction and velocity of flow. Positioning the scanning plane parallel and in proximity (about 1 cm) to the valvular plane, flow can be visualized in its systolic and diastolic phase. The planimetry of the vessel (aorta) or of the valvular plane that is performed on the cine Gradient Echo images allows to measure automatically the ortho-dromic flow and the anti orthodromic fraction in the parametric images (Fig. 7.57) [10-12]. This method of quick execution, which is seemingly easi-er than the precedent, requires good orthogonal alignment to the flow.

The measurements obtained through this technique provide absolute val-ues (ml/beat), with an added value to the exam as compared to other non-invasive imaging techniques.

Likewise, in stenosing pathologies MRI offers the possibility of accurately visualizing the anatomy of the valve and the transvalvular flow. The operator can obtain a mapping of residual volume and the transvavular gradient [13-17]

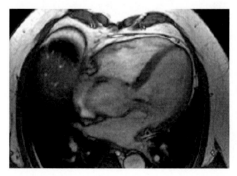

Fig. 7.56. Image in Fast cine FIESTA on the long horizontal axis of the heart showing the aortic valve regurgitation and dilatation of the aortic root

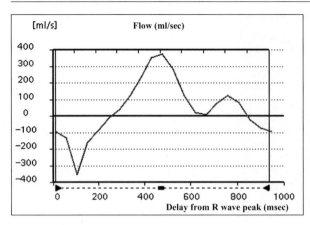

Fig. 7.57. Volume-time curve of transmitral flow obtained by Phase Velocity encoding. The negative values of flow in the systolic phase indicate a mild mitral regurgitation

by combining the morphological images in both SE T1 "black blood" and in cine (for example, SPGR) and applying the simplified equation of Bernoulli as for Echocardiography to valves computed on PC images. In the case of mitral stenosis, movement of the valve is evidenced in a similar way to that in Echocardiography (doming shape of the valve during the diastolic phase, anomalous opening, etc.) (Fig. 7.58).

Moreover, it must be considered that MRI allows a better evaluation of the ventricular function and mass, superior to any other technique, as well as a very detailed visualization of the ascending aorta (see related chapters).

The survey, therefore, should always be completed with the measurements above in order to broaden the study and obtain a more general cardiological picture.

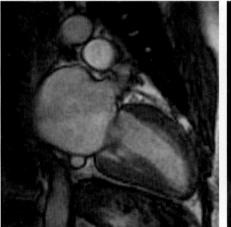
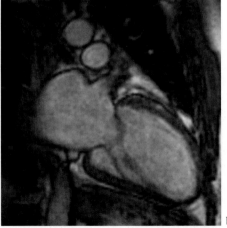

a   b

Fig. 7.58 a, b. Mitral stensosis. Images on the long vertical axis of the heart. (a) End-diastolic image showing thickening of the valvular leaflets. (b) End-diastolic image with reduced opening of the mitral that evidences a "doming" morphology

7.4.3 Study of prosthetic valves

One of the most frequent requests made to operators in MRI cardiovascular labs concerns the safety of submitting patients with prosthetic valves to MRI. It must be underlined that when there is an abundance of metal components, the void signal produced by these components invalidates the possibility of using MRI for their evaluation (Figs. 7.59, 7.60). On the contrary, when the metal components are practically absent (as in stentless biological valves) the MRI exam is similar to that performed on a native valve.

It is extremely rare to encounter patients with valvular prostheses non-compatible to MRI. The last incompatible prostheses (Star-Edwards) were implanted back in the early sixties [18-20].

7.4.4 Current limitations

The current limitations of MRI in the study of valvular diseases are the spatial and temporal resolution below optimal levels, and the need for regular cardiac rhythm. This latter element, as in the case of valve disease that is often associated to atrial fibrillation (such as mitral disease), can determine a significant deterioration of the images. In reality, spatial resolution would not appear to limit the technique too much, since in certain kinds of sequences it yields a resolution on plane <1 mm with a slice thickness of 4-5 mm. Also temporal resolution does not represent a significant limitation in general, except for the study of very fluctuating valves or valves that have a very rapid movement throughout the cardiac cycle.

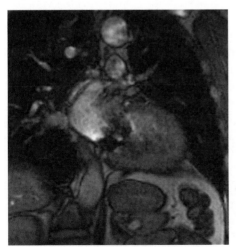

Fig. 7.59. Patient with a biological prosthesis, with a supporting metal structure, in mitral position. Image in Fast cine SPGR evidences a large void of the signal, which does not allow to assess valve function

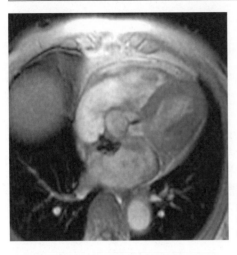

Fig. 7.60. Patient with a metal prosthesis to correct inter atrial patency (umbrella). The presence of the device does not allow to evaluate the eventual residual shunt

7.4.5 Imaging procedure

In practice, there is no standardized procedure for the study of valvular diseases. Some important notions can be, however, acknowledged from data in literature [21].

For a study of the mitral or the tricuspid, the praxis is to acquire images on the long horizontal axis, using 3 to 5 parallel slices so to cover the entire valvular plane.

As for the aortic and pulmonary valves, it is common practice to obtain images parallel to the valvular plane and in planes perpendicular to the latter, proximally and distally.

For all valves, and when phase velocity encoding images are requested, the planes are positioned at about 1 cm from the valve, proximally and distally.

The sequences generally used are the SE T1 "black blood" and Fast cine SPGR. When available, also ultrafast sequences (SSFP) can be used. From the data reported in literature it is evident that when the SPGR sequence is used, the TE must be set as closely as possible at 8 msec so to avoid underestimating the entity of the regurgitation. Sometimes, in order to obtain this result it is necessary to reduce the sampling bandwidth. In the case of phase contrast images it is crucial to set the maximum velocity to be used for phase encoding, compatible with the velocity of the flow under study and be, as much as possible, oriented orthogonal to transvalvular flow.

The diagnostic procedure is considerably advantaged when the study of the valve is flanked by a study of ventricular function, of wall thickness, and of ventricular mass.

For the study of the origin and the coursing of the coronaries, see Paragraph 7.5; noteworthy is the fact that using the 3D techniques available today for imaging of the coronary arteries, this latter part of the study requires only an additional 15 minutes.

References

1. Schwitter J (2000) Valvular heart disease: assessment of valve morphology and quantification using MR. Herz 25:342-355
2. Kizilbash AM, Hundley WG, Willett DL et al (1998) Comparison of quantitative Doppler with magnetic resonance imaging for assessment of the severity of mitral regurgitation. Am J Cardiol 81:792-795
3. Hundley WG, Li HF, Willard JE et al (1995) Magnetic resonance imaging assessment of the severity of mitral regurgitation. Comparison with invasive techniques. Circulation 92:1151-1158
4. Arai AE, Epstein FH, Bove KE, Wolff SD (1999) Visualization of aortic valve leaflets using black blood MRI. J Magn Reson Imaging 10:771-777
5. Pollak Y, Comeau CR, Wolff SD (2002) Staphylococcus aureus endocarditis of the aortic valve diagnosed on MR imaging. Am J Roentgenol 179:1647
6. Reynier C, Garcier J, Legault B et al (2001) Cross-sectional imaging of post endocarditis paravalvular myocardial abscesses of native mitral valves: 4 cases. J Radiol 82(6 Pt 1):665-669
7. Caduff JH, Hernandez RJ, Ludomirsky A (1996) MR visualization of aortic valve vegetations. J Comput Assist Tomogr 20:613-615
8. Suzuki J, Caputo GR, Kondo C, Higgins CB (1990) Cine MR imaging of valvular heart disease: display and imaging parameters affect the size of the signal void caused by valvular regurgitation. Am J Roentgenol 155:723-727
9. Sondergaard L, Lindvig K, Hildebrandt P et al (1993) Quantification of aortic regurgitation by magnetic resonance velocity mapping. Am Heart J 125:1081-1090
10. Fujita N, Chazouilleres AF, Hartiala JJ et al (1994) Quantification of mitral regurgitation by velocity-encoded cine nuclear magnetic resonance imaging. J Am Coll Cardiol 23:951-958
11. Karwatowski SP, Brecker SJ, Yang GZ et al (1995) Mitral valve flow measured with cine MR velocity mapping in patients with ischemic heart disease: comparison with Doppler echocardiography. J Magn Reson Imaging 5:89-92
12. Kozerke S, Schwitter J, Pedersen EM, Boesiger P (2001) Aortic and mitral regurgitation: quantification using moving slice velocity mapping. J Magn Reson Imaging 4:106-112
13. Heidenreich PA, Steffens J, Fujita N et al (1995) Evaluation of mitral stenosis with velocity-encoded cine-magnetic resonance imaging. Am J Cardiol 75:365-369
14. Casolo GC, Zampa V, Rega L et al (1992) Evaluation of mitral stenosis by cine magnetic resonance imaging. Am Heart J 123:1252-1260
15. Sondergaard L, Hildebrandt P, Lindvig K et al (1993) Valve area and cardiac output in aortic stenosis: quantification by magnetic resonance velocity mapping. Am Heart J 126:1156-1164
16. Kilner PJ, Manzara CC, Mohiaddin RH et al (1993) Magnetic resonance jet velocity mapping in mitral and aortic valve stenosis. Circulation 87:1239-1248
17. Sondergaard L, Stahlberg F, Thomsen C et al (1993) Accuracy and precision of MR velocity mapping in measurement of stenotic cross-sectional area, flow rate, and pressure gradient. J Magn Reson Imaging 3:433-437
18. Randall PA, Kohman LJ, Scalzetti EM, Szeverenyi NM, Panicek DM (1988) Magnetic resonance imaging of prosthetic cardiac valves in vitro and in vivo. Am J Cardiol 62:973-976
19. Sievers B, Tintrup K, Franken U, Kickuth R, Trappe HJ (2002) Cardiovascular magnetic resonance of bioprosthetic mitral valve. Heart Vessels 17:86-88
20. Soulen RL, Budinger TF, Higgins CB (1985) Magnetic resonance imaging of prosthetic heart valves. Radiology 154:705-707
21. Arrive L, Najmark D, Albert F et al (1994) Cine MRI of mitral regurgitation in planes angled along the intrinsic cardiac axes. J Comput Assist Tomogr 18:569-575

7.5 Coronary arteries

ALESSANDRO PINGITORE, MASSIMO LOMBARDI, PAOLO MARCHESCHI, PIERO GHEDIN

7.5.1 Introduction

Coronary atherosclerosis is the principal physiopathological substrate of ischemic syndromes, the most frequent cause of natural death and morbidity in western countries. At present, selective coronary angiography is the only validated technique for the direct evaluation of coronaries. It is an invasive technique and requires the use of ionizing radiation and of iodinated contrast agents, which have a significant organ toxicity (especially nephrotoxicity). Although the procedure has low risk for major events, it is still an invasive technique that should be performed only in the case of a motivated clinical suspicion. For these reasons, the screening and evaluation of the patient with coronary disease today is performed with indirect and non-invasive techniques of induction, of myocardial ischemia (treadmill or cycloergometer stress test, stress echo, scintigraphy, stress-MRI, etc.) that allow to evidence alterations of perfusion, of contractile function, or simply the electrocardiographic alterations that belong to the myocardial ischemic cascade. The development of non-invasive angiographic techniques – among which multi-detector Computed Tomography (CT), Electron Beam Tomography (EBT) and MRI – could deeply modify the diagnosis and management of the patient with coronary disease. The multi-detector CT and EBT have the inconvenience of utilizing high doses of radiation and require the administration of a iodinated contrast agent; yet both techniques are rather accurate in quantifying coronary calcium – which is, among other things, a risk factor in the characterization of patients with suspected coronary disease [1]. Indeed, thanks to its most recent developments, multi-detector CT seems to be close to clinical use, although large trials which show the real accuracy of this method in unselected patients are still not available.

7.5.2 Magnetic Resonance of coronaries: angiographic approach

Angiography in the different arterial districts of the body (endocranial vessels, supraortic vessels, aorta, renal aa., arteries of the limbs, etc.) by MRA is becoming a widespread method in clinical practice. The diagnostic capacity of MR is based on the administration of a contrast agent and the acquisition of 3D images (CEMRA) with an excellent SNR. However, the visualization of the coronaries with this technique is difficult and not proposable due to the small dimensions of the structure (less than 5 mm), the contorted and variable coursing, and especially due to the rotational and translational movement caused by cardiac and respiration activity. For this reason, purposely

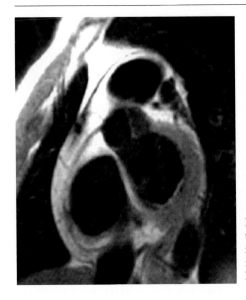

Fig. 7.61. T1 "black blood" image. The visualization of the coursing of the right coronary is facilitated by the contrast produced by perivascular fat, which appears hyperintense in respect to the highly hypointense vascular lumen

designed techniques are being developed for imaging this vascular district and overcoming the related obstacles. The sequences used so far can be classified according to their technical options in "black blood" and "white blood" sequences, two or three dimensional, breath-hold or free breathing, with or without contrast medium [2-8].

"Black blood" techniques completely cancel-out the signal from blood through the application of a double inversion pulse (double inversion recovery), the first of which non-selective at 180°, and the second selective on the scanning plane at 180°. The first pulse inverts the magnetization field throughout the body, blood included. The second re-inverts the magnetization of the tissues on the scanning plane. The final result in the image is the annulment of the signal emitted from blood, whereby the lumen of the vessel is black in contrast to the more or less intense signal of the wall (Fig. 7.61). A presaturation signal (inversion recovery) can be added to the technique to cancel out the signal from adipose tissue (triple IR); otherwise a selective pulse (Fat Sat or CHESS) for fat suppression can be applied so that the cardiac tissue appears enhanced compared to the neighboring fatty tissue. The limit to this approach lies in the fact that it is 2D; consequently in "black blood" imaging several attempts must be made to find a single plane on a long tract of the coronary vessel being studied. Furthermore, "black blood" techniques are prone to artifact due to flow, which can degrade the image significantly.

Images in "white blood" can be obtained by several acquisition techniques (Gradient Echo, echo planar, spiral, etc.) that have the advantage of being faster, with an excellent contrast between the vascular lumen and the sur-

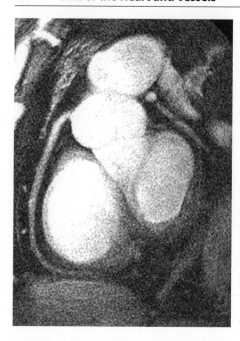

Fig. 7.62. 2D image in Fast GRE with filling of K-space in a spiral manner and fat subtraction. The vessel appears hyperintense and surrounded by hypointense tissue

rounding fat, which can be easily canceled. These techniques collect most favor because of their option of three-dimensional acquisitions, which enables the operator to center the coronary vessel more easily. However, these techniques cannot visualize the arterial wall, but only evidence the lumen (Fig. 7.62).

Breath-held sequences reduce artifacts caused by respiratory movement. The main drawback of these techniques is, however, the necessity of acquiring the entire signal in a very short time: this requires the maximum collaboration on behalf of the patient who has to perform several breath-holdings. Free-breathing sequences are acquired during diastole through the synchronization with ECG, and minimize respiratory movement through the use of a breathing trigger that limits signal acquisition to only one phase of the respiratory cycle (expiratory phase). This acquisition technique is known as Navigator Echo. The substantial difference between Navigator Echo and respiratory synchronization lies in the kind of trigger used. Navigator Echo analyses a real echo signal formed by two successive RF pulses (90° and 180°) generally in the right hemi thorax; these pulses excitate a small volume from which the operator can visualize the position of the right hemi-diaphragm by evidence of the tissue border between liver and pulmonary parenchyma, which are respectively hyper and hypointense. The intrinsic advantage of the technique is that it does not require collaboration on behalf of the patient, who is asked to breath regularly. In addition Navigator Echo allows to monitor, and thus synchronize, the scan with the respiratory cycle the best way

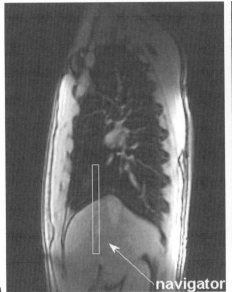
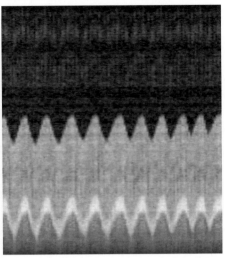

Fig. 7.63 a, b. (a) Tracker for controlling the position of the hemi-diaphragm and detect its cranial-caudal position. (b) Monitoring of the cranial-caudal position of the right hemi-diaphragmatic excursion at the level of the tracker. Once the operator has selected the ideal position (in expiration) and set the spatial limits for the acquisition, the system automatically selects the position in which to acquire the signal. The acquisition is always done in diastole (ECG trigger not shown in figure)

possible, limiting the acquisition to the exact moment in which the diaphragm reaches a preselected position along its cranio-caudal movement. This method can eliminate almost all breathing artifacts (Fig. 7.63a, b).

The most important limits of this method are the long acquisition time (5-10 minutes) and the easier occurrence of artifacts and, thereby, a worse signal noise ratio. The free-breathing navigator technique has been applied to two- and three-dimensional sequences (Fig. 7.64).

The two-dimensional sequences were the first to be introduced in both "black blood" and in "white blood". Their intrinsic limit is determined by the anatomy of the coronary arteries that course on a single plane only for limited extensions – if we exclude the right coronary that can sometimes be visualized entirely from the origin up to the crux. Also the reconstructions derived from these images are full of artifacts.

Compared to 2D sequences, 3D have the advantage of acquiring a volume of significant thickness (2-15 cm) that includes the area in which the vessels course, which eliminates the problem of anatomical variability of these vessels. In recent years, research has been developing exclusively 3D sequences, but at the moment there is no technique excelling above others, as each presents limits that reduce its diagnostic efficacy.

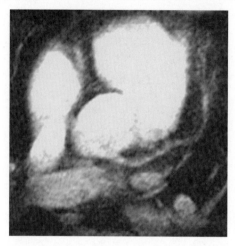

Fig. 7.64. 3D image of the left coronary obtained with the navigator technique in free breathing

7.5.3 How to improve SNR and CNR

Contrast medium greatly improves the SNR and CNR, providing a better definition of the coronaries from the surrounding tissues (Fig. 7.65). At present, clinical practice employs gadolinium-based contrast agents that remain confined inside the capillary bed for an extremely short time. The contrast medium transiently reduces the T1 of blood from 1200 msec to less than 100 msec. Ongoing studies are testing the use of contrast agents that have specific char-

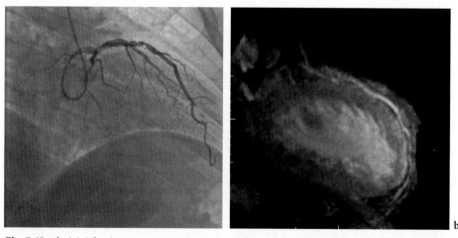

a   b

Fig. 7.65 a, b. (a) Selective coronary angiography of the anterior descending artery that evidences a stenosis at the beginning of the medium third. (b) 3D FIESTA image in breath-hold (acquisition time 20 sec) after the administration of a contrast medium (GdDTPA-BMA, gadiodamide, 0,1 mol/kg) that evidences the stenosis of the coronary lumen at the same level

acteristics that constrain them inside the vasculature (blood pool), remarkably improving the SNR.

SNR and CNR can also be improved by using sequences capable of amplifying the differences in signal due to the relaxation characteristics of tissues. This can be achieved by applying, for example, preparation pulses that suppress the signal from surrounding tissues. One of the suggested preparation pulses consists of a preparation prepulse (T2 prep), which cancels out tissues with a low relaxation time, such as the cardiac muscle (T2=50 msec), venous haematic flow (T2 with saturation of O2 at 20%=3 msec) and adipose tissue, while the signal from arterial blood (T2=250 msec) is not modified [9].

7.5.4 Feasibility of coronary angiography by MR

The feasibility of coronary angiography by MRI varies according to the coronary and to the arterial segments considered, being higher for the Left Main (LM) and for the proximal segments of the Left Anterior Descending a. (LAD) (respectively, 95-100% and 80-90%), the Right Coronary a. (RC) (90-95%), the Circumflex Coronary a. (CX) (60-75%), as compared to the distal segments of these arteries and of the secondary branching (in total 40-60%) (Fig. 7.66). Consequently, the diagnostic accuracy is good for the proximal and medium segments, while it cannot be evaluated for distal segments and secondary branching. Conversely, there are no substantial differences of diagnostic accuracy among the various sequences tested, which have evident limits of temporal and spatial resolution; in the best of cases acquisition time is 100 msec per heartbeat, and the voxel is approximately 1 mm³. Recent multicenter data (3D free-breathing) of comparison between invasive angiography and MRA have evidenced an 84% feasibility for 7 coronary segments (LM and proximal and middle segments of LAD and RC and proximal segment of CX) with the identification of 83% of the significant stenoses [10].

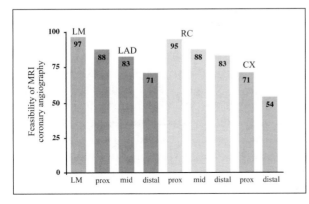

Fig. 7.66. Feasibility of coronary angiography utilizing 2D spiral FGRE (personal data on 54 patients). LM=Left Main; LAD= Left Anterior Descending Artery; RC=Right Coronary Artery, CX= Circumflex Coronary Artery; Prox=proximal segment; middle=middle segment; distal=distal segment

7.5.5 Study of the coronary wall by MRI

Atherosclerosis is a degenerating process of the arterial wall that is characterized by fatty deposits within the wall at first, and by composite plaques in its final stage [11].

In clinical practice, the identification of a stenosis is performed by invasive angiography, which in reality is no more than a luminogram, unable to lead to a histological characterization of the atherosclerotic plaque or to visualize the arterial wall, and to evidence any initial injuries within that same wall. Ultrasounds and MRI can visualize the wall directly and are therefore able to identify its alterations. The thickening of the intima and media is an accurate marker of sub-clinical atherosclerosis and is predictive of ischemic events, either in the brain or in the heart [12]. In post mortem studies, the study of coronary vessels has evidenced that vessel remodeling depends on a number of factors – such as the entity of flow, endothelial reactivity, etc. – and that it can develop outward from the vessel lumen (which thus appears patent or even dilated) and lead to the development of the plaque [13]. If an important cause of a chronic ischemic event is the severity of the atherosclerotic plaque, the precipitating factor of an acute ischemic event is the rupture of a vulnerable plaque [14]. The vulnerability of the plaque is not strictly linked to the severity of the stenosis, but rather to the components of the plaque itself [15]. The cellular and structural characteristics of a vulnerable plaque are: the abundance of inflammatory cells, a wide lipidic core, and a thinned fibrous cap. The fissuring of the cap activates a local thrombolytic process (at the level of the plaque), which in turn determines a rapid growth of the plaque that becomes clinically evident with an acute ischemic syndrome. Another destabilizing factor is neoangiogenesis inside the plaque [16].

At the level of the carotid, MRI has demonstrated to be a good method for visualizing early atherosclerotic injuries corresponding to lesions of type I and type II (collection of foam cells and fatty streaks), and type III (preatherome with extra cellular lipid collection) according to the classification by the American Heart Association [17, 18].

Tissue characterization by MRI is based on characteristics of relaxation and of proton density (PD) of the single components of the plaque [13, 19-22]. In T_1-weighted SE images, tissues with a short T_1 have a hyperintense signal as compared to those with a long T_1. Vice versa, tissues with a short T_2 appear hypointense as compared to those with a long T_2. The signal intensity in PD depends on the tissue density of the protons, therefore in the images in PD the tissues richer of protons have a hyperintense signal, while calcifications have a low concentration of protons and appear hypointense. The lipid plaques have both a short T_1 and a short T_2, therefore they are hyperintense in T_1-weighted images and hypointense in T_2, while in Fast SE

T2 fat is hyperintense. Fibrous plaques have a quite similar signal intensity in T1- and T2-weighted images; the signal intensity is lower compared to lipidic plaques in T1-weighted images. The areas of hemorrhage have a signal that is variable in time, in function of the metabolic state: deoxy-hemoglobin > met-hemoglobin > hemosiderin. An important fibrosis will thus determine a highly hypointense border between the lumen and the atherome [24-26].

The studies on tissue characterization of the plaque have been mostly performed on carotid plaques because of the easy access to these vessels (Fig. 7.67). The characterization of the walls and of the coronary plaques is made difficult by the same factors that make difficult its angiographic visualization. It has been proposed to use a Spin Echo T2-weighted sequence with double presaturation stimulus to visualize the coronary wall, which resulted to be on average 1mm thick with a lumen surface of 9.3 mm² in the control subjects. In patients with known coronary disease, the thickness of the coronary is significantly greater (on average 1.5 mm) and the surface of the lumen is significantly less (7.0 mm² on average) [27]. These data confirm why atherosclerosis is a degeneration of the vessel wall that affects the entire vessel, and not only at the site of the plaque, which only appears to be the point of maximum development of the degenerative process. Hence, the study of the wall, and not the luminogram alone, represents a complementary path for performing a study of atherosclerosis that can characterize initial atherosclerotic lesions, as well as artery vessel remodeling (silent at conventional angiography), and for identifying the atherosclerotic plaques, which are unstable and at high risk of rupture.

7.5.6 Study of coronary reserve

The coronary reserve expresses the vasodilatation capacity of coronary vasculature in response to cardiac metabolic demand. Thanks to this mechanism of auto-regulation, coronary flow can increase up to 5 times the baseline value. In presence of a coronary stenosis, the vasodilatatory reserve guarantees an adequate blood flow at basal conditions and when faced with a limited increase of the cardiac energetic demand. This limit progressively diminishes with the growing severity of the stenosis, and thus with the reduction of the lumen until the complete exhaustion of the coronary reserve.

The relation between flow and coronary stenosis is not linear at baseline conditions nor during maximum vasodilatation. Coronary flow decreases only in the presence of a stenosis over 85%, while the coronary reserve begins to decrease – even if slightly – in presence of a stenosis of about 35-40%. This reduction becomes evident in the presence of stenoses of over 70%, and when the stenosis is over 90% the reserve goes down to zero [28]. In consideration

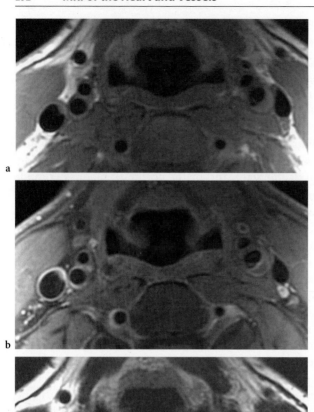

a

b

c

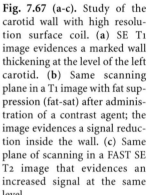

Fig. 7.67 (a-c). Study of the carotid wall with high resolution surface coil. (a) SE T1 image evidences a marked wall thickening at the level of the left carotid. (b) Same scanning plane in a T1 image with fat suppression (fat-sat) after administration of a contrast agent; the image evidences a signal reduction inside the wall. (c) Same plane of scanning in a FAST SE T2 image that evidences an increased signal at the same level

of the scarce correlation between flow and coronary stenosis, in particular for moderate injuries, the physiological meaning of a coronary stenosis has important clinical implications [29, 30]. As for the other districts, it is possible to measure coronary flow using a Phase Contrast sequence (see Chapter 3) (Fig. 7.68). The values of coronary reserve as measured by PC images (ratio of flow in maximum vasodilatation obtained with adenosine over baseline flow) closely correlate with the severity of the stenosis and with the coronary reserve evaluated invasively. Considering a limit value for coronary reserve of 1,7, the sensitivity and specificity for the diagnosis of coronary stenoses >70% are respectively 100 and 83% [31]. The same sequence can be applied to the diagnosis of restenosis in presence of a coronary stent.

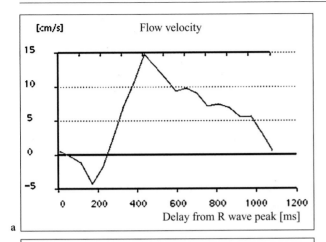

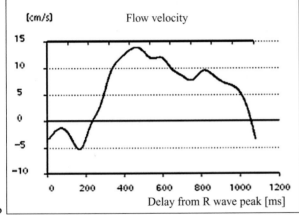

Fig. 7.68 a, b. (a) Measure of the velocity of blood flow at the level of the proximal anterior descending coronary artery by Phase Encoding Velocity technique. **(b)** Measurement at the level of the proximal right coronary artery

7.5.7 Scanning planes for coronaries (in 2D or 3D small slab)

7.5.7.1 Right coronary artery

Basically there are two approaches. Starting from an image on the horizontal long axis of the heart, in which the atrio-ventricular groove is visible, a plane is traced parallel to interventricular septum. The image obtained is an oblique coronal where the right coronary is visible in its short axis both cranially and over the diaphragm. The scanning planes useful for viewing the entire coronary pass through these two sections of the vessel. If the coronary is lying on a single plane, as often happens, the vessel is visualized from its origin to the origin of the posterior descending a. at the level of the crux.

In an alternative approach the scanning planes are positioned directly over the image on the long horizontal axis of the heart, parallel to the atrio-ventricular groove.

7.5.7.2 Left main (LM) and left anterior descending artery (LAD)

Starting from the sagittal scout passing through the aortic root, a number of images are obtained in coronal. Such planes must be positioned recalling that on a sagittal plane the origin of the left coronary a. is posterior and high above the profile of the aorta. Once the LM has been identified, para-axial planes are positioned between the inferior margin of the pulmonary trunk and the superior profile of the cardiac silhouette. From the para-axial images obtained it is possible to view the LM, and the LAD from the origin up to the middle and sometimes the distal tract. The circumflex a. is visible in particular in the proximal half. From this projection it is possible to trace another scanning plane parallel to the coursing of the LAD (Fig. 7.65).

7.5.7.3 Circumflex artery (CX)

Adopting as scout an image on the coronal plane with evidence of the aortic root and of the left main, trace a para-axial plane inclined downwards in antero-posterior orientation that intersects the aortic root perpendicularly and passes through the origin of the LM.

7.5.8 Bypass and STENT

The application either of SE or GRE sequences, and especially CEMRA, allows an accurate evaluation of the morphology of both arterial and venous grafts (Fig. 7.69). The main limit of the sequence employed so far is the difficulty in evaluating the region of conjunction between the bypass and the native coronary vessel in constant movement with the heart, which induces an unavoidable loss of phase coherence during the acquisition time (15-20 seconds). However, with this approach it has been demonstrated that it is possible to visualize 98% of bypasses and give their accurate description with an 88% specificity [33].

The measurement of blood flow by means of the Phase Contrast sequence can provide further information on the hemodynamic effect of a stenosis of the graft. Such information, as in the case of native coronaries, is perhaps more important than visualizing its anatomy. With this method, the flow through the venous bypasses appears biphasic with a preponderant diastolic component. The systolic flow can be explained by the high compliance of the venous duct that is much higher than that of the native coronary and which influences the flow particularly in the proximal tract of the venous bypass. Conversely, in the distal tract flow is stalled by the high coronary resistances [34]. The flow in the bypasses can also be measured after adenosine for the evaluation of the flow reserve calculated as the ratio of flow after adenosine

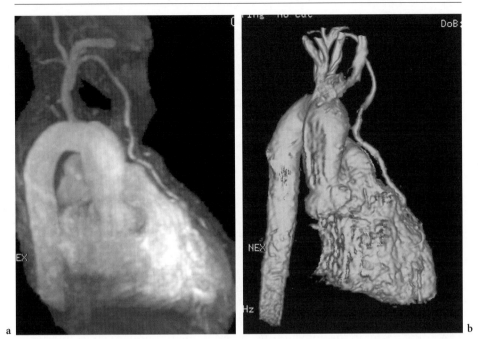

Fig. 7.69 a, b. (a) 3D CEMRA Image of bypass (left internal mammary-left anterior descending artery). The image allows to appreciate the alterations in by pass profile at proximal and distal levels. (b) Same image after volume rendering postprocessing

over baseline flow. Once the bypass has been visualized, the scanning plane of the contrast sequence is positioned perpendicularly to the proximal tract of the graft. The flow reserves diminish significantly in the stenotic bypass (1.8±0.9) compared to the patent bypass (2.5±0.7) [35]. Other hemodynamic parameters that can be evaluated are systolic and diastolic velocity, the velocity reserve that is the ratio between the max velocities measured after adenosine and at the baseline. These parameters have been evaluated for the study of the functionality of arterial and venous bypasses, resulting accurate for the identification of significant stenoses [36]. These hemodynamic parameters can also be calculated for the evaluation of intra stent restenosis. The scanning plane is positioned in this case 5 mm distally to the stent. The measurement of flow occurs downstream from the area of stent implantation so to avoid artifacts produced by the stent, which make these measurements impracticable. In these patients, coronary reserve has been demonstrated to be 3±0.6 in presence of stenoses <50%, and 1.1±0.3 when the stenosis is >70%. Considering a threshold value of coronary reserve of 2.0, sensitivity and specificity for the diagnosis of stenosis are respectively 100 and 89% [32]. The measurement of the coronary flow in revascularized vessels has the advantage of being a non-invasive solution, of not using contrast medium, and of being reproducible over time. Considering the reserve of velocity expressed as the ratio of max velocities after adenosine respect to baseline, reserve velocity is much lower in the presence of an intra stent restenosis >75% (1.10±0.22) than in absence of restenosis (1.78±0.16) or of stenoses below 75% (1.46±0.22) [37]. Recently a study has demonstrated the safety of MRI in 111 patients within the first 8 weeks following the implantation of the stent [38].

7.5.9 Anomalies in the coursing of coronaries

The anomalies in the coursing of the coronaries concern the origin and the proximal tract of the main coronary arteries and have an incidence of 0.3-0.8% within the population studied. Generally, the origin of the right coronary a. occurs in the right aortic sinus while, the origin of the left coronary occurs in the left aortic sinus. The circumflex artery rarely originates from the right aortic sinus directly. The coursing of the proximal tract of abnormal coronaries, either right or left, can be posterior, anterior (Fig. 7.70) septal or inter-arterial. In the posterior coursing the coronary passes posterior to the ascending aorta; in the anterior one, it wraps the pulmonary cone anteriorly; in the septal or sub-pulmonary it courses in the interventricular sulcus; in the inter-arterial one, it courses between the aorta and the pulmonary artery. Among these types of coursing, the inter-arterial coursing is the most dangerous (Fig. 7.71) because it is associated to myocardial infarction and sudden death. The anatomical relation between coronary, aorta, and pulmonary trunk is hence fundamental for the prognostic impact. MRI has a good feasibility in

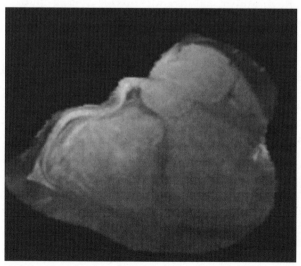

Fig. 7.70. 3D FIESTA image in breath-hold after administration of contrast medium (Gd-DTPA-BMA 0.1 mmol/kg). Anterior position origin of the right coronary in a patient with bicuspid aortic valve

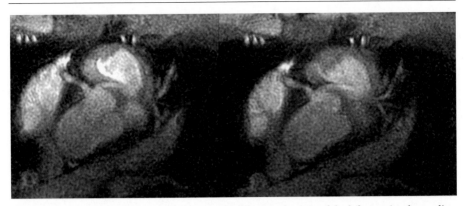

Fig. 7.71. Images obtained by 2D spiral FAST GRE. Abnormal origin of the left anterior descending coronary artery of the right valvular sinus, close to the origin of the right coronary. The vessel then courses between the pulmonary artery and the aorta

the evaluation of the proximal tract of the coronary arteries and, importantly, visualizes directly the relationships between the great vessels (aorta and pulmonary trunk, and the main branching of the pulmonary aorta) and the Left Main and the proximal segment of the main coronary branching.

7.5.10 Conclusions

The combined evaluation of dimensions, morphology, biochemical composition, and functional value of the atherosclerotic plaque makes MRI a potentially complete technique for the study of coronary atherosclerosis, which can provide additional information as compared to conventional angiography. The non-invasiveness of the method also allows serial evaluations and thus longitudinal studies on the evolution of atherosclerosis in vivo, from the initial phases of wall thickening until the formation of the plaque. However, a further development of technology and clinical trials is necessary before this non-invasive approach can be proposed as a routine diagnostic tool.

References

1. O'Rourke RA, Brundage BH, Froelicher VF et al (2000) American College of Cardiology/ American Heart Association Expert Consensus Document on Electron-beam computed tomography for the diagnosis and prognosis of coronary artery disease: Committee Members Circulation 102:126-140
2. Manning WJ, Edelmann RR (1993) A preliminary report comparing magnetic resonance angiography with conventional angiography. N Engl J Med 328:828-832

3. van Geuns RJ, de Bruin HG, Rensing BJ et al (1999) Magnetic resonance imaging of the coronary arteries: clinical results from three dimensional evaluation of a respiratory gated technique. Heart 82:515-519

4. Hundley WG, Clarke GD, Landau C et al (1995) Noninvasive determination of infarct artery patency by cine magnetic resonance angiography. Circulation 91:1347-1353

5. Regenfus M, Ropers D, Achenbach S, Kessler W, Laub G, Daniel WG, Moshage W (2000) Noninvasive detection of coronary artery stenosis using contrast-enhanced three-dimensional breath-hold magnetic resonance coronary angiography. J Am Coll Cardiol 36:44-50

6. Oshinski JN, Mukundan S, Dixon WT, Parks DJ, Pettigrew RI (1996) Two-dimensional coronary MR angiography without breath holding. Radiology 201:737-743

7. Post JC, van Rossum AC, Hofman MB, de Cock CO, Valk J, Visser CA (1997) Clinical utility of two-dimensional magnetic resonance angiography in detecting coronary artery disease. Eur Heart J 18:426-433

8. Sardanelli F, Molinari G, Zandrino F, Balbi M (2000) Three-dimensional, navigator-echo MR coronary angiography in detecting stenoses of the major epicardial vessels, with conventional coronary angiography as the standard of reference. Radiology 214:649-650

9. Botnar RM, Stuber M, Danias PG, Kissinger KV, Manning WJ (1999) Improved coronary artery definition with T2-weighted, free-breathing, three-dimensional coronary MRA. Circulation 99:3139-3148

10. Kim WY, Danias PG, Stuber M et al (2001) Coronary magnetic resonance angiography for the detection of coronary artery disease. N Engl J Med 345:1863-1869

11. Libby P (2001) The vascular biology of atherosclerosis. In: Braunwald, Zipes, Libby (eds) Heart Disease, pp. 995-1009

12. Furberg CD, Byington RP, Riley W (1995) B-mode ultrasound: a noninvasive method for assessing atherosclerosis. Cardiovascular Medicine. In: Willerson JT, Cohn JN (eds). New York, NY: Churchill Livingstone, pp. 1182-1187

13. Ward MR, Pasterkamp G, Yeung AC, Borst C (2000) Arterial remodeling: mechanisms and clinical implications. Circulation 102:1186–1191

14. Langfield M, Gray-Weale AC, Lusby RJ et al (1989) The role of plaque morphology and diameter reduction in the development of new symptoms in asymptomatic carotid arteries. J Vasc Surg 9:548-557

15. Falk E (1992) Why do plaque rupture? Circulation 86 (Suppl III): III-30-III42

16. McCarthy MJ, Loftus IM, Thompson MM et al (1999) Angiogenesis and the atherosclerotic carotid plaque: an association between symptomatology and plaque morphology. J Vasc Surg 30:261-268

17. Cai JM, Hatsukami TS, Ferguson MS, Small R, Polissar NL, Yuan C (2002) Classification of human carotid atherosclerosis lesions with in vivo multicontrast magnetic resonance imaging. Circulation 106:1368-1373

18. Pohost GM, Fuisz AR (1998) From the microscope to the clinic: MR assessment of atherosclerotic plaque. Circulation 98:1477-1478

19. Choundhury RP, Fuster V, Badimon JJ, Fisher EA, Fayad ZA (2002) MRI and characterization of atherosclerotic plaque: emerging applications and molecular imaging. Arterioscler Thromb Vasc Biol 22:1065-1074

20. Fayad ZA, Fuster V, Fallon JT, Jayasundera T, Worthley SG, Helft G, Aguinaldo G, Badimon JJ, Harma SK (2000) Noninvasive in vivo human coronary artery lumen and wall imaging using black-blood magnetic resonance imaging. Circulation 102:506-510

21. Shinnar M, Fallon JT, Wehrli S, Levin M, Dalmacy D, Fayad ZA, Badimon JJ, Harrington M, Harrington E, Fuster V (1997) The diagnostic accuracy of ex vivo MRI for human atherosclerotic plaque characterization. Arterioscler Thromb Vasc Biol 17:542-546

22. Toussaint JF, LaMuraglia GM, Southern JF, Fuster V, Kantor HL (1996) Magnetic resonance

images lipid, fibrous, calcified, hemorrhagic, and thrombotic components of human atherosclerosis in vivo. Circulation 94:932-938

23. Hatsukami TS, Ross R, Polissar NL et al (2000) Visualization of fibrous cap thickness and rupture in human atherosclerotic carotid plaque in vivo with high resolution magnetic resonance imaging. Circulation 102:959-964

24. Yuan C, Mitsumori LM, Ferguson MS, Polissar NL, Echelard D, Ortiz G, Small R, Davies JW, WS Kerwin, Hatsukami TS (2001) In vivo accuracy of multispectral magnetic resonance imaging for identifying lipid-rich necrotic cores and intraplaque hemorrhage in advanced human carotid plaques. Circulation 104:2051-2056

25. Corti R, Osende JI, Fayad ZA, Fallon JT, MD, Fuster V, Mizsei G, Dickstein E, Drayer B, Badimon JJ (2002) In vivo noninvasive detection and age definition of arterial thrombus by MRI. J Am Coll Cardiol 39:1366-1373

26. Yuan C, Kerwin WS, Ferguson MS, Polissar N, Zhang S, Cai J, Hatsukami TS (2002) Contrast-enhanced high resolution MRI for atherosclerotic carotid artery tissue characterization. J Magn Reson Imaging 15:62-67

27. Botnar RM, Stuber M, Kissinger KV, Kim WY, Spuentrup E, Manning WJ (2000) Noninvasive coronary vessel wall and plaque imaging with magnetic resonance imaging. Circulation 102:2582-2587

28. Gould KL, Lipscomb L (1974) Effects of coronary stenoses on coronary flow reserve and resistence. Am J Cardiol 34:50

29. Ferrari M, Schnell B, Werner GS, Figulla HR (1999) Safety of deferring angioplasty in patients with normal coronary flow velocity reserve. J Am Coll Cardiol 33:82-87

30. Kern MJ, de Bruyne B, Pijls NH (1997) From research to clinical practice: current role of intracoronary physiologically based decision making in the cardiac catheterization laboratory. J Am Coll Cardiol 30:613-620

31. Hundley WG, Lange RA, Clarke GD (1996) Assessment of coronary arterial flow and flow reserve with magnetic resonance imaging. Circulation 93:896-902

32. Hundley WG, Hillis D, Hamilton CA, Applegate RJ, Herrington DM, Clarke GD, Braden GA, Thomas MS, Lange RA, Peshock RM, Link KM (2000) Assessment of coronary arterial restenosis with phase contrast magnetic resonance imaging measurements of coronary flow reserve. Circulation 101:2375-2381

33. Galjee MA, van Rossum AC, Doesburg T, van Eenige MJ, Visser CA (1996) Value of magnetic resonance imaging in assessing patency and function of coronary artery bypass grafts: an angiographically controlled study. Circulation 93:660-666

34. Bedaux WLF, Hofman MBM, Vyt SLA, Bronwaer JGF, Visser CA, van Rossum AC (2002). Assessment of coronary artery bypass graft disease using cardiovascular magnetic resonance determination of flow reserve. J Am Coll Cardiol 40:1848-1855

35. Langerak SE, Vliegen HW, Jukema W, Kunz P, Zwinderman AH, Lamb HJ, van der Wall EE, de Roos A (2003) Value of magnetic resonance imaging for the noninvasive detection of stenosis in coronary artery bypass grafts and recipient coronary arteries. Circulation 107: 1502-1508

36. Nagel E, Thout T, Klein C, Schalla S, Bornstedt A, Schnackenburg B, Hug J, Wellnhofer E, Fleck E (2003) Noninvasive determination of coronary blood flow velocity with cardiovascular magnetic resonance in patients after stent deployment. Circulation 107:1738-1743

37. Gerber TC, Fasseas P, Lennon RJ, Valeti VU, Wood CP, Breen JF, Berger PB (2003) Clinical safety of magnetic resonance imaging early after coronary artery stent placement. J Am Coll Cardiol 42:1295-1298

38. Paetsch I, Huber ME, Bornstedt A et al (2003) Reliable detection of coronary stenoses with contrast enhanced, 3D free breathing coronary MR angiography using a gadolinium based intravascular contrast agent. Circulation 108, IV, 488

7.6 Tumors and masses of the heart and of the pericardium

Virna Zampa, Massimo Lombardi

7.6.1 Introduction

Primitive tumors of the heart and of the pericardium are very rare. Of these, approximately 75% are benign and 25% are malignant. Tumors of the myocardium occur more often than pericardial ones. Table 7.6 reports the most common benign and malignant tumors in descendant order of frequency.

The most common benign tumor among adults is the mixoma, while rhabdomyoma is the most common among children (40%), and rhabdomyoma and theratoma are the most common in infants.

The most common malignant tumors in adults and rarest in children are represented by angiosarcomas (33%), by rhabdomiosarcomas (24%), by mesotheliomias (15%), and by fibro sarcomas (10%).

The introduction of MRI in the study of the cardio-vascular apparatus has notably modified the diagnostic strategy of the para or intra-cardiac masses.

This technique provides a complete multiplanar and non-invasive evaluation of the lesions involving the cardiac chambers, pericardium and extra cardiac structures, assuming a relevant role in providing diagnostic information useful for surgical planning. The details to be assessed are: morphology, dimensions, location, extension, topographic relation, presence of infiltration in the surrounding tissues, and signal characteristics that can contribute to histopathological characterization (presence of adipose tissue, necrosis, hemorrhage, calcification, mixoid tissue, vascularization, etc.).

In reality, the histopathological characterization of lesions is rarely possible except for the lipomatose forms (subtraction or suppression of fat). Often the diagnosis is based upon indirect and probabilistic findings that address the diagnosis towards a kind of tumor rather than another.

Table 7.6. The most common tumors of the heart and of the pericardium

Benign tumors	Malignant tumors
Myxoma	Angiosarcoma
Lipoma	Rhabdomyosarcoma
Papillary fibroelastoma	Mesothelioma
Rhabdomyoma	Fibrosarcoma
Fibroma	Lymphoma
Hemangioma	Extraskeletal osteosarcoma
Theratoma	Neurogenic sarcoma
Mesothelioma of the AV node	Malignant theratoma

Table 7.7. Characteristics of the MRI signal from different tissues in the T₁- and T₂-weighted images

Tissue	T₁	T₂	Contrast agent
Liquid	Low (—-)	High (+++)	absent
Myxoid	Low (—-)	High (+++)	scarce
Collagen	Low (—)	Low/High (—/++) *	scarce*
Adipose	High (+++)	High (++)	absent
Necrosis	Low (—)	High (+++)	absent
Fibrous	Low (—)	Low/High (—/++) *	scarce*
Calcium	Low (—-)	Low (—-)	absent
Vascularized	Low (—)	High (++)	marked

* The type of signal and the capture depends on the vascularization and the cellularity of such tissues

A correct characterization of the cardiac and paracardiac mass requires integrated information that is obtainable with the different MRI sequences available. In other words, to characterize a cardiac or para-cardiac mass it is necessary to obtain images in T₁, T₂, IR (STIR) or, T₁ and T₂ with spectral suppression of the fat, in GRE T₂* (for eventual calcifications or hemorrhages inside the mass), and in T₁ after contrast medium (0.1 mmol/kg). Furthermore, it is suggested to obtain images for the study of the movement of the wall involved (cine SPGR, SSFP, etc.). Often a study of the dynamic impregnation of the contrast medium is performed utilizing GRE T₁-weighted sequences (very short TR and TE).

Such studies are generally quite lengthy and at times bring the physician very close to the nature of the malignancy. Table 7.7 reports the characteristics of the signal of the various tissue components useful for a diagnostic orientation.

7.6.2 Benign atrial tumors

The benign lesions most frequently affecting the atrial chambers are the myxoma and the lipoma.

The **myxoma** originates from the endocardium as a polipoid mass that is generally peduncolated (90%), but may also present a large base of implantation and smooth or, more rarely, villous surfaces [1].

The most typical site is the atria (left atrium 75%, right atrium 18%, right ventricle 4%, left ventricle 3%).

A typical location of the myxoma of the left atrium is the interatrial septum at the level of the fossa ovalis; the pedunculus allows the tumoral mass

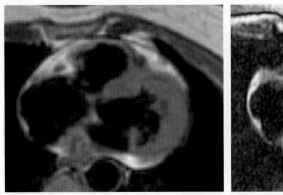
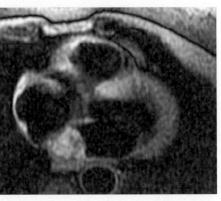

a   b

Fig. 7.72 a, b. (a) A SE T1 image showing a myxoma in the left atrium, which typically generates from the interatrial septum. (b) An FSE-IR image showing the slightly hyperintense lesion in which hypointense areas due to fibrous and calcified components can be evidenced

to move freely in the atrial chamber and sometimes to protrude into the left ventricle, in the diastolic phase, through the mitral valve.

Clinically, it can be asymptomatic or mimic a mitral stenosis. When the site of origin is not typical, the differential diagnosis with masses of other nature is more difficult.

Typically, the myxoma presents an in-homogeneous signal due to the presence of fibrous, necrotic, hemorrhagic, and sometimes calcified tissue inside (Fig. 7.72a, b). In the context of mass tumors, there are inevitably findings of hemorrhagic areas (81% of cases), of thrombosis, or areas containing catabolites of hemoglobin (e.g. hemosiderin), all responsible for the heterogeneous signal [2]. If the quantity of myxoid tissue is abundant, the lesion will have an elevated signal in the T2-weighted images (Fig. 7.73), whereas if the fibrous component prevails the mass will show a hypointense signal.

The presence of calcification is a common finding (56%) and is more frequent in the myxomas of the right atrium. Calcium is responsible for the areas of low signal [3] in the context of the lesion, which is more noticeable in GRE T2* images. The drop of signal may also be caused by the effects of magnetic susceptibility, correlated to the presence of iron [4]. On the other hand, the hemorrhagic areas exhibit an elevated indicator in both T1 and T2 sequences [5].

It is proven that the enhancement of the tumor is correlated to its histology and that the zones which do not capture a signal correspond to necrosis or cystic areas. [6]

The differential diagnosis includes thrombotic masses (Fig. 7.74) and other less common lesions, such as the cardiac sarcomas and the papillary fibroelastoma. The thrombi of the left atrium are notably less frequent than the myxomas and frequently associated to an enlargement of the chambers.

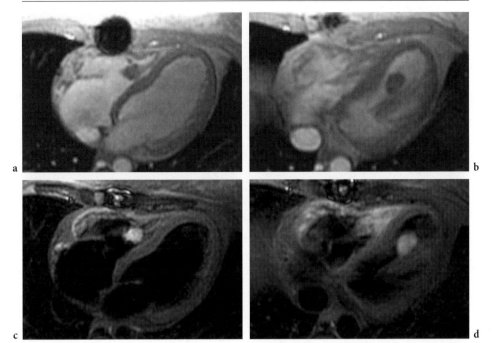

a   b

c   d

Fig. 7.73 a-d. Intraventricular myxomas in a patient already subjected to a previous intervention of exeresis of a myxomatose mass inside the left atrium. (**a, b**) Cine-MR images evidencing two hypointense ventricular myxomas. (**c, d**) IR images in which the structures appear markedly hyperintense due to the myxomatose components. (Note the artifact caused by the presence of ferromagnetic material at level of the sternum)

These usually originate from the posterior and lateral atrial wall or from the auricola and are associated to atrial fibrillation and mitral valvular disease. The thrombi of the left ventricle, common in patients with ventricular dysfunctions secondary to anterior infarction of the myocardium or to dilatative cardiomyopathy, develop in the regions where the intracavity haematic flow is slower (Fig. 7.74) and where myxomas are rarely encountered.

MRI images without contrast agent generally do not help in differentiating the myxoma from the thrombus, because both can present heterogeneity of the signal in SE images and low intensity in the GRE sequences [7]. The administration of a contrast determines an enhancement of the signal of the myxoma, while thrombotic formation usually does not show modifications (Fig. 7.75) [8] except in rare cases of thrombotic formations that have become vascularized.

Sarcomas usually invade the pericardium and adjacent structures and can give mediastinal metastasis [9]. The papillary fibroelastoma usually interests the mitral or aortic valves and is generally of smaller dimensions [10].

The **lipoma** is a relatively rare cardiac tumor (14% of benign tumors); it

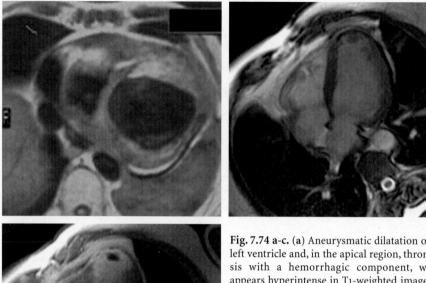

a

b

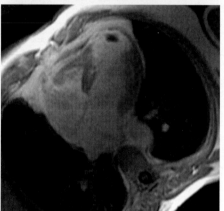

c

Fig. 7.74 a–c. (a) Aneurysmatic dilatation of the left ventricle and, in the apical region, thrombosis with a hemorrhagic component, which appears hyperintense in T1-weighted images. In b and c another case of intra-ventricular thrombus in a patient with previous myocardial infarction. In the image obtained with ultrafast cine sequence (FIESTA) **(b)** the thrombotic material appears iso-intense to the myocardium but well in contrast with the high signal of the intracavity blood flow. **(c)** In the IR-GRE sequence, after administration of the contrast medium, the mass appears markedly hypointense while the region of necrotic myocardium appears hypeintense

can have the shape of the properly said lipoma (Fig. 7.76a) (encapsulated or surrounded by myocardium) and of lipomatosis of the interatrial septum (Fig. 7.76b). The latter consists of non-capsulated adipose tissue, which extends into the epicardial fat. Half of the cardiac lipomas are subendocardial, the other half have a subepicardial and mesocardial location [11]. The left atrium and ventricle are the most frequent locations.

The lesion presents the characteristics of the MRI signal typical of the adipose tissue: elevated intensity of the signal in the T1- and T2-weighted images. The techniques of fat suppression easily demonstrate the adipose nature of the tissue.

The **papillary fibroelastoma** is made up of fibrous tissue, smooth elastic fiber and muscular cells. The structure is usually small, circular and adherent to the atrium-ventricular or semi lunar valves. In literature there are no descriptions on the behavior of the MRI signal for this lesion, and the diagnosis is generally based on Echocardiography.

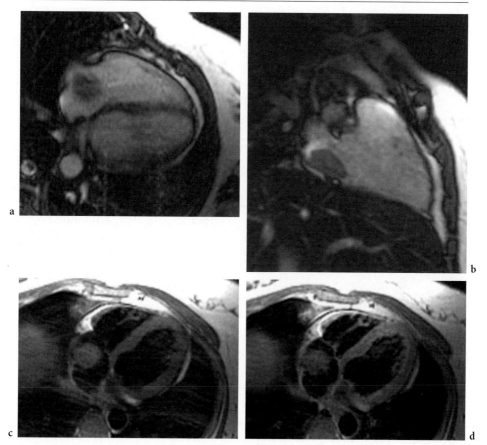

Fig. 7.75 a-d. (a, b) Thrombus of the right atrium, well evidenced in ultrafast (FIESTA) images, surrounded by the hyperintense flow signal. In T1 images, before (c) and after (d) administration of contrast medium, there is no significant enhancement of the signal within the thrombotic material. This is a highly specific finding for differential diagnosis

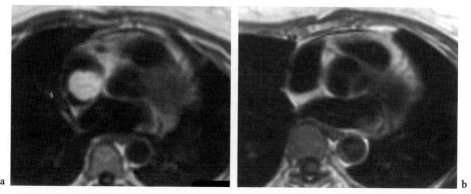

Fig. 7.76 a, b. Lipoma of the right atrium (a) and lipomatosis of the interatrial septum (b). Despite the morphological differences, both lesions are characterized by a hyperintense signal in T1-weighted images, which is typical of the fatty tissue

7.6.3 Benign ventricular tumors

The primitive tumors of the ventricle are very rare in adults. The most frequent tumors of the left ventricle are the fibroma and the rhabdomyoma, which are more common in the pediatric years.

The **rhabdomyoma**, frequent in children, first appears as multiple nodules within the cardiac cavity, which protrude into the cavity or at an intramural location.

The **fibroma** is the most frequent benign tumor of the left ventricle of the adult. It is usually intramural and it appears as an area of irregular hypertrophy of the septum, of the apex, or of the free wall and displays a hypointense signal in the T2 sequence. After administration of a contrast medium, the morphology appears as formed by a hypointense core surrounded by an iso intense "shell" [12] (Fig. 7.77).

Myxomas, fibromas, and rhabdomyomas can be found in the right ventricle.

7.6.4 Malignant tumors

The malignant tumors of the heart are less frequent (25%) than the benign ones and more frequent in the right sections than in the left. Autoptic studies report an incidence of 0.001-0.28% [13]. Primitive malignant tumors of the heart are extremely rare and constitute a diagnostic dilemma, as they are asymptomatic until they reach significant dimensions and, even in these cases, the symptoms are usually aspecific. The introduction of sophisticated imaging techniques has introduced the possibility of detecting such lesions in patients before being compromised and, sometimes as a casual finding, contributing to the characterization of the lesions and to the choice of the therapeutical strategy.

The angiosarcoma is the most frequent (37%) of the malignant tumors of the heart [1]. It originates from endothelial cells, most frequently in the right atrium, with involvement of the pericardium, and with a frequent complica-

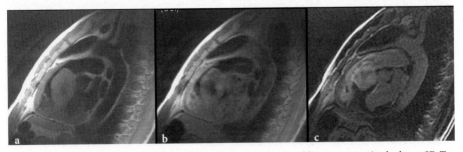

Fig. 7.77 a-c. Fibroma of interventricular septum. Images in oblique parasagittal plane. SE T1-weighted images before (**a**) and after contrast administration (**b**). In (**c**) image obtained by IR-GRE sequence after contrast administration

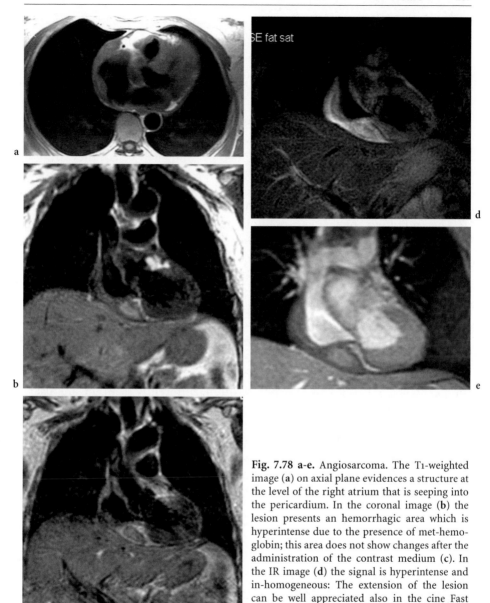

Fig. 7.78 a-e. Angiosarcoma. The T1-weighted image (a) on axial plane evidences a structure at the level of the right atrium that is seeping into the pericardium. In the coronal image (b) the lesion presents an hemorrhagic area which is hyperintense due to the presence of met-hemoglobin; this area does not show changes after the administration of the contrast medium (c). In the IR image (d) the signal is hyperintense and in-homogeneous: The extension of the lesion can be well appreciated also in the cine Fast SPGR image (e)

tion caused by pericardial effusion – often of haematic origin. Despite the invasion of this structure, discovering tumor cells in the pericardial liquid is not always immediate.

Two forms of angiosarcoma are described in literature: a well-defined mass protruding into atrial cavity with preservation of the septum, or an infiltrating mass extended along the pericardium (Fig. 7.78). The presence of hemorrhage and necrosis is frequent and responsible for the heterogeneous signal typical of this lesion, which usually presents areas of elevated intensity in the T1-weighted sequences because of the presence of methemoglobin in relation to the hemorrhagic phenomena (Fig. 7.78b). In the cases of pericardial infiltration, contrast agent uptake is characterized by a linear morphology around vascular structures.

Non-differentiated sarcomas (0-24% of all the malignant tumors) [1] are malignant lesions that are named according to their histological characteristics (pleiomorphic sarcoma, with rounded or elongated cells); they are not properly typical, and are negative to multiple markers in immuno-histochemical tests. The prognosis is generally unfavorable. In a recent study, 81% of sarcomas originate in the left atrium.

The pathology appears as a polipoid mass, isointense to the myocardium in MR images, with thickening of the myocardium in the site of infiltration or with an aspect similar to the angiosarcoma with pericardial infiltration.

The rhabdomyosarcoma (4-7%) is a tumor that originates from the muscular striated fibers. Two forms are distinguished: embryonal neoplasia that appears in infancy, in children and young adults, and the sarcoma of the adult, which is very rare in the heart. Despite the low incidence, this neoplasm represents the most frequent form of malignant cardiac tumor in childhood. It can show up anywhere in the myocardium, and more frequently than other sarcomas it involves the valvular systems (Fig. 7.79). These tumors are often multicentric and can involve the pericardium. Differently from the angiosarcoma, the myocardium is always involved and the pericardium often presents nodular masses, rather than laminar ones.

The characteristics of the MR signal are variable (isointensity to the myocardium, hyperintensity in T2 relative to cystic-like or necrotic areas).

Osteosarcomas (3-9%) are a heterogeneous group of tumors containing malignant cells that produce bone and sometimes fibrous or cartilaginous tissue.

Differently from the metastatic osteosarcoma that often starts off in the right atrium, the primitive cardiac osteosarcoma most often involves the left

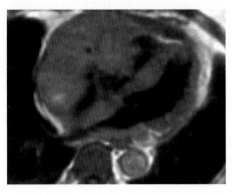

Fig. 7.79. Rhabdomyosarcoma. Large malignant neoplasia involving the right section of the heart with evident infiltration into the myocardial wall, the valve system and the pericardium. The infiltrating feature and the size confirm the aggressive nature of the lesion

atrium. It is aggressive, and has a dramatic prognosis. The demonstration of a bony component can be appreciated more simply through CT images.

The leiomyosarcoma (8-9%) originates from the bundles of smooth muscle cells that delimit the subendocardial space. It can also originate from the cells of the arteries and pulmonary veins and spread to the cardiac structures. It has a predisposition for the left atrium and in particular at the level of the posterior wall. The patients are typically in their fourth decade, slightly younger as compared to age groups affected by other sarcomas.

As in other cases, MRI features are aspecific: lobulated masses, irregular, and multiple in 30% of cases with a tendency to invade the pulmonary veins or the mitral valve, showing an intermediate signal in T1 and a high one in T2.

The fibrosarcoma (5%) is a rare tumor that, as other sarcomas, prefers the left atrium. It can show an infiltrative pattern into the pericardium by direct invasion or by nodules, which primarily affect the visceral pericardium; it can also form directly from the pericardium with aspects that recall the mesothelioma: it can appear heterogeneous in MR images.

The liposarcoma is an extremely rare tumor that contains lipoblasts and tends to originate in the atria, although it has also been described in the ventricles and in the pericardium. It can involve the pericardium with a nodular aspect or cause pericardial effusion. Differently from the benign lipoma, the adipose component in the primitive liposarcoma of the heart is scarce or absent.

The primitive cardiac lymphoma is a tumor prevalently constrained to the heart and to the pericardium. The diagnosis is based on findings of the pericardial liquid, although a biopsy is usually necessary. Despite the rare occurrence of the tumor, it is important to include this tumor in the differential diagnostic of cardiac masses, since early chemio-therapic treatment can give excellent results [14]. The most frequently affected site is the right atrium; the pericardial effusion is often present and abundant. Compared to other malignant tumors, necrosis in this tumor is less frequent as well as the involvement of the cardiac chambers and the valvular structures. It can appear as a polipoid mass or as an infiltrating mass with undefined borders. The MRI signal is hypointense in T1 and hyperintense in T2, but has also been reported as iso-intense respect to the myocardium; the enhancement pattern is variable (homogeneous, in-homogeneous, mild) (Fig. 7.80).

7.6.5 Para-cardiac masses

MRI is very efficient in documenting the extra cardiac extension of primitive tumors of the heart, providing the information needed to establish the most appropriate surgical approach. Likewise, it demonstrates the engagement on behalf of the extra-cardiac masses with excellent anatomical detail. Therefore, when there is the suspicion of a secondary involvement of the

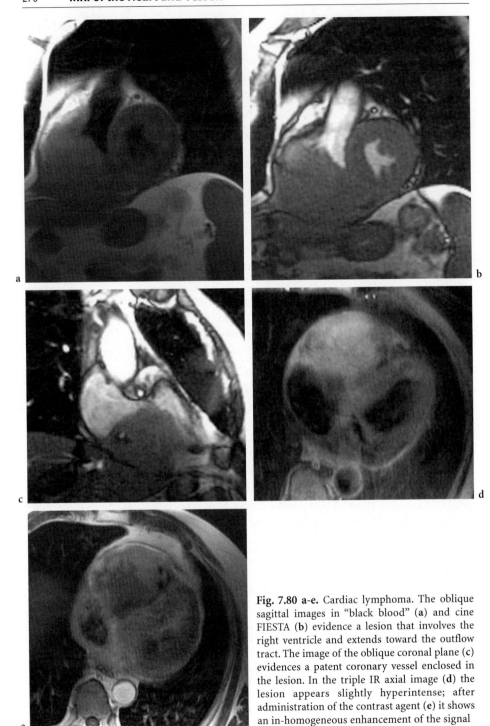

Fig. 7.80 a-e. Cardiac lymphoma. The oblique sagittal images in "black blood" (**a**) and cine FIESTA (**b**) evidence a lesion that involves the right ventricle and extends toward the outflow tract. The image of the oblique coronal plane (**c**) evidences a patent coronary vessel enclosed in the lesion. In the triple IR axial image (**d**) the lesion appears slightly hyperintense; after administration of the contrast agent (**e**) it shows an in-homogeneous enhancement of the signal

heart, the physician generally requests an MRI study. Moreover, the metastases of the heart and of the pericardium are much more common than primitive tumors; the tumors that more often affect the heart and pericardium are the lung carcinoma, the mammary gland carcinoma, melanoma, lymphoma, and leukemia. The metastases appear as a pulmonary or mediastinal mass that directly invades the heart, or like masses that protrude into the left atrium through the pulmonary veins, or under the form of pericardial nodules and/or as myocardial nodules (Fig. 7.81). The high MRI contrast resolution distinguishes the tumor from the myocardium, and the tumor or thrombus from flow artifacts much more easily than other techniques, and in some cases even helps in tissue characterization. To give an example, one may consider the metastases from a melanoma that present a hyperintense signal in T1 due to the metal-bound melanin with a paramagnetic effect [15].

7.6.6 Pitfall

Several anatomical structures can mimic a cardiac mass; to avoid falling into an erroneous diagnosis it is necessary to be aware of the site, dimensions, form and motility of these normal findings (pseudo-masses).

The moderating band of the right ventricle crosses the ventricular cavity; it originates from the septum-marginal trabecula and courses obliquely all the way to the base of the anterior papillary muscle. It may be erroneously interpreted as a thrombus, mural mass or hypertrophy of the interventricular septum.

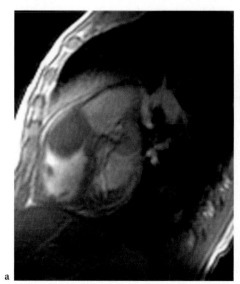

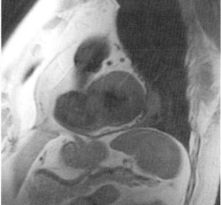

a   b

→

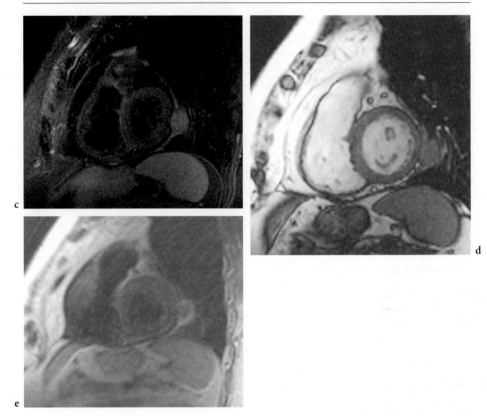

Fig. 7.81 a-e. (a) Metastasis in the right ventricle outflow tract, originated from a mammary tumor. The neoplastic lesion is well contrasted by the hyperintensity of the flow in the cine-SPGR sequence; the expansion of the lesion and its relation to the pericardium are also well evident. Pericardial metastasis caused by tumor of the lung in images T1 (b), triple IR (c) and cine-FIESTA (d). The images evidence the pericardial involvement of the lesion with no infiltration into the myocardium. The image, after administration of contrast medium (e) evidences enhancement of the signal in the peripheral layer of the neoplastic mass

The Eustachian valve of the right atrium is a clinical feature found in adults, and is a residue of the embryonic right sinus venosus; this is visible at the junction between the inferior vena cava and the posterior atrial wall. The Chiari's net is found in the right atrium in approximately 2-3% of healthy subjects and may be erroneously interpreted as a thrombus, tumor, vegetation of the tricuspid valve or rupture of the cordae tendineae.

References

1. Burke A, Virmani R (1996) Tumors of the heart and great vessels. Atlas of tumor pathology. 3rd series, fasc 16. Washington, DC: Armed Forces Institute of Pathology

2. Grebenc ML, Rosado-de-Christenson ML, Green CE, Burke AP, Galvin JR (2002) Cardiac myxoma: imaging features in 83 patients. Radiographics 22(3):673-689
3. Burke AP, Virmani R (1993) Cardiac myxoma: a clinicopathologic study. Am J Clin Pathol 100:671-680
4. Seelos KC, Caputo GR, Carrol CL, Hricak H, Higgins CB (1992) Cine gradient refocused echo (GRE) imaging of intravascular masses: differentiation between tumor and nontumor thrombus. J Comput Assist Tomogr 16:169-175
5. Masui T, Takahashi M, Miura K, Naito M, Tawarahara K (1995) Cardiac myxoma: identification of intratumoral hemorrhage and calcification on MR images. AJR Am J Roentgenol 164:850-852
6. Matsuoka H, Hamada M, Honda T e al (1996) Morphologic and histologic characterization of cardiac myxomas by magnetic resonance imaging. Angiology 47:693-698
7. Gomes AS, Lois JF, Child JS, Brown K, Batra P (1987) Cardiac tumors and thrombus: evaluation with MR imaging. AJR Am J Roentgenol 149:895-899
8. Funari M, Fujuta N, Peck WW, Higgins CB (1991) Cardiac tumors: assessment with Gd-DTPA enhanced MR imaging. J Comput Assist Tomogr 15:953-958
9. Araoz PA, Eklund HE, Welch TJ, Breen JF (1999) CT and MR imaging of primary cardiac malignancies. RadioGraphics 19:1421-1434
10. Edwards FH, Hale D, Cohen A et al (1991) Primary cardiac valve tumors. Ann Thorac Surg 52:1127-1131
11. Puvaneswary M, Edwards JRM, Bastian BC, Khatri SK (2000) Pericardial lipoma: US, CT and MRI findings. Australas Radiology 44:321-324
12. Kiaffas MG, Powell AJ, Geva T (2002) Magnetic resonance imaging evaluation of cardiac tumor characteristics in infants and children. Am J Cardiol 89(10):1229-1233
13. McCallister HA, Jr (1979) Primary tumors of the heart and pericardium. Curr Probl Cardiol 4:1-51
14. Ceresoli FL, Ferrei AJM, Bucci E e al (1997) Primary cardiac lymphoma in immunocompetent patients: diagnostic and therapeutic management. Cancer 80:1497-1506
15. Chiles C, Woodard PK, Gutierriez R, Link KM (2001) Metastatic involvement of the heart and pericardium: CT and MR imaging. Radiographics 21:439-449

7.7 Congenital heart disease

PIERLUIGI FESTA

7.7.1 Introduction

In recent years MRI has become a powerful diagnostic tool for the study of congenital heart disease thanks to technological advances that have created extremely Fast MRI machines yielding images with a large Field Of View (FOV) and a high resolution on any plane of space. Improvement of therapy has increased life expectancy for patients with congenital heart disease, and thus the population of individuals, who now benefit from this non-ionizing and non-invasive diagnostic technique throughout long term follow-ups, is steadily increasing.

Hence, with no doubt MRI represents an indispensable diagnostic presidium for those centers dedicated to the treatment and follow-up of patients with congenital heart disease.

7.7.2 Techniques

The study of pediatric patients generally requires a high spatial resolution hence the operator must employ a surface coil appropriate for the patient's weight. In addition, the dimensions of the FOV must be optimized, the slice thickness has to be reduced, and the matrixes employed have to allow a high spatial resolution. Often these changes in the scanner setting are counterproductive in terms of a reduction of SNR, but the obstacle can be overcome by modulating other parameters, such as the number of excitations (NEX), which however prolongs the acquisition time. The high heart rate, which is typical in children, can compensate in part this temporal limit. However, this elevated frequency requires a high temporal resolution in the cine techniques (Fast SPGR, SSFP). The TR is thereby very short and it is important to optimize the filling of K-space for each patient so as to obtain a better quality of the image. Therefore, as it appears obvious from this premise, the good outcome of the exam is based on the exasperation of the very principles that allow to achieve an optimal compromise between spatial and temporal resolution, acquisition time, and SNR.

7.7.2.1 Intra and extra cardiac anatomy

The sequences usually used for the morphological study of the heart are breath-hold (10-15 seconds) Fast SE ("black blood") synchronized with the ECG; these sequences yield images with high spatial resolution (less than 1 mm) and with good contrast between tissues. Moreover, they are relatively less affected by the presence of artificial material used in many biomedical devices in use today (e.g. metallic stitches, valvular prosthesis, stents, spirals, etc.).

The morphological study also relies on cine images (Fast SPGR and SSFP, etc.) in "bright blood" and breath-hold (12-25 seconds). Over the last few years these sequences have greatly improved in terms of spatial resolution. The latter sequences are extremely useful for studying defects of septation, postsurgery intracardiac tunnels, transvalvular flows with turbulence secondary to regurgitation or stenosis, the outflow of both ventricles, the arterial-venous conducts, and lastly for studying vessel dynamics.

In the study of vessels, MRA with 3D CEMRA (see Chapter 2) covers an important role for providing anatomical and topographic 3D information. In case of 3D CEMRA, it is recommended to perform two or three sequential acquisitions: an early phase to delimit the pulmonary arteries and a second phase to picture the systemic circulation and if necessary, a third phase to visualise the venous vessels. However, as in younger patients the differentiation and of single phases is not always possible due to the high velocity of circulation, and the beginning of acquisition needs to be optimized with a preventive bolus test or using an interactive method such as fluoro triggering, etc. [1].

The postprocessing phase covers a fundamental importance and should be performed by trained personnel with specific experience in this field [2].

7.7.2.2 Ventricular function

The techniques and sequences used for the evaluation of the ventricles are substantially the same as those used for the study of non-congenital cardiac diseases in adults. The sequences usually employed are in cine, properly optimized to body size and heart rate.

The main differences from the exams performed on adults concern slice thickness and the scanning planes: in children, thickness is kept under 5-6 mm and the planes must be adapted to a highly variable heart morphology.

The right ventricle can be studied extensively by MRI and is particularly suitable in patients affected by congenital heart disease [3]. As the ventricle occupies a retrosternal position and has a complex geometry, transthoracic Echocardiography generally yields sub-optimal results. Yet, there is a close correlation between results obtained with 3D Echocardiography and MRI [4]. In some cases (e.g. patients with single ventricle pre and postFontan) tagging can provide detailed information on function and regional deformation, in addition to that provided by the traditional cine techniques [5].

7.7.2.3 Flow analysis

Phase Contrast imaging is an accurate and reproducible technique for the analysis and quantification of blood flows. The employment of Phase Contrast sequence (PC) allows to acquire important information on the physiopathology of the congenital heart disease under study. Indeed, it is widely used for the measurement of the systemic and pulmonary outputs and thus the calculation of the shunt (QP/QS) (Fig. 7.82) [6, 7]. PC is also applied in the differential calculation of left and right pulmonary flows, of the systemic veins and of other vessels. In addition, it is appreciated for providing an accurate quantification of the regurgitation volume through the cardiac valves.

7.7.3 Cardiac MRI exam in congenital heart disease

7.7.3.1 Preparation of the pediatric patient

To obtain the best control of breathing and movements, it is very important for the operator to motivate the young patient in order to obtain a good collaboration. The presence of a parent or a relative in the magnet room can make the patient feel more comfortable, and thus should be encouraged. Cases of true claustrophobia are extremely rare among children.

Generally surface coils that can cover the entire chest are employed. However, in the case of patients under 10 kg, a skull coil may be used in place of specific low body-weight coils when the proper instrument is not available within the lab facilities. Patients younger than 6-8 years of age are generally

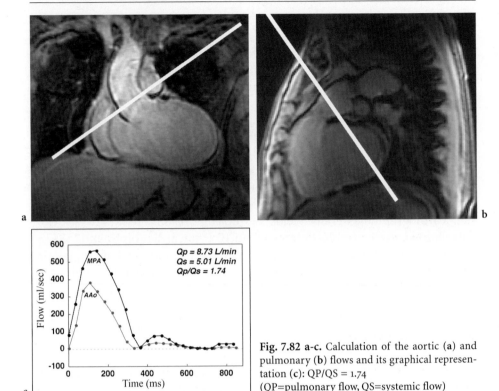

Fig. 7.82 a-c. Calculation of the aortic (a) and pulmonary (b) flows and its graphical representation (c): QP/QS = 1.74 (QP=pulmonary flow, QS=systemic flow)

sedated during the MRI study. The age limit for undergoing an MRI exam awake is not fixed and depends on the patient's ability to collaborate and on the length of the study. The sedation of newborns or small infants weighing less than 7 kg can be performed by means of chloral hydrate per os, or ketamine i.v. (under one year of age). For all other patients, i.v. propofol is a valid option. In patients who are hemodynamically unstable, the method of choice is endo-tracheal tubing with the patient under anesthesia, so that the operator can achieve a higher control over the airways and a better quality of the exam: in fact, although the method requires a greater organizing effort and specialized personnel, it allows extended periods of controlled apnea, which avoids artifacts arising from respiratory motion.

7.7.3.2 General principles

The study of complex cardiac disease requires the acquisition of scout images on the three planes (sagittal, coronal, axial) so that the heart and any extra cardiac structure of interest can be identified; however, in many cases it may be particularly useful to associate this procedure to a free-breathing TOF 2D localizer, along with an adequate number of axial images that cover the entire mediastinum as a reference for future acquisitions.

The MRI exams for complex heart disease obviously change based on the anatomical and pathological characteristics of the disease and on the surgical corrections previously performed.

7.7.4 Extracardial defects of the mediastinal vessels

MRI is advantaged in the study of abnormalities of mediastinal vessels by the wide FOV that allows to locate all the structures inside the mediastinum itself, airways included.

Historically the study of aortic coarctation was the first clinical application of MRI in pediatric cardiology back in the eighties.

7.7.4.1 Aortic coarctation (AoCo)

In most cases aortic coarctation is a stenosis located in the proximal region of the descending aorta, close to the ductus arteriosus or the arterial ligament. AoCo can be treated surgically or with a percutaneous intervention with dilatation and, eventually, implantation of stents based on the age and anatomical characteristics of the patient.

The queries to which a MRI study of a AoCo must respond are: anatomy and diameter of the aortic arc and the isthmus and origin of the supraortic trunks; characterization and localization of the stenosis; and calculation of the aortic flow at different levels up to the diaphragm to evaluate the entity of the collateral vasculature [9]. By employing the PC images to measure the maximum velocity of flow (v) the operator can calculate the pressure gradient (ΔP) at the level of the stenosis, applying the modified Bernoulli's law ($\Delta P=4V^2$) in a similar manner as with Echo-Doppler. However, it must be remembered that PC can be inaccurate in evaluating highly turbulent flow as in the case of isthmic stenosis of the aorta; moreover, the equation above cannot be applied indistinctively to all cases of accelerated flow, independent on the degree and location of the stenosis [10].

In the follow-up of the AoCo treated by surgery (Fig. 7.83a) or by angioplasty, MRI is extremely useful for excluding residual defects or complications such as aneurysms (Fig. 7.83b).

MRI strategy
- Localizer on three planes and eventually using a 2D axial TOF free-breathing for the assessment of the entire aorta on the short axis (Fig. 7.84).
- Study of the bi-ventricular function and of the bi-ventricular myocardial mass according to the procedures described in Paragraphs 7.1 and 7.2.

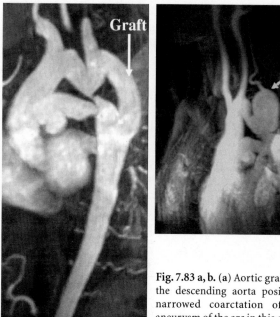

Fig. 7.83 a, b. (a) Aortic graft joining the arc and the descending aorta positioned to correct a narrowed coarctation of an isthmus; (b) aneurysm of the arc in this case complicating the surgical repair

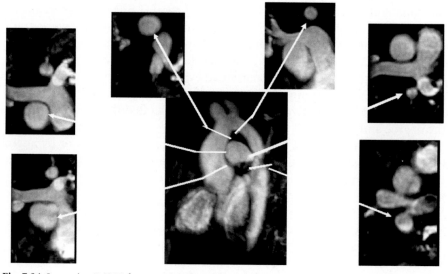

Fig. 7.84. Image in 2D TOF for assessing the caliber of the aorta

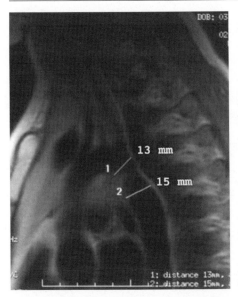

Fig. 7.85. Image in FSE "black blood" for the study of aortic coarctation

- Images in Fast SE on the oblique sagittal plane for the anatomic characterization of the arc and the coarctation (Fig. 7.85). It must be noted that quite often the curving of the arc is distorted and may sometimes interfere with the visualization of the entire arc on a single plane; this is overcome by making a number of oblique acquisitions.
- Images in cine (Fast SPGR and SSFP, etc.) in oblique sagittal projection for visualizing the turbulent flows secondary to obstructions or distortions of the arc or the isthmus and for assessing the prescription of the images in PC used to measure the velocity and flow of the aorta at different levels.
- MRA with injection of contrast medium (CEMRA) for a 3D view of the vessels in its entire extension (Figs. 7.86, 7.87).

7.7.4.2 Vascular rings. Abnormalities of the pulmonary arteries and of the aortic arc

Certain anomalies of the aortic arc and of the pulmonary arteries may cause vascular rings (Fig. 7.88a). When the ring is incomplete, it is commonly referred to as a sling. Several vascular structures, especially the pulmonary ones, can determine vascular slings (Fig. 7.88b). In the case of a significant compression of the trachea (and of the esophagus) respiratory distress can ensue and eventually even lead to dysphagia. This condition is often asymptomatic and discovered by chance [10].

These anomalies can be isolated or associated to other congenital heart defects. Sometimes it is possible to encounter the dilatation of one or both

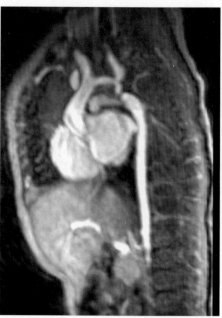

Fig. 7.86. MRA of the aorta. Rare example of the coarctation of the arc

Fig. 7.87. MRA of isthmic coarctation associated to hypoplasia in an infant of 3 months of age

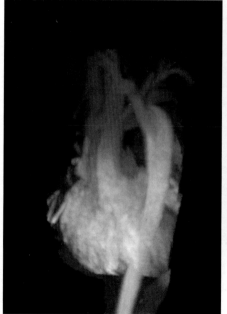

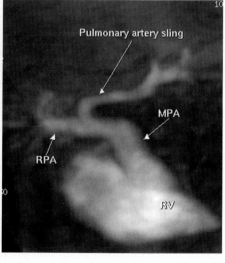

Fig. 7.88 a, b. (a) Double aortic arc. **(b)** Pulmonary artery sling: the left pulmonary artery origins more distally and courses around the trachea. MPA=Main Pulmonary Artery; RPA=Right Pulmonary Artery; RV=Right Ventricle

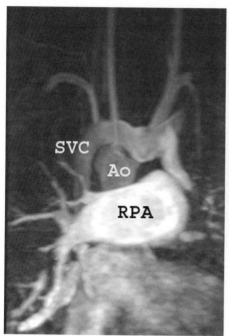

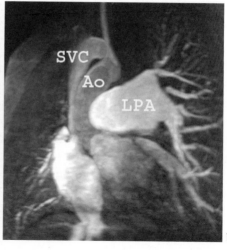

Fig. 7.89 a, b. Large aneurysm of the right (a) and left (b) pulmonary artery reconstructed by MIP postprocessing. RPA= Right Pulmonary Artery; SVC=Superior Vena Cava; AO=Aorta; LPA=Left Pulmonary Artery

pulmonary arteries. Generally these situations are asymptomatic and found while performing an Echo-Doppler or a chest X-Ray. In few cases, aneurysms of the pulmonary arteries have also been described (Fig. 7.89).

MRI strategy
- Localizer on three planes accompanied by an axial 2D TOF free-breathing (as for AoCo).
- Contiguous images on axial planes in Fast SE at the level of the tracheal-bronchial tree and of vessels of the mediastinum.
- Images in cine (Fast SPGR, SSFP, etc.) in oblique projection in the case vascular obstructions are suspected.
- CEMRA for 3D visualization of vessels.

7.7.4.3 Anomalous Pulmonary Venous Return (APVR)

Whenever there is a total anomalous pulmonary return (in the systemic vein or directly in the right atrium) from both lungs, the condition is severe and is generally diagnosed in the very first weeks of life. Conversely, when the anomalous pulmonary return is partial, the condition behaves, from a physiopathological point of view, as an Interatrial Defect (IAD) with left-right shunt and is hardly symptomatic during the first years of life.

7.7.4.3.1 Total Anomalous Pulmonary Venous Return (TAPVR)

There are several types of TAPVR: supra cardiac, intra-cardiac, sub-cardiac or mixed. If all the drainage of the pulmonary veins has been clearly investigated by Echo-Doppler, surgical correction is suggested without any further investigations. Invasive angiography may be required in case of doubt; otherwise a MRI study may complete the picture with additional useful information, also in the case of newborns or very small infants.

7.7.4.3.2 Partial Anomalous Pulmonary Venous Return (PAPVR)

As for the total anomalous venous return, in this case there are also several types of PAPVR.

1. *IAD simulating the sinus venosus + anomalous pulmonary venous return to the Superior Vena Cava (SVC)* (the most frequent PAPVR). A defect in the septum that separates the SVC from the superior right pulmonary vein. Although this vein preserves a normal localization (normal connection), it drains into the left atrium (anomalous drainage) because of the communication with the SVC at the level of the SVC right atrium connection [12] (Fig. 7.90).
2. *Superior pulmonary vein into SVC without IAD and sinus venosus.* In this case the right superior pulmonary vein drains directly into the SVC, but at a slightly higher point compared to the previous case.
3. *Right pulmonary vein into right atrium.* All the right pulmonary veins drain in the right atrium. The number of the pulmonary veins varies, most often from two to three. This condition is often associated with an IAD (Fig. 7.91).

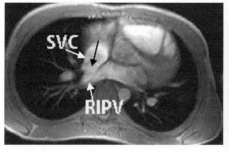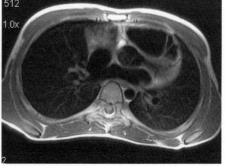

Fig. 7.90 a, b. IAD of the sinus-venous type in a SPGR image (**a**) and FSE (**b**); the black arrow points to the incomplete septum that divides the pulmonary veins from the root of the superior vena cava. SVC=Superior Vena Cava; RIPV=Right Inferior Pulmonary Vein

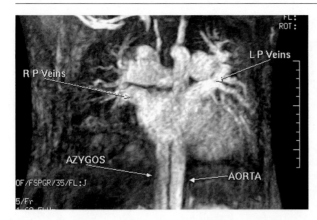

Fig. 7.91. Anomalous right pulmonary vein return into the right atrium (MIP of MRA). LP=Left Pulmonary; RP=Right Pulmonary

4. *Anomalous return of the right Pulmonary vein into the Inferior Vena Cava (IVC) (scimitar syndrome).* The entire pulmonary venous flow drains into the inferior cava vein through a collector that is oriented down towards the diaphragm coursing parallel along the right border of the pericardium with an increasing diameter, which curves centrally to drain at the level of the connection of the inferior vena cava and the right atrium. The condition is often accompanied by hypoplasia of the right lung, which can cause a shift toward the right side of the mediastinum (Fig. 7.92).

5. *Anomalous left pulmonary vein return.* The entire left pulmonary venous flow is connected to the innominate vein through the persistence of a vertical vein. It is rare that the superior pulmonary vein be involved alone (Fig. 7.92).

In addition to these anomalies, there are also other more rare kinds of anomalous pulmonary venous returns that are extensively treated in other specific readings [13].

MRI strategy
- Localizer on three planes, often accompanied by an axial TOF in free breathing used as templates for following acquisitions (as for AoCo).
- Study of the bi-ventricular function for quantifying the volume overload of the right ventricle.
- PC images at the level of the ascending aorta and of the pulmonary artery to calculate respectively the systemic and pulmonary outputs, and thus the shunt expressed as ratio of the two flows (QP/QS).
- CEMRA for 3D visualization of vessels.

Whenever there is a concomitance of PAPVR + interatrial sinus venosus defect, it is advisable to acquire fast cine images in coronal and axial planes at the level of the root of SVC in order to have a better visualization of the septal defect between the SVC and the right superior pulmonary artery (Fig. 7.90).

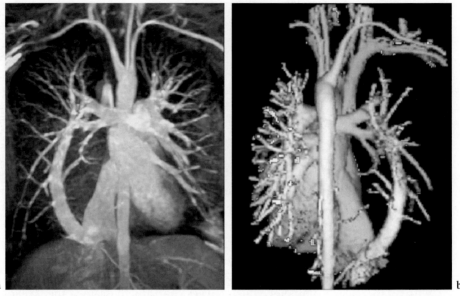

a   b

Fig. 7.92 a, b. Scimitar syndrome seen by MRI from the anterior (**a**) and posterior (**b**) view with two different postprocessing methods: MIP (**a**) and volume rendering (**b**). (Courtesy of Dr. Tal Geva, Boston Children Hospital, Department of Pediatric Cardiology)

7.7.5 Simple isolated cardiac defects

7.7.5.1 Atrial Septal Defect (ASD)

ASD can be found at different sites and is the most frequent cause of left-right shunt. Its most common manifestations are ASD type ostium secundum and the patency of the Fossa Ovalis. These defects may be treated by implanting an occlusive device percutaneously. The procedures in use today require a detailed knowledge on the anatomy, size and location of the defect. The size of the defect is generally measured by Transesophageal Echography (TEE) [14]; however, also MRI provides excellent anatomical details and, additionally, an excellent estimate of the shunt [7].

MRI strategy
- Localizer on three planes.
- Study of bi-ventricular function with images in cine on parallel planes on the short axis of the ventricles.
- PC images at the level of the aorta and pulmonary a. for the calculation of the QP/QS as for the PAPVR.
- Images in fast SE and fast cine on the long horizontal axis and on the short axis with planes passing through the aortic valvular ring for visualizing the ASD and the eventual left atrium-right atrium jet; the operator must keep in mind the extremely thin and mobile structure of the interatrial

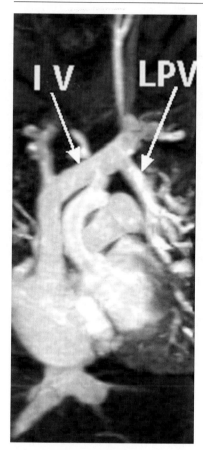

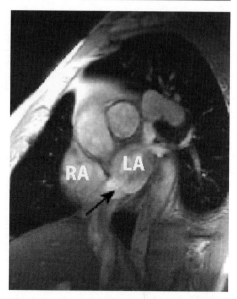

Fig. 7.94. Inter-atrial defect ostium secundum type: the arrow indicates the communication between the left and the right atrium. RA=Right Atrium; LA=Left Atrium

Fig. 7.93. Anomalous left pulmonary vein return with drainage into the anonymous trunk. IV=Innominate Vein; LPV=Left Pulmonary Vein

septum. Furthermore, the jet especially in the case of broad low-velocity defects has a slow speed. Hence, the procedure requires images with a high SNR, and in the case of Fast SPGR requires images with a TE of approx 8 msec in order to evidence the jet better (Fig. 7.94).

7.7.5.2 Ventricular septal defect (VSD)

The isolated interventricular defect is a common heart disease that involves a left-right shunt, and in the case of wide VSD, elevated pulmonary artery pressures. In other cases the VSD is accompanied by other anomalies, the most common: infundibular stenosis of the pulmonary valve, aortic regurgitation, aortic coarctation and sub-aortic stenosis. In other cases the VSD is part of a larger picture of malformations, such as Fallot's tetralogy, defect of the artio-ventricular

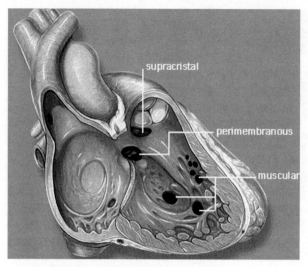

Fig. 7.95. Sites where interventricular defects most frequently occur

canal, complex univentricular heart disease. The isolated VSD is classified according to its location in the interventricular septum (Fig. 7.95): defect of the membranous septum (the most common), of the infundibular septum, of the trabecular-muscular septum, inflow septum. The therapeutic indication towards the closing of the defect depends on the entity of the shunt and its location.

MRI strategy
– Localizer on three planes.
– Study of bi-ventricular function with images in cine on parallel planes on the short axis of the ventricles.
– PC images for calculation of the QP/QS as for PAPVR or ASD.

It may be useful to underline that the shunt of the VSD is mainly systolic and causes an increase in left volume of the heart (not of the right as with ASD), despite the fact it is left-right (as for ASD); hence, the amount of blood passing through the VSD is directly poured into the pulmonary vessels, entailing an increase in pulmonary output and thus with a burden of the pulmonary venous return on the left ventricle.

Interventricular defects and their jets are located with Fast Cine SPGR, which allow to identify also other structures (e.g. the aortic valve) that could have relevant implications in a future closure by means of a transcutaneous device (Fig. 7.96).

7.7.5.3 Bicuspid aortic valve

Bicuspid aortic valve is by far one of the most common valve defects. The MRI exam is an extremely valid tool in the study and follow-up of this anom-

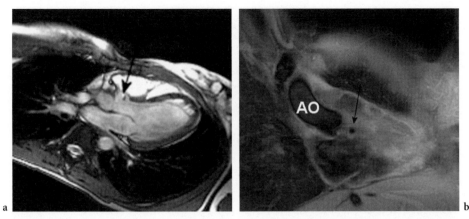

Fig. 7.96 a, b. Small interventricular peri-membranous defect visualized on the long axis in GRE image (**a**) and oblique frontal aspect in FSE image (**b**). The arrow indicates the defect. AO=Aorta

aly; its main aims are the evaluation of the valve's anatomy (Fig. 7.97a) [15], of the wall and caliber of the ascending aorta, the quantification of the aortic regurgitation, and the evaluation of the origin of the coronaries [15]. The quantification of the regurgitation is fundamental in the decision-making process. In virtue of its accuracy and non-invasiveness, MRI is the most recent and promising diagnostic tool in this field [16].

MRI strategy
–   Localizer on three planes.
–   Study of bi-ventricular function with images in cine on parallel planes on the short axis of the ventricles.
–   Images in cine according to a plane on the long axis of the left ventricle at the level of the outflow for visualizing the jet of the aortic regurgitation (Fig. 7.97b, c).
–   Acquisitions in PC at the level of the ascending aorta few mm over the plane of the aortic semilunar valves [16] (Fig. 7.97b, c) for quantification of the aortic regurgitation. The eventual presence of a very turbulent antero-grade flow (e.g. when there is an associated stenosis) can reduce the accuracy of the measurement.
–   Images in cine on the short axis at the level of the valvular plane for the study of the anatomy of the valve and the sinuses, especially to visualize the opening dynamics.
–   Images in Fast SE and if required 2D TOF of the ascending aorta for measuring the dimensions of the ascending aorta itself.
–   2D or 3D acquisition (e.g. 3D FIESTA with fat suppression) at the level of the aortic sinuses for the study of the root of the coronaries.

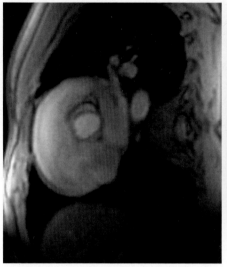

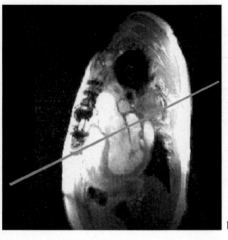

b

a

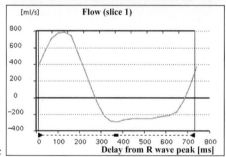

c

Fig. 7.97 a-c. (a) Bicuspid aortic valve upon opening, visualized in a SPGR image; (b) PC evaluation of the aortic regurgitation; (c) graphic representation of thoracic flow: in diastole the curve is negative, the area underneath between the line of zero and the curve represents the volume of regurgitation. Fractional regurgitation = regurgitant flow volume/anterograde volume

7.7.6 Defects of the atrio-ventricular connection

7.7.6.1 Endocardial Cushions Defects (ECD)

This is a relatively common congenital heart disease, which is very diffused among individuals affected by trisomy-21. It is characterized by the lack of septal tissue immediately above and under the atrio-ventricular plane, in the region that is generally occupied by the septum in the normal heart. The lack of tissue over the plane of the A-V valves produces an interatrial defect as with the ostium primum type. The lack of tissue below the plane produces an interventricular defect of variable degree, if not total, according to how the atrio-ventricular valve is implanted on the interventricular septal crest. There can be one or two orifices or any intermediate situations. Hence the defect of the endocardial cushions includes a wide array of defects ranging from the most simple in which there is an IAD without a interventricular defect to the presence of two atrio-ventricular orifices and a cleft of the anterior mitral leaflet (partial defect of the atrio-ventricular canal), to the more complex

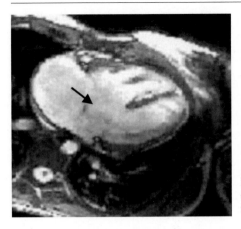

Fig. 7.98. Common atrio-ventricular canal in GRE: the arrow indicates the common atrio-ventricular valve

cases with a common orifice of atrio-ventricular canal, IAD and a large interventricular defect (complete defect of the atrio-ventricular canal). These hearts are also generally characterized by an anomalous position of the aortic valve that is not positioned as usual on the atrio-ventricular plane but is dislocated in a superior, anterior position. The physiopathology obviously depends on the prevailing type of malformation and varies according to the presence and size of the interventricular defect and on the presence or absence of regurgitation of the atrio-ventricular valve.

Echocardiography is the diagnostic tool of choice and in most cases is enough to indicate a surgical intervention with no further exams. However, it is possible that the ventricles be unbalanced by the hypoplasia of one of them, requiring a more accurate volumetric and spatial evaluation. In these selected cases, MRI can provide additional information (Fig. 7.98).

MRI strategy
- Localizer on three planes.
- Study of the bi-ventricular function with images in cine on parallel planes on the short axis of the ventricles.
- Evaluation of the left outflow with cine images.

7.7.6.2 Ebstein's malformation

This is a relatively rare anomaly (about 0.3% of all congenital heart disease) [17] that affects the tricuspid valve, which is dysplastic with a vast array of variants.

Classically the septal leaflet, and sometimes also the anterior one, is displaced downward in the right ventricle making the identification of the ring difficult and causing "atrialization" of the basal wall.

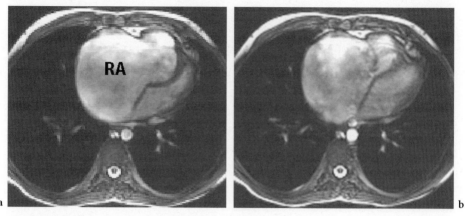

Fig. 7.99 a, b. Ebstein's malformation: image in GRE in diastole (a) and in systole (b) in which the large right atrium is well illustrated. RA=Right Atrium

The anterior leaflet is generally more extended than usual, and can present a constrained movement depending on the relationship with the cords and the papillary muscles, which also conditions the sealing of the valve, and depending on the surgical strategy. It is often associated with a right-left shunt because of the elevated pressure of the right atrium, which can entail cyanosis. Ebstein's malformations can be diagnosed by Echocardiography, and MRI can rarely add some anatomical details in view of an indication toward a planning for surgery (Fig. 7.99a, b).

MRI strategy
- Localizer on three planes.
- Study of the bi-ventricular function with images in cine on parallel planes on the short axis of the ventricles.
- Images in PC for calculating the QP/QS as for ASD.
- Images in Fast cine and in Fast SE, axial and coronal, in order to visualize the septal and posterior leaflets [18] and quantify the portion of "atrialized" right ventricle.

7.7.7 Tronco-conal defects

7.7.7.1 Fallot's Tetralogy (FT) and Pulmonary Atresia + VSD

Fallot's tetraology is the most classical among the tronco-conal congenital cardiac diseases. It is characterized by the anterior leftward deviation of the conal (or infundibular) septum that determines an interventricular defect due to the so-called "abnormal alignment". The anterior deviation of the conal septum causes on one hand the typical aortic overlapping on the interventricular defect, on the other the stenosis of the right ventricle outflow tract that can even reach total pulmonary atresia in the case of an extreme deviation. Thus FT and pulmonary atresia + VSD are the expression of different degrees of the same congenital defect. Also in this case, the diagnosis is typically performed by Echocardiography, but sometimes in view of the surgical correction, a hemodynamic examination is also necessary in order to define pulmonary vascularization, the anatomy of pulmonary arteries and the origin of the coronaries, whenever Echocardiography is not satisfactory. At present, MRI is not employed in clinical practice as a routine in presurgical planning of FT, but potentially can answer all the surgical queries above [19].

7.7.7.2 Truncus arteriosus

Also called common aortic-pulmonary trunk. This is a cardiac disease in which a single large artery (arterial trunk) origins from the base of the heart from a single semilunar valve also known as trunk valve. The coronaries and the medium pulmonary artery (or both pulmonary arteries without interposition of a medium pulmonary artery) generate from the arterial trunk, proximal to the brachio-cephalic trunks. Under the trunk valve there is always a VSD.

In view of surgical planning, Echocardiography allows to portray an exhaustive anatomical picture in most cases. In complex cases (when the pulmonary artery is not visible) angiography (either invasive or with MRI) becomes necessary.

presurgery MRI strategy
- Localizer on three planes.
- Study of bi-ventricular function with images in cine on parallel planes on the short axis of the ventricles.
- Study of the aortic valve (or of the trunk) by "black blood" images on the short axis and images in cine and in PC for the quantification of eventual regurgitation.
- Evaluation of the origin and the proximal coursing of the coronaries.
- MRA for visualizing the anatomy of pulmonary vessels.

7.7.7.3 Trunk-conal defects (postsurgery)

The surgical correction of this group of cardiac disease is aimed at re-establishing the continuity between the right ventricle and the pulmonary trunk (by means of patches, or valvulate and non-valvulate ducts) and the closure of the VSD.

At present, MRI is the most complete non-invasive technique for the follow-up of patients with this condition and is likely to become the method of choice in the near future. The aims of an MRI study are to assess the continuity between outflow of the right ventricle and the pulmonary artery, evaluate the anatomy of the pulmonary tree and any pulmonary regurgitation (Fig. 7.100), and above all the function and volumes of the right ventricle [6].

Recently, it has been underlined that the MRI study of the functional relation of the two ventricles in presence of an overload of volume and/or pressure of the right ventricle provides precise information on the timing for a second intervention for reducing the overload on the right ventricle [21].

MRI strategy
- Localizer on three planes.
- Study of bi-ventricular function with images in cine on parallel planes on the short axis of the ventricles.
- Study of the right outflow tract by cine images on sagittal oblique and coronal planes.
- Acquisition of PC images at the level of the pulmonary infundibulus for quantifying the pulmonary flow and regurgitation.
- 3D CEMRA for visualizing the pulmonary anatomy.

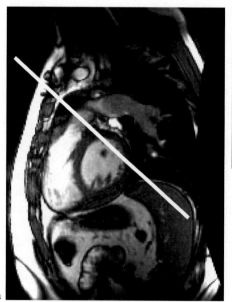

a

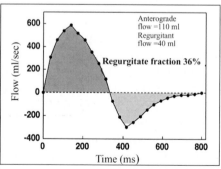

b

Fig. 7.100 a, b. A corrected tetralogy of Fallot: evaluation of the regurgitation by PC (a); the flow curve and the calculation of the regurgitant fraction (b)

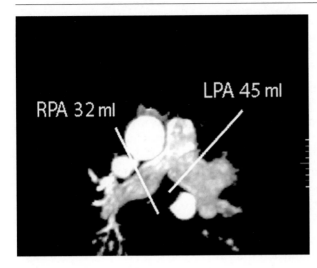

RPA 32 ml

LPA 45 ml

Fig. 7.101. Calculation of the differential pulmonary flow in a corrected tetralogy of Fallot, by means of PC mapping; the numbers indicate the flow in cc/heart beat. RPA=Right Pulmonary Artery; LPA=Left Pulmonary Artery

In the presence of stenoses or distortions of the pulmonary branches, Fast SE "black blood" images on the pulmonary arteries can be useful for studying the anatomy in detail, while acquisitions in PC at the level of the pulmonary branches provide a more accurate quantification of the flow in the single pulmonary branches allowing a functional analysis on the hemodynamics effects of the stenosis (Fig. 7.101).

7.7.8 Defects of the ventricular-arterial connections (postsurgery)

7.7.8.1 Transposition of the great arteries (simple TGA), TGA+ VSD

TGA is a relatively frequent cardiac disease (5-6% of congenital heart disease) [22] that consists in a ventricular-arterial discordance: the right ventricle is connected to the aorta and the left ventricle is connected to the pulmonary artery. The survival of newborns affected by this pathology is exclusively possible due to the presence of a shunt at the level of the interatrial septum, and the rate is 20% at one year if not treated [23]. The surgical treatment varies according to the base anatomy: arterial switch with transposition of the coronaries, tunneling of the left ventricle toward the aorta and connection of the right ventricle to the pulmonary artery with the aid of a conduit or homograft (Rastelli procedure) or with a patch and without interposition of conduits (direct ventriculo-arterial connection, or Réparation à l'Etage Ventriculaire – REV); or atrial switch (Mustard or Senning procedure). This last technique consists in crossing the atrial flows in such a way that the oxygenated blood coming from the pulmonary veins drains into the right ventricle and thereby in the aorta, while the systemic venous blood is directed toward the left ventricle and thus to the pulmonary artery. This latter option has been almost completely abandoned since the ventricle loses functionality in the long term when subjected to systemic pressures. Hence in patients with operated TGA, MRI is performed specifically according to the technique that has been used in the procedure.

In the case of the Mustard or Senning procedure, MRI aims to study the function of the right ventricle (systemic ventricle) [24] and the patency of the two new atria surgically built by means of patches [25]. In the case of arterial switch, the study aims to assess the left ventricular function and the anatomy of the proximal pulmonary segments that can be stenosed because of stretching following the surgical procedure. In the case of the Rastelli procedure or REV the study especially evaluates the connection between the right pulmonary ventricle and the eventual pulmonary regurgitation, the anatomy of the pulmonary arteries and the left outflow.

MRI strategy (mustard/senning)
- Localizer on three planes with 2D axial TOF.
- Study of the bi-ventricular function with images in cine on parallel planes on the short axis of the ventricles.
- Images in cine on the new atrial conduits on oblique planes [25] (Fig. 7.102).

MRI strategy (arterial switch)
- Localizer on three planes with 2D axial TOF.
- Study of the bi-ventricular function with images in cine on parallel planes on the short axis of the ventricles.

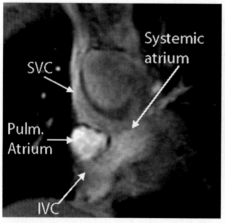 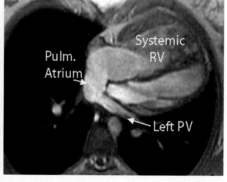

Fig. 7.102 a, b. Correction of transposition of the great vessels by Mustard procedure. (**a**) New systemic atrium that collects the blood coming from the two cava veins. (**b**) New pulmonary atrium in connection with the right ventricle connected to the aorta. SVC=Superior Vena Cava; IVC=Inferior Vena Cava; RV = Right Ventricle

- 3D CEMRA of the pulmonary tree and, if required, the acquisition of images in Fast SE "black blood" and in PC (as in postsurgery Fallot) in case of regurgitation and/or pulmonary stenosis.

MRI strategy (REV/ Rastelli)
- Procedure as for arterial switch, putting special attention on the connection right ventricle>pulmonary artery, with PC images at the level of the pulmonary infundibulus for quantifying the eventual pulmonary regurgitation.
- Images in cine for the evaluation of the surgically rebuilt left outflow.

7.7.9 Complex defects (presurgery and postsurgery)

One of the peculiar aspects of the complex cardiac diseases arises from the extreme variability of the cardiac segments. One of the main tasks of the diagnostic path consists in the correct identification of the cardiac structures.

7.7.9.1 Atrio-ventricular and ventricular-arterial discordance (TGA congenitally correct)

The congenitally correct transposition of the great arteries is a cardiac anomaly characterized by a discordant atrioventricular connection (the right atrium is connected to a morphologically left ventricle, while the left atrium is connected to a morphologically right ventricle) associated to a discordant ventricular-arterial connection (transposition of the great arteries). Thus the circulations are correctly in series (from which the term of "congenitally correct"). The atria can be in situs solitus or in situs inversus. If there is a situs solitus, the left ventricle (that is connected to the right atrium) is generally located on the right, slightly lower and posterior to the morphologically right ventricle; the outflow that is connected to the pulmonary artery does not cross the outflow of the right ventricle, hence the two large arteries are parallel to one another. The aorta that originates from the infundibulus of the morphologically right ventricle is located anteriorly and to the left of the pulmonary a. (Fig. 7.103). The most frequently associated anomalies are sub-pulmonary stenosis and the VSD [13].

Subjects with congenitally correct TGA without associated anomalies show normal hemodynamics, but have a lower life expectancy because of the presence of a morphologically right ventricle subjected to systemic pressures. This condition favors the development of ventricular failure eventually favored by the presence of significant regurgitation at the level of the atrioventricular morphologically tricuspid valve.

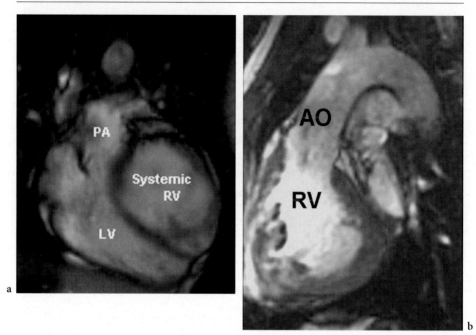

Fig. 7.103 a, b. Correct transposition of the great vessels. (**a**) Morphologically Left Ventricle (LV) is connected to the Pulmonary Artery (PA). (**b**) The morphologically right ventricle (RV) is connected to the aorta (AO)

MRI strategy

- Localizer on 3 planes, preferably by employing 2D TOF images such as the axial localizer.
- Study of bi-ventricular function. The standard procedure for locating the vertical axis of the ventricle cannot be applied in this case as in all other cases of complex heart disease, because of the unusual disposition of the ventricles. There are however several alternative methods in use today. The images by Fast GRE in real time (approx 200 msec per image) allow an interactive change of the scanning plane until the correct angulation is reached. The spatial parameters obtained are then transferred to images of higher quality for the continuation of the study. In alternative it is possible to use 2D TOF images in axial projection to be used as a scout for the following acquisitions. Once the projection on the long horizontal axis of the ventricles has been identified, the operator positions the planes orthogonal to this one for the study of the volume and of the ventricular mass.
- Images in cine on two axes perpendicular to the outflow of the morphologically left sub-pulmonar ventricle to exclude any sub-pulmonary stenosis.
- Images of Phase Contrast on the aorta and pulmonary artery for the calculation of the respective outputs.

7.7.9.2 Isomerisms and single ventricles

Complex malformations represent a wide group of cardiac diseases that become manifest with extremely variable anatomic pictures. Sometimes these malformations are associated to isomerisms and heterotaxy syndrome (incorrect lateral position defects). The diagnostic characterization of these cardiac diseases relies on the sequential analysis, which consists in defining the anatomy segment by segment and the connection of the cardiac chambers. Echocardiography in the newborn almost always meets the requirements of an adequate sequential analysis; however, in adults MRI is an instrument of great diagnostic potential [26].

MRI strategy
- Localizer on three planes, eventually using the 2D TOF as axial localizer. The localizer images on coronal plane are utilized also for locating the bronchial site (Fig. 7.104), and those on the axial plane for locating the atrial appendages as markers of the atrial site.
- Cine images on the three main axes to better locate the disposition and anatomy of the ventricles, which is very variable. This method, also allows to locate the VSD in space along with its relation to the great vessels in view of the planning of a correct surgical strategy (Fig. 7.105).
- Cine images for locating eventual stenoses of the ventricles outflows.
- PC acquisitions of the medium pulmonary aorta for the calculation of the systemic and pulmonary outputs, of the single pulmonary arteries in the case of stenoses and eventual calculation of the differential pulmonary flow (right and left pulmonary arteries).
- 3D MRA according to CEMRA for the study of the pulmonary artery and systemic and pulmonary venous returns (Fig. 106). This diagnostic insight covers a fundamental role for the planning of surgical strategies according to the principle of Fontan.

7.7.9.3 Isomerisms and single ventricles (postsurgery)

The surgical history of patients affected by complex congenital heart diseases is almost always, when feasible, the conversion towards the procedure of Fontan. This procedure consists in dividing the systemic and pulmonary circulations also in patients with a single functioning ventricle, detouring all or part of the systemic blood directly to the pulmonary arteries, bypassing the heart. In this way, the existing ventricle is employed in pumping the blood to the aorta, while the pulmonary flow is guaranteed by the low resistance of the pulmonary circulation, by the negative intra-thoracic pressure determined by the breathing action and expiration forces of the ventricle. There are many

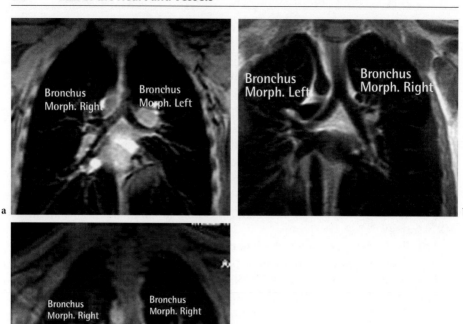

Fig. 7.104 a-c. Determination of the bronchial situs. (a) Situs solitus: the bronchi are positioned correctly. (b) Situs inversus: the morphologically right bronchus is positioned to the left and vice-versa. (c) Right isomerism: both bronchi have morphology on the right

variations to the original procedure which was devised in the seventies, based on the different techniques for identifying anastomoses between the vena cava and the pulmonary artery, and on whether or not the right atrium was included [13].

The cardiologic evaluation of these patients is especially aimed at the calculation of the ventricular function. A good ventricular function is a fundamental condition for the correct functioning for the Fontan hemodynamic system. However, given the extremely variable geometry of these ventricles, the echocardiographic evaluation is not totally accurate, while MRI, eventually associated to stress MRI (dobutamine), has revealed to be a valid instrument even in the search of improving the knowledge on the dynamics of these pre and post Fontan ventricles [5, 27, 28]. In the case in which the aorta origins from the accessory ventricle (e.g. double entrance

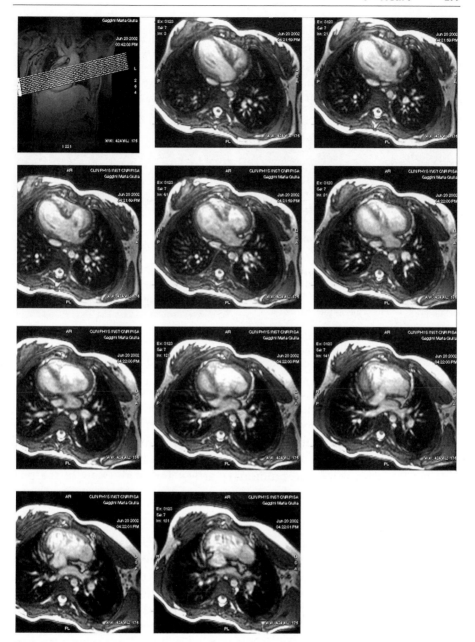

Fig. 7.105. Heart with criss-cross disposition: the two right and left inlets are perpendicular to each other

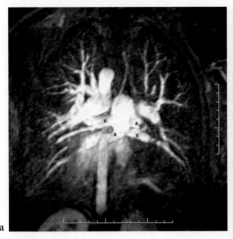

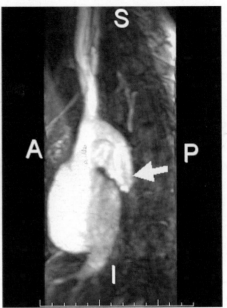

a

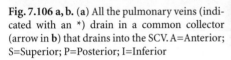

Fig. 7.106 a, b. (a) All the pulmonary veins (indicated with an *) drain in a common collector (arrow in **b**) that drains into the SCV. A=Anterior; S=Superior; P=Posterior; I=Inferior

b

in the left ventricle and transposition of the great vessels), it may be necessary to exclude the eventual presence of a "restrictive" IAD, which would involve a sub-aortic stensosis as the aortic flow would be limited by the interventricular defect. Other aims for an MRI study in patients operated using the Fontan procedure are the visualization of the anastomoses between the cava veins and pulmonary artery and of the flow of the pulmonary tree [29].

MRI strategy
- Localizer on three planes eventually using a 2D TOF as axial localizer.
- Images in cine for the study of the ventricular study, proceeding as in the cases of complex cardiac diseases. In some cases it may be useful to obtain some images in cine during the pharmacological inotropic stimulus (dobutamine) in order to exclude dynamic stenoses [28].
- 3D CEMRA to exclude eventual obstacles or stenoses of anastomoses between the cava veins and pulmonary artery, of the pulmonary arteries up to the pulmonary veins (Fig. 7.107).
- PC acquisitions at the level of the superior and inferior cava veins and of the single pulmonary arteries to evaluate the differential pulmonary flow. These are flows with venous characteristics, hence slower and more sensitive to respiratory variations since they are not supported by the myocardial pump.

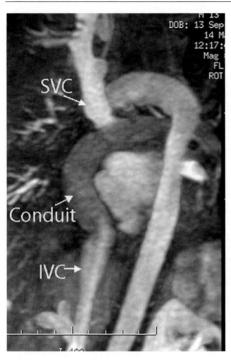

Fig. 7.107. Example of Fontan reconstruction: the Inferior Vena Cava (IVC) is directly connected to the pulmonary circle by means of a extra cardiac conduit; the Superior Vena Cava (SVC) is directly anastomized to the pulmonary artery

References

1. Haliloglu M, Hoffer FA, Gronemeyer SA (1999) Application of three dimensional gadolinium-enhanced MRI angiography in children Proc. Int Soc Magn Reson Med 7:1222
2. Vick GW (2000) Three and four-dimensional visualization of magnetic resonance imaging data sets in pediatric cardiology. Pediatr Cardiol 21:27-36
3. Jauhiainen T, Järvinen VM, Hekali PE (2002) Evaluation of methods for MR imaging of human right ventricular heart volumes and mass. Acta Radiol 43:587-592
4. Fujimoto S, Mizuno R, Nakagawa et al (1998) Estimation of the right ventricular volume and ejection fraction by transthoracic three-dimensional echocardiography. A validation study using magnetic resonance imaging. Int J Card Imaging 14:385-390
5. Fogel MA, Gupta KB, Weinberg PM et al (1995) Regional wall motion and strain analysis across stages of Fontan reconstruction by magnetic resonance tagging. Am J 269(3 Pt 2):H113.
6. Powell AJ, Geva T (2000) Blood flow measurement by magnetic resonance imaging in congenital heart disease. Pediatr Cardiol 21:47-58
7. Powell AJ, Tsai-Goodman B, Prakash A et al (2003) Comparison between phase-velocity cine magnetic resonance imaging and invasive oximetry for quantification of atrial shunts. Am J Cardiol 91:1523-525, A9
8. Chernoff DM, Derugin N, Rajasinghe HA e al (1997) Measurement of collateral blood flow in a porcine model of aortic coarctation by velocity-encoded cine MRI. Magn Reson Imaging 7:557-563
9. Oshinski JN, Parks WJ, Markou CP et al (1996) Improved measurement of pressure gradients in aortic coarctation by magnetic resonance imaging. J Am Coll Cardiol 28:1818-2186
10. Freedom cong. Heart Disease 1997: textbook of Angiocardiography. Armonk NY

11. Van Praagh S, Carrera ME, Sanders SP et al (1994) Mayer JE, Van Praagh R. Sinus venosus defects: unroofing of the right pulmonary veins-anatomic and echocardiographic findings and surgical treatment. Am Heart J 128:365-379

12. Cardiac Surgery (Kirkling/Barratt-Boyes) (1993) Churchill-Levingston

13. Zhu W, Cao QL, Rhodes J et al (2000) Measurement of atrial septal defect size: a comparative study between three-dimensional transesophageal echocardiography and the standard balloon sizing methods. Pediatr Cardiol 21:465-469

14. Beerbaum P, Korperich H, Esdorn H et al (2003) Atrial septal defects in pediatric patients: noninvasive sizing with cardiovascular MR imaging. Radiology 228:361-369

15. Arai AE, Epstein FH, Bove KE et al Visualization of aortic valve leaflet using black blood MRI. J Magn Reson Imaging 10:771-777

16. Chatzimavroudis GP, Oshinski JN, Franch RH et al (1998) Quantification of the aortic regurgitant volume with magnetic resonance phase velocity mapping: a clinical investigation of the importance of imaging slice location. J Heart Valve Dis 7:94-101

17. Nora JJ, Nora AH, Toews WH (1974) Letter: Lithium, Ebstein's anomaly, and other congenital heart defects. Lancet 2:594-595

18. Choi YH, Park YK, Choe YH (1994) MR imaging of Ebstein's anomaly of the tricuspid valve. Am J Roentgenol 163:539-543

19. Geva T, Greil GF, Marshall AC et al (2002) Gadolinium-enhanced 3-dimensional magnetic resonance angiography of pulmonary blood supply in patients with complex pulmonary stenosis or atresia: comparison with x-ray angiography. Circulation 106:473-478

20. Helbing WA, de Roos (2000) A clinical applications of cardiac magnetic resonance imaging after repair of tetralogy of Fallot. Pediatr Cardiol 21:70-79

21. Davlouros PA, Kilner PJ et al (2002) Right ventricular function in adults with repaired tetralogy of Fallot assessed with cardiovascular magnetic resonance imaging: detrimental role of right ventricular outflow aneurysms or akinesia and adverse right-to-left ventricular interaction. J Am Coll Cardiol 40:2044-2052

22. Christofer A Loffredo (2000) Epidemiology of cardiovascular malformation. American Journal of Medical Genetica (Semin Med Genet) 97:319-325

23. Liebman J, Cullum L, Belloc NB (1969) Natural history of transposition of the great arteries. Anatomy and birth and death characteristics. Circulation 40:237-262

24. Lorenz CH, Walker ES, Graham TP et al (1995) Right ventricular performance and mass by use of cine MRI late after atrial repair of transposition of the great arteries. Circulation 92 (9 Suppl):II233-9

25. Fogel MA, Hubbard A, Weinberg PM (2001) A simplified approach for assessment of intracardiac baffles and extracardiac conduits in congenital heart surgery with two- and three-dimensional magnetic resonance imaging. Am Heart J 142:1028-1036

26. Geva T, Vick GW 3rd, Wendt RE et al (1994) Role of spin echo and cine magnetic resonance imaging in presurgical planning of heterotaxy syndrome. Comparison with echocardiography and catheterization. Circulation 90:348-356

27. Fogel MA, Weinberg PM, Fellows KE et al (1993) Magnetic resonance imaging of constant total heart volume and center of mass in patients with functional single ventricle before and after staged Fontan procedure. Am J Cardiol 72:1435-1443

28. Tulevski II, van der Wall EE, Groenink M et al (2002) Usefulness of magnetic resonance imaging dobutamine stress in asymptomatic and minimally symptomatic patients with decreased cardiac reserve from congenital heart disease (complete and corrected transposition of the great arteries and subpulmonic obstruction). Am J Cardiol 89:1077-1081

29. Rebergen SA, Ottenkamp J, Doornbos J et al (1993) Postoperative pulmonary flow dynamics after Fontan surgery: assessment with nuclear magnetic resonance velocity mapping. Am Coll Cardiol Jan 21:123-131

8   Pericardium and mediastinum

Virna Zampa, Giulia Granai, Paola Vagli

8.1 Pericardium

8.1.1 Introduction

Indications for a Magnetic Resonance Imaging (MRI) study of pericardial disease usually follow the findings of echocardiographic screening. Indeed, Computed Tomography (CT) and MRI are employed when the clinical symptoms are not in agreement with the echocardiographic findings, or when Echocardiography is inadequate because of technical limitations, or whenever a more specific characterization of the findings has been requested. In the specific case of expanding lesions involving the pericardium, MRI is always the best choice for diagnostic investigation: in fact transthoracic Echocardiography, just as Transesophageal Echocardiography (TEE), is constrained by a limited Field Of View (FOV); CT is penalized by inevitable artifacts (especially when it is not synchronized with ECG) and, except for detection and measurement of calcifications, it seems to be inferior to MRI in characterizing the injury; furthermore, it scarcely differentiates effusions from epicardial thickenings. Therefore, MRI is generally preferred although it may give sub optimal results when pericardial disease is accompanied by arrhythmia.

8.1.2 Normal anatomy

The pericardium is formed of two layers that fold over the heart chambers, enveloping them all the way to the base of the great vessels. Its anchoring points to the sternum, spine and diaphragm limit excursion of this sac during movement of the body.

The visceral pericardium, formed by a single layer of mesothelial cells, is closely adherent to the cardiac surface, except in those areas where fatty tissue is interposing (in variable amounts from one individual to another). The fatty tissue is more abundant at the level of sulci and surrounds the vessels that run across the myocardium. The parietal layer often has a thick fibrous component and is separated from the visceral layer by a small quantity of serous liquid (15-50 ml).

The folds of the pericardium over the cardiac structures create recesses, which are: the oblique sinus, located behind the left atrium and separated from the pericardial cavity; the anterior-superior recess, which surrounds the aorta and the pulmonary a. (the distension of this structure allows to confirm the presence of pericardial effusion in the cases where it is difficultly identified); the transverse sinus, located dorsally to the ascending aorta, which can erroneously be misinterpreted for aortic dissection. In fact in order to avoid such errors, it is important for the operator to have extensive knowledge on the anatomy of these structures.

The best images of the pericardium are acquired by cardiac gating. In absence of abundant pericardial fluid, the two pericardial layers are visualized in SE images as a thin single line with no signal, interposed between the high intensity of the mediastinal and subepicardial adipose tissue, and the intermediate signal of the myocardium. The best visualization of the pericardium is obtained in systole, about 200 msec after the R wave. In the regions near the lungs, such as in the postero-lateral region of the left ventricle, the sac is difficultly distinguishable from the pulmonary parenchyma.

The normal pericardium has a thickness of 2 mm [1]; measurements should be made on an image, on axial plane, that simultaneously represents the right atrium and the left and right ventricles. In more caudal images, pericardial thickness may be overestimated: either due to the ligamentous insertion of the diaphragm into the pericardium or to the images in axial view with tangential position to the inferior border of the heart and the relative pericardium.

8.1.3 Congenital disease

Congenital abnormalities of the pericardium are rare; they are classified in: congenital absence or defects of the pericardium such as pericardial cysts, diverticoli, and theratomas.

The total absence of the pericardium is rare. The disease most frequently affects the left ventriculum (70%); in half of the cases the entire left portion is missing and there are partial defects in the remaining portions. In one third of cases, pericardial defects accompany other congenital defects (tetralogy of Fallot, defect of the atrial septum, patency of arterial ductus, bicuspid aortic valve, hiatus hernia, or bronchogenic cysts). Partial defects can lead to hernia of the heart or to compression on the coronary. Usually, the total absence of the pericardium remains asymptomatic. It can be supposed from the standard radiographic exam of the chest, which evidences the unusual contour of the heart that reveals the more defined borders of its segments. The absence of the pericardium, which generally folds between

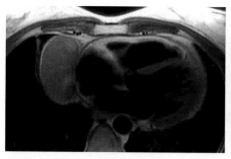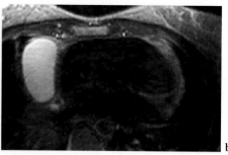

a   b

Fig. 8.1 a, b. Pericardial diverticulus on the anterior-right border of the heart (postsurgery diagnosis). The lesion gives an intermediate signal in "black blood" images (**a**), and hyperintensity in T2 (**b**) as typical for liquid lesions. In this case, the communication with the pericardial is not visible, which makes differential diagnosis with pericardial cyst impossible

the aorta and pulmonary artery makes the edges of pulmonary artery more visible. Often the partial lack of the pericardium is accompanied by a shift of the heart to the left, sometimes with a blurred profile of the left ventricle.

MRI directly visualizes the altered pericardial anatomy and accurately demonstrates the extension of the defect, therefore providing a definite diagnosis.

Pericardial cysts have a congenital origin and develop separated isles of pericardial tissue during the embryonic stage; they are enveloped and do not have any connection to the pericardial space. Seventy percent of cysts are located on the right side and 90% of them are found within cardio-phrenic sulci; those located at other sites cannot be distinguished from bronchogenic or thymic cysts.

At MRI, pericardial cysts appear as para-cardiac masses with low signal intensity in the T1-weighted images and with high signal intensity in T2-weighted images. They show no internal septation, are homogeneous and with no changes after contrast agent administration, and are surrounded by a thin line of low intensity signal from the pericardial tissue. On rare occurrences, they may contain protein-rich fluid, which gives an elevated intensity on T1-weighted images.

The pericardial diverticulum (congenital, or in consequence of a hernia through a defect of the parietal pericardium) contains a layer of pericardium and communicates with the pericardial cavity, with the result that its volume changes with the volume of the pericardial fluid. The signal characteristics are similar to those given by cysts and sometimes indistinguishable due to the impossibility of seeing an extremely small-sized passage (Fig. 8.1).

Theratomas and intra-pericardic bronchogenic cysts represent the most frequent benign tumoral lesions of the pericardium. MRI can be useful in demonstrating the relationship of the mass with contiguous anatomical structures and in characterizing the nature of the lesions.

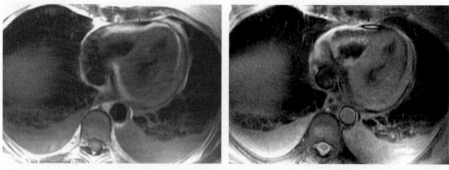

a   b

Fig. 8.2 a, b. Haematic pericardial effusion due to heart rupture, complicating Acute Myocardial Infarction. In the T1-weighted (**a**) and triple IR (**b**), the effusion appears in-homogeneous due to the presence of partially organized haematic matter with medium intensity. Bilateral pleural effusion

8.1.4 Pericardial effusion

Pericardial effusion derives from the obstruction of venous or lymphatic drainage of the heart, or from an altered capillary permeability that occurs in consequence to one of a range of causes (heart or kidney failure, infections, neoplasia, trauma, etc.).

MRI is very sensitive in detecting localized pericardial effusions, even of small dimensions; these deposits usually have an elliptic shape and are recognizable in a posterior-lateral position to the right atrium and the left ventricle. Non-complicated effusions present the typical MRI signal emitted from liquids, while effusions rich of protein matter or of haematic nature show an increase in signal intensity in T1-weighted images (Figs. 8.2, 8.3). In particular, blood deposits usually yield a hyperintense signal in T1-weighted images and a low signal in cine-GRE images [1].

The shift of fluid in systole and diastole can be detected by cine-MRI, thus differentiating small effusions from limited pericardial thickenings [2].

8.1.5 Constrictive pericarditis

MRI represents the technique of choice in the evaluation of a patient with suspected constrictive pericarditis. If not idiopathic, the most common causes of this condition are heart surgery, radiotherapy, infections, connective disease, uremia, and neoplasia. In constrictive pericarditis the thickness of the pericardium, which can be measured directly by MRI, should be equal to 4 mm or thicker [2]; pericardial thickening can eventually be limited to the heart's right section alone, or even to a less extended region. Such evaluation may become difficult in the presence of a concomitant effusion. The presence of calcium, typical of this pathology cannot be directly proved by MRI

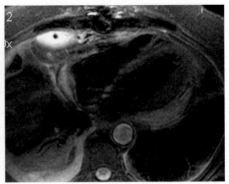

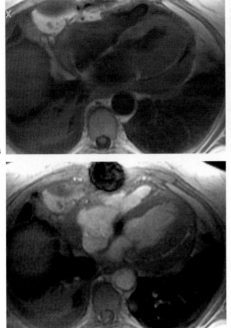

Fig. 8.3 a-c. Patient with previous cardio-surgical intervention complicated by purulent pleuro-pericarditis. In the axial "black blood" images (a), triple IR (b), and cine-FIESTA (c) underscore the pleural and pericardial deposit, the latter partially organized and hypointense in cine images. In addition there is purulent material in the left paracardial region with small gaseous bubbles

because the absence of signal from calcium is the same as that created by a thickening of the pericardium. A CT investigation is therefore mandatory.

The diagnosis of constrictive pericarditis is based on coexisting anamnestic, clinical and anatomical criteria (tubular left ventricle, dilatation of the right atrium and of the superior vena cava) and evidence of a thickening of the pericardium (Fig. 8.4).

It must be underlined that the detection of thickenings and calcifications of the pericardium are not indicative of constrictive pericarditis if there are no coexisting symptoms and clinical signs.

8.1.6 Hematoma

MRI is particularly useful in the diagnosis of pericardial hematoma due to the peculiar signal characteristics emitted from the catabolites of hemoglobin, which can lead the operator to the nature and the date of the bleeding. Hematomas in a sub-acute phase show a heterogeneous signal with high intensity areas in T1 and T2 images. The organized chronic hematomas present areas of low signal intensity which are seen better in GRE images in relation to calcifications and hemosiderin.

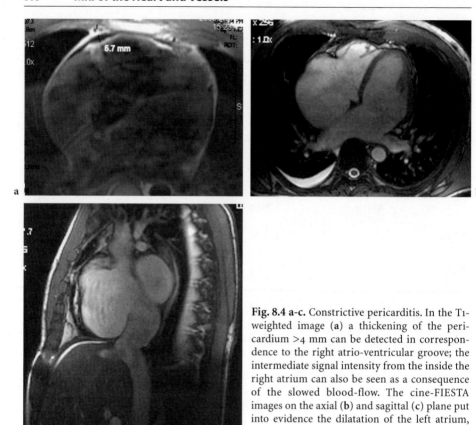

Fig. 8.4 a-c. Constrictive pericarditis. In the T1-weighted image (**a**) a thickening of the pericardium >4 mm can be detected in correspondence to the right atrio-ventricular groove; the intermediate signal intensity from the inside the right atrium can also be seen as a consequence of the slowed blood-flow. The cine-FIESTA images on the axial (**b**) and sagittal (**c**) plane put into evidence the dilatation of the left atrium, the tubular aspect of the right ventricle, and the dilatation of the inferior vena cava

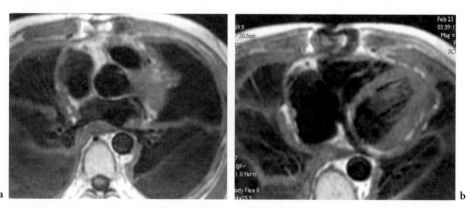

Fig. 8.5 a, b. Pericardial mesothelioma. The broad thickening of the pericardium in T1-weighted images (**a, b**) and the neoplastic involvement of the pleura

The absence of flow and the detection of the contrast agent are the elements that differentiate the hematoma from pseudoaneurysms and masses of other nature.

Pericardial tumors are treated in detail ahead in the chapter on cardiac tumors. Here, special mention should be given, however, to the malignant primary mesotheliome of the pericardium that can manifest itself as an isolated effusion, and only on occasions is associated to nodules with a specific signal characteristics (Fig. 8.5). In the case of pleural mesotheliome it is not rare to incur in a case of a direct invasion.

8.2 Mediastinum

8.2.1 Introduction

This part of the chapter deals with indications and limits of applying MRI to non-vascular pathology of the mediastinum and in particular to tumors. MRI represents a useful complement to CT whenever it becomes necessary to establish through multiplanar vision the exact spatial relation between masses and surrounding structures. Despite the fact that continuous methodological and technological developments have lead to a marked improvement of image quality, MRI is not a routine procedure in the study of the mediastinum, where instead CT is the technique of choice. Yet, in the evaluation of mediastinal masses, MRI can provide information on the tissue components of a lesion that, together with shape, dimension, and geographic location represents the base for differential diagnostics of the tumoral pathology of this district.

The most frequent cases in which MRI is suggested are: tumors of nervous origin, pre-operatory evaluation of mediastinal tumors, and patients with contraindications to iodinated contrast.

8.2.2 Technological and methodological aspects

The mediastinum is an anatomical district located between the two pleural cavities, the diaphragm and the superior thoracic outlet, and includes several anatomical structures, among which the heart and the great vessels. The artifacts caused in these regions by breathing and flow can be reduced by synchronizing the acquisition with cardiac and respiratory cycles, or by making the acquisition during breath-holds.

Synchronization with heart beat is performed with the application of electrocardiographic triggering: to obtain an adequate R wave, specific MRI electrodes are positioned on the rib cage or on the patient's back as in the study of the heart.

According to the clinical aim, the technique employs either a body coil, a surface coil, or a phased array – whichever is the most suitable for increasing the Signal-to-Noise Ratio (SNR).

To study the mediastinum, it is advisable to begin by acquiring a first series of T1-weighted coronal images with a large thickness for a first impression on the conditions of the mediastinum and of the chest; this will help position the subsequent axial acquisitions. The integration of the two planes allows the analysis of those regions of the mediastinum that are difficult to evaluate with other techniques, such as the aorto-pulmonary window or the sottocarenal region.

T1 and T2 axial images, with a thickness ranging according to the diagnostic query, are synchronized with the cardiac and/or respiratory cycle; the flow signal is saturated to minimize the artifacts. The fast sequences or the Turbo T2-weighted sequences, that have substituted conventional T2 SE thanks to their much shorter acquisition times, are acquired with prospective respiratory gating. This allows the acquisition of data during the expiratory phase, eliminating the artifacts caused in most part by the subcutaneous adipose tissue. In conventional T1-weighted acquisitions, respiratory compensation is used instead; this procedure retrospectively reorganizes the encoding lines of K-space in a manner that eliminates the artifacts.

The study of flow is performed with GRE sequences. Thanks to the use of a very short TR, the images can be acquired in breath holding or, if the patient is not compliant, in free breathing by using an ECG trigger approach (cine-MRI).

At present, ultrafast sequences such as SSFP are available and are prevalently used for kinetic studies that allow to perform acquisitions in breath hold (See Chapter 7).

Finally, for the study of the sovraclavear o retrosternal region, the use of a sagittal scanning plane is recommended.

8.2.3 Clinical applications

The main application of MRI for the study of the mediastinum is in cases of tumoral pathologies, with the aim of obtaining a more accurate characterization of the mediastinal masses of various nature.

Primitive tumors of the mediastinum are represented by a heterogeneous group of neoplastic, congenital, and inflammatory alterations; approximately 2/3 of the lesions are of benign nature. The lesions, sub-grouped according to their location, are:

– *Anterior mediastinum* (posterior to the sternum and anterior to the heart and vessels)
  Thymic pathologies, mediastinal goiter, parathyroid adenoma, lymphangioma, dysontogenetic tumors.

- *Medium mediastinum* (includes heart and vessels, trachea and bronchi) Cysts (bronchogenic, henterogenic, pericardial), carcinoma of the esophagus.

- *Posterior mediastimun* (delimited frontally by the heart and extending to the thoracic vertebrae) Neurogenic tumors, lymphomas which are ubiquitous in this district.

Tumors of the thymus are the most frequent tumors of the anterior mediastinum. There are no characteristic MRI signal features that aid in differentiating these lesions from other mediastinal expansive lesions. In T1-weighted images thymomas have a signal similar to that of muscle and a high signal in T2-weighted images, sometimes inhomogeneous due to the presence of cystic, necrotic, or hemorrhagic components (Fig. 8.6). The spreading of the tumor beyond the capsula and infiltration of neighboring structures are indicative criteria of malignancy of the lesion (invasive thymoma, Fig. 8.7); a multinodular aspect of the lesion in T2 is more frequently described with invasive thymomas.

MRI is sometimes used in the pre-surgical phase and in the posttherapy follow-up of the tumoral pathology of the thymus, to get a better contrast resolution than that provided by CT, especially in the evaluation of the invasion of surrounding structures.

Carcinomas of the thymus are a heterogeneous group of malignant epithelial neoplasias that have a local invasiveness and metastasic potential. They are masses with scarcely defined limits, infiltrating, often associated to pleural and pericardial effusion. The differential diagnosis with invasive thymoma in absence of metastasis and enlarged lymph nodes is difficult.

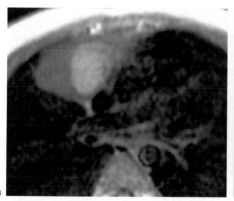 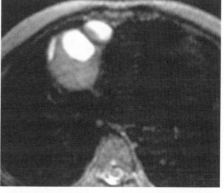

a   b

Fig. 8.6 a, b. Thymoma. The lesion presents a hemorrhagic component that can be recognized in the T1-weighted image (a) for its hyperintensity and the presence of a cystic component, which is well defined in the T2-weighted image (b)

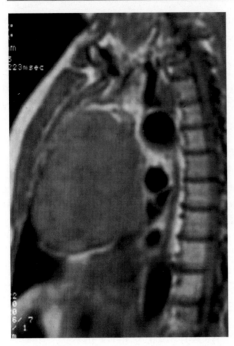

Fig. 8.7. Invasive thymoma. Voluminous thymic neoformation that has invaded the mediastinal fat and extends to the anterior chest wall

The thymic carcinoid is a rare neoplasia with characteristics similar to those of carcinoids of other districts; endocrine alterations are found in 50% of cases (often the Cushing syndrome), while the classical form has low incidence. It manifests itself as a lobulate mass with cystic and necrotic areas, sometimes with pointy dystrophic calcifications, and often tends to local invasiveness. Metastases of lymph nodes are reported in 73% of cases [3].

The thymolipoma is a rare benign tumor with slow growth, mostly in young adults. It manifests itself as an encapsulated mass formed by adipose and thymus tissue that often extends to the antero-inferior mediastinum and is characterized by the fact it changes shape with movement of the body. MRI reveals the classical combination of parenchymal and fatty tissue; if the latter is prevailing, this structure may not be distinguishable from a lipoma.

The use of MRI for the study of thyroidal masses is rare; sometimes the study of large goiters plunged into the mediastinum is requested to get a better picture (than that provided by CT images) of the altered anatomy and on the relationship between the goiter and the neighboring structures.

A true utility of MRI is found instead in the evaluation of parathyroid adenomas located within the mediastinum, which is a district of difficult exploration by means of echo-Doppler; also CT, which is limited to axial scanning, provides a less elegant and clear representation of the cervical-thoracic outlet. The examination of the neck is performed with a surface coil, a small FOV (16-36 cm), and a thin scanning thickness (3-5 mm) because of the small size that the ademomas usually have. The study of the mediastinal region implies the use of larger FOV (28-36 cm) and of coils suitable for this district.

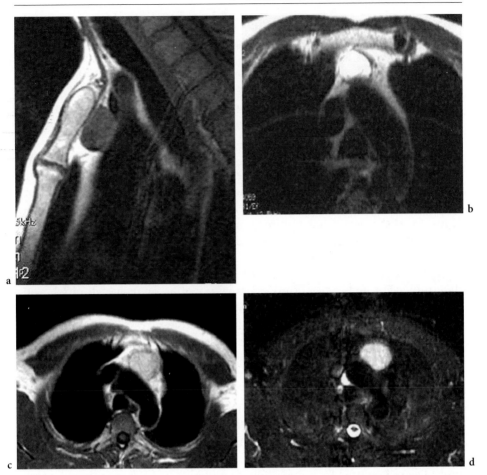

Fig. 8.8 a-d. Typical parathyroid adenoma. Typical signal features by the retrosternal lesion: low intensity in T1 sagittal image (**a**), and a high intensity in the T2-weighted axial image (**b**). A different case with atypical signal features: high signal intensity in T1 (**c**) and STIR (**d**) sequences

The "typical" parathyroid adenoma is characterized by a low and high signal, respectively in the T1- and T2-weighted images (Fig. 8.8a, b), and has a marked enhancement after administration of the contrast agent. There have also been cases of adenomas with low signal in T2 [4] or hyperintense in the T1-weighted images (Fig. 8.8c, d).

The diagnostic accuracy of MRI reaches high values especially if the anatomical findings correlate to the functional findings of scintigraphy [5].

Dysontogenic tumors represent 10-15% of the primitive masses in the mediastinum and are usually found in young adults. They occur more frequently in the anterior mediastinum (only 5% in the posterior); in 80% of the cases they are benign.

A theratoma is a capsuled tumor characterized by the coexistence of solid areas and cystic areas; it contains elements of various origin: ecto-(teeth and hairs), meso-(bone), and endodermic (intestinal and pancreatic tissue). The presence of solid tissue is described in almost all theratomas; the presence of liquid component in 76%, and calcium in 54%; these elements together are present in 36% of cases, while 15% are purely cystic [6]. A liquid/fat level is considered highly indicative of these lesions, yet quite rare [7]; in these pathologies it is important to adopt techniques for fat suppression to discriminate the adipose component from a macro-hemorrhagic area, which are both hyperintense in T1.

In MRI images the aspect varies according to the composition of the tumor: cystic areas, fat, liquid/fat levels, focal and linear calcifications, and ossifications are peculiar to these lesions; the pleiomorphic aspects of such tumors allow a differential analysis with lesions of the thymus or lymphomas. However, MRI is less reliable in recognizing calcification compared to CT.

Immature tumoral forms (seminomas: malignant tumors of germinal cells) do not have specific characteristics and their malignancy is hypothesized based on their tendency to infiltrate other surrounding structures and the presence of metastases. Tumoral masses can be scarcely delimited; calcifications are rarer and a capsule enhanced by contrast medium is usually observed. In these cases it is important that serologic results (such as values of AFP, β-HCG) and imaging features correlate. Indeed, the values of AFP and β-HCG are positive in case of malignant tumor of the germinal cells, and only 10% of subjects with seminoma have high values of β-HCG, while AFP values are always in normal range.

Congenital cystic lesions (bronchogenic, esophageal duplication, neurohenteric, pericardial and thymic) represent 15-20% of the mediastinal masses: they are spherical lesions, well delimited by a capsule, with liquid contents, and delimited by epithelium. In MR images they appear characterized by the typical signal emitted by liquids (low T1 and high T2). Cysts with non-serous liquid contents given by the presence of proteins, hemorrhage, calcium, or mucous can yield higher attenuation values with CT (>20 HU), and perhaps do not appear in T1-weighted MR images with the typical signal of liquid. Such lesions preserve however a high intensity in T2-weighted images, which is extremely useful, together with the feeble wall enhancement by the contrast medium, for a differential diagnosis with solid masses [8] (Fig. 8.9).

The mediastinal lympho-angioma represents 0.7-4.5% of tumors in the mediastinum and is typical of the newborn and infants. It is formed by multiple cyst-like formations, sometimes snake-like, typically located in the region of the neck or axilla. Approximately 10% later extend to the mediastinum [9]. These tumors are grouped according to the size of the lymphatic vessels into: simple (capillaries), cavernous, or with cysts. The latter are the most common.

In MR images the lympho-angioma is characterized by signal heterogeneity in T1 images, the high intensity signal in T2 (indicative of liquid contents), and by marked enhancement of septa after administration of the contrast

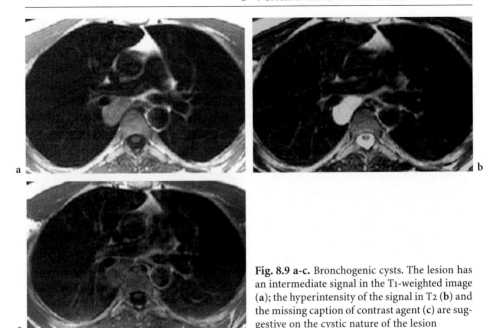

Fig. 8.9 a-c. Bronchogenic cysts. The lesion has an intermediate signal in the T1-weighted image (**a**); the hyperintensity of the signal in T2 (**b**) and the missing caption of contrast agent (**c**) are suggestive on the cystic nature of the lesion

agent. The recognition of the septa inside the lesion is more immediate with MRI than with other techniques.

MRI represents the technique of choice in the study of neurogenic tumors (10% of the mediastinum masses in adults, 30% in children) that are typically located in the posterior mediastinum, owing to the more sophisticated and reliable demonstration it offers on the relations of the tumor with the conjugation foramens, the spinal canal, spinal chord, and bone [10]. The age of the patient and the growth pattern are the pivotal elements for establishing the benign or malignant nature of the lesion. The tumors originating from the peripheral nerves and from myelin coating are more common in the adult (schwannoma, neurofibroma and neurogenic sarcoma); those originating from the sympathetic ganglia are more common in children (ganglioneuroma, ganglioneuroblastoma, neuroblastoma).

The schwannoma or neurinoma grows eccentrically from the nerve of origin, compressing the fibers of the nerve; it has a pseudo-capsule, and MRI generally shows a high central signal intensity in relation to the cystic degeneration and an outer component with lower signal intensity, in T2-dependant images; usually the enhancement following the administration of a contrast medium is marked (Fig. 8.10).

Contrarily to the neurinoma, the neurofibroma grows centrally to the nerve which remains trapped in the mass; it is non-capsulated and usually presents a high signal in T2, at times with a 'salt and pepper' or 'target' aspect;

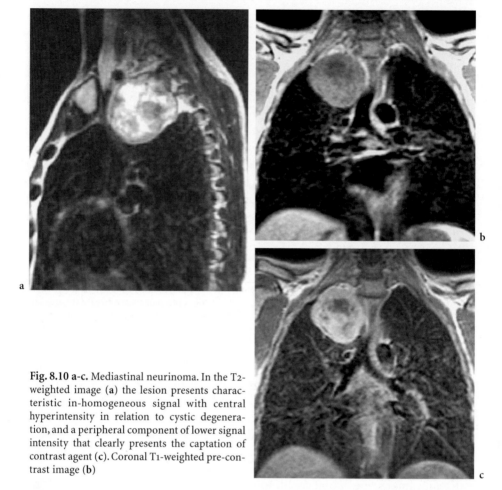

Fig. 8.10 a-c. Mediastinal neurinoma. In the T2-weighted image (**a**) the lesion presents characteristic in-homogeneous signal with central hyperintensity in relation to cystic degeneration, and a peripheral component of lower signal intensity that clearly presents the captation of contrast agent (**c**). Coronal T1-weighted pre-contrast image (**b**)

it has a central fibrous area of low signal intensity enhanced after contrast administration, and a distal area of high signal and a mixed contents that does not show enhancement after administration of the contrast. This aspect is not found in all cases and can resemble a neurinoma, but is however a sign of benignancy. The cystic degeneration is more rare than in the case of neurinoma. Both tumors can grow inside the conjunction foramens and extend into the spinal canal.

Radiological imaging offers a scarce aid in diagnosing the malignant form of peripheral nerves; criteria suggesting malignancy (dimensions, surrounding oedema, hemorrhage-related lack of homogeneity and necrosis, invasion of the adipose planes, involvement of lymph nodes and bones, pleural effusion) are non-specific and with no absolute value.

The ganglioneuroma is a benign tumor that affects teenagers and young adults; they are undistinguishable from other neurogenetic tumors even if a spiraloid aspect has been described as typical in T1-weighted images, which corresponds to layers of Schwann cells and collagen fibers, and heterogeneous hyperintensity of the signal in T2-weighted images.

The high intensity of the signal in T2 is related to the abundant mixoid component, and scarce cellular and fiber component; on the other hand an intermediate signal indicates hypercellularity, an abundant fibrous component and a scarce mixoid component (Fig. 8.11). In dynamic studies, enhancement is not homogenous, but rather delayed and gradually increases over time [11].

The ganglioneuroblastoma affects children of older age groups in respect to the neuroblastoma and is less common. It can appear as a large round mass or small and elongated. The larger masses show minimal or no signal change after administration of the contrast medium. Most neuroblastomas occur in children below 5 years of age and origin in the suprarenal glands, 15-30% in the mediastinum. The extradural invasion of the spinal canal is frequent, sometimes asymptomatic and can be accurately demonstrated by MRI.

Lymphomas (especially that of Hodgkin), represent one of the most frequent neoplasias of the mediastinum both as an isolated manifestation and as a disease associated to a systemic involvement. CT continues to be the technique of choice in the staging of this pathology as it can also evaluate an eventual involvement of the pulmonary parenchyma. The use of MRI for

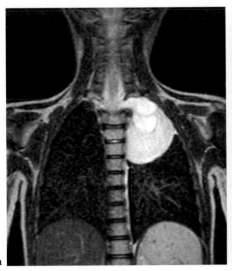
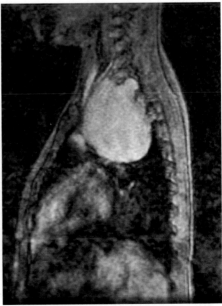

a

b

Fig. 8.11 a, b. Ganglioneuroma. The lesion appears markedly in-homogeneous; there is a recognizable mixoid component at the center, and a peripheral portion of fibrous nature, rich of cells with intermediate intensity. The relationship of the mass with the intervertebral foramen is well visible in the coronal (**a**) and the sagittal (**b**) images

evaluating the activity of the disease of the lymphomatose residues treated with chemo- and radiotherapy is still argued and non-reliable.

A study [12] that analyzed the changes of the signal from the masses subjected to treatment after the introduction of a contrast agent demonstrates that in cases of total remission, enhancement of the residual mass decreases until reaching the enhancement of muscular tissue; a marked enhancement and a growth in size represent fundamental points in the diagnosis of persistence or reactivation of the disease.

References

1. Wang Zf, Gautham PR, Reddy P et al (2003) CT and MR imaging of pericardial disease Radiographics 23:167-180
2. Smith WHT, Beacock DJ, Goddard AJ et al (2001) Magnetic resonance evaluation of the pericardium. Br J Radiol 74:384-932
3. Strollo DC, Rosado-de-Christenson ML, Jett JR (1997) Primary mediastinal tumors. Part I. Tumors of the anterior mediastinum. Chest 112:511-522
4. Auffermann W, Gooding GAW, Okerland MD et al (1988) Diagnosis of recurrent hyperparathyroidism: comparison of MR imaging and other imaging techniques. AJR 150:1027-33
5. Gotway MB, Reddy GP, Webb R et al (2001) Comparison between MR imaging and 99m Tc MIBI scintigraphy in the evaluation of recurrent or persistent hyperparathyroidism. Radiology 218:783-790
6. Moeller KH, Rosado-de-Christenson ML, Templeton PA (1997) Mediastinal mature teratoma: imaging features. Am J Roentgenol 169:985-990
7. Fulcher AS, Proto AV, Jolles H (1990) Cystic teratoma of the mediastinum: demonstration of fat/fluid level. Am J Roentgenol 154:259-260
8. Jeung MY, Bernard G, Gangi A et al (2002) Imaging of cystic masses of the mediastinum. Radiographics 22:79-93
9. Faul JL, Berry GJ, Colby TV et al (2000) Thoracic lymphangiomas, lymphangiectasis, lymphangiomatosis, and lymphatic dysplasia syndrome. Am J Respir Crit Care Med 161:1037-1046
10. Strollo DC, Rosado-de-Christenson ML, Jett JR (1997) Primary mediastinal tumors. Part II. Tumors of the middle and posterior mediastinum. Chest 112:1344-1357
11. Zhang Y, Nishimura H, Kato S et al (2001) MRI of ganglioneuroma: histologic correlation study. J Comput Assist Tomogr 25(4):617-623
12. Rahmouni A, Divine M, Lepage E et al (2001) Mediastinal lymphoma: quantitative changes in gadolinium enhancement at MR imaging after treatment. Radiology 219 (3):621-862

9 Thoracic aorta

Massimo Lombardi

9.1 Introduction

The study of the thoracic aorta represents one of the most frequent requests to cardiovascular Magnetic Resonance Imaging (MRI) labs. The study of the vessel can be performed by MRI along its entire coursing with a detail and accuracy that equals at least that of Transesophageal Echography (TEE) and spiral Computed Tomography (CT). The relatively modest use of MRI compared to these other techniques is mainly due to its scarce diffusion and, consequently, the reduced familiarity of clinicians to its use.

In the study of the thoracic aorta, MRI represents a very elegant solution, with some significant advantages over the two techniques mentioned above.

The advantages that MRI has as compared to TEE are the wider field of view, greater topographical detail, and especially its non-invasiveness. Transesophageal Echography maintains its supremacy especially in cases of urgency or with a scarcely collaborative patient, but is less efficient than MRI in the study of the ascending aorta and the arch of the aorta and requires a highly skilled operator to follow the tortuous coursing of the vessel, as often happens. Moreover, TEE is a semi-invasive technique that is usually not well tolerated by the patient.

The advantages of MRI over CT can be summarized in a better capacity of visualizing the ascending aorta – which is an important diagnostic detail as for example in the cases of type A dissection of the Stanford classification – and in the fact that MRI does not require the use of an iodinated contrast medium and, obviously, the use of non-ionizing radiation. Compared to spiral CT, MRI still suffers from a somewhat complex execution and, in many cases, from the lack of collaboration of the patient, in addition to its absolute and relative contraindications. Obviously the choice of the methodology strictly depends on the equipment and expertise available.

Altogether, MRI demonstrates excellent diagnostic accuracy and represents one of the two techniques of choice, along with spiral CT, for the study in stable patients, while TEE and spiral CT are still preferred in acute cases or scarcely collaborative patients [1].

9.2 Patient preparation

The study of the thoracic aorta foresees the use of surface coils, in particular phased array coils: whenever available, they should be preferred as they yield a much better Signal-to-Noise Ratio (SNR). In alternative to these two systems, also body coils may be used. In the case the disease to be examined concerns an area expanding beyond the thoracic district (as with aortic dissection or an aneurysmal pathology extending under the diaphragm) multi-station imaging or surfing techniques can be used. In such cases an "ad hoc" coil is employed; otherwise, a surface coil is positioned in the station that requires the best SNR, while the body coil is used for the other remaining stations.

Some sequences (as dynamic sequences) require a cardiac trigger; generally it is sufficient to use the peripheral pulse on the patient's finger as triggering, while ECG is used with sequences that expressly require it, or when the operator plans to visualize the aortic valve during the same session.

9.3 Imaging techniques

In the study of the thoracic aorta, we may rely on both static sequences (Spin Echo, Fast-Spin Echo, Inversion Recovery) and dynamic sequences such as SPGR, and, more recently, on ultrafast sequences such as SSFP. Futhermore, 3D angiographic sequences that imply contrast agent administration, such as contrast enhanced MRA (CEMRA), are relatively easy to obtain and extremely useful [2-4].

The aims of the static techniques are to establish in detail topographic relationships and characterize the vessel walls. In the SE T1-weighted sequences the presaturation pulse cancels out the signal coming from blood, thereby producing a clear contrast between circulating blood and the wall tissue. It is necessary to have an ECG or peripheral pulse trigger. The TE generally varies between 20 and 30 msec, while TR depends on the heart rate. With the Fast SE T1-weighted techniques (those suggested today), which presuppose additional RF pulses, it is possible to reduce the acquisition time of each image to 10-20 sec and, therefore, obtain it in breath-hold, gaining a marked improvement in image quality. The fast techniques allow to obtain also T2-weighted images in inversion recovery, a fact which further improves the capacity of describing anatomical and histopathological details of the vessel wall. The slice thickness should be between 5-8 mm and the matrix should allow a high spatial resolution. The sequence must be thoroughly optimized for each patient and be performed by a skilled operator.

The combination of the images in T1, T2 and IR is the ideal solution for detecting the presence of intraluminal thrombosis, intra-wall hemorrhage, or wall oedema as in the case of acute artheritic processes. It is advisable to associate the images in para-sagittal projection (parallel to the course of

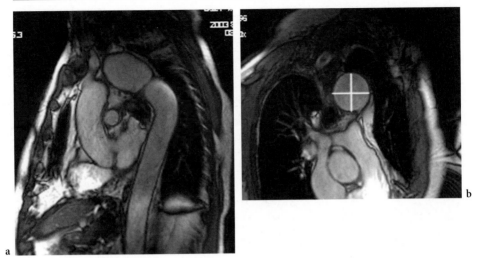

Fig. 9.1 a, b. (a) Image of the para-sagittal projection of the thoracic aorta with ultrafast dynamic sequence (SSFP, FIESTA). (b) Short axis images of the vessel at the level of the aneurysm right after the emergency of the left subclavian artery

the aortic arc) to images orthogonal to the vessel's major local axis (Fig. 9.1a, b).

Dynamic techniques as GRE (TE 20-40 msec) and especially breath-held Fast SPGR (TE 2-3 msec, TR 4-8 msec) and ultrafast techniques (SSFP) permit a very useful imaging of the vessel for evidencing flow turbulences or dynamic wall alterations (as for intimal flaps, which require a high temporal resolution). In addition, dynamic techniques facilitate the measurement of the external as well as endoluminal diameters of the vessel.

Phase Contrast (PC) images can be used to quantitatively evaluate endovascular flows, which can turn extremely useful in cases such as aortic coarctation, aortic dissection, or aortic valvular regurgitation.

Although images obtained with ultrafast techniques like SSFP are more contrasted and with higher definition, they are much more prone to artifacts, which sometimes make SPGR preferable.

For sizing, it is better to use parasagittal planes parallel to the aortic arc (Fig. 9.1a) or planes obtained orthogonally to the longitudinal axis of the segment being examined (Fig. 9.1b).

Static images, and in part dynamic images, are indispensable for evaluating wall morphology and details like intraluminal thrombosis that often accompany aortic pathologies, while dynamic images – and even more so 3D angiographic images – are suggested for evaluating the lumen, and for identifying in case of aortic dissection the entrance site (eventually using virtual navigation techniques) (Fig. 9.2a, b).

Today, CEMRA is considered an indispensable technique in the MRI study of many aortic pathologies. As in all the "white blood" techniques based on

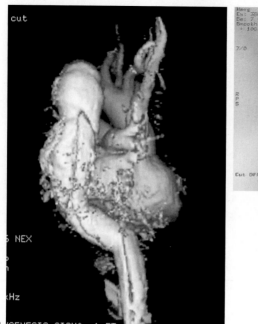
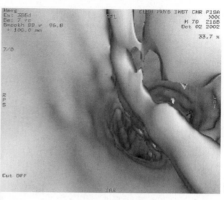

Fig. 9.2 a, b. (a) Reconstruction according to the volume rendering approach of aortic dissection type B. (b) Virtual navigation inside the dissected aorta with evidence of communication between true lumen and false lumen

the Time Of Flight (TOF) concept, signal intensity of flowing blood is exalted by the entrance of fresh magnetized spins into the sampled volume, while stationary tissues are saturated by the rapid application of RF pulses. However, in CEMRA sequences, signal intensity does not strictly depend on inflow of blood with a non-null magnetic moment, but mostly depends on the shortening effect of T_1 induced by the contrast medium. In other words, the presence of contrast medium can induce a signal increase that is independent from the velocity of flow. Hence, it is understood that CEMRA presupposes signal acquisition once the contrast medium has reached an optimal level in the segment being examined. The coordination between the arrival of the contrast agent in situ and the beginning of the acquisition is achieved in several ways.

In addition to the well-known *best guess* approach that uses the presumed time elapsing between the start of the injection of the contrast medium and the beginning of data acquisition, there are basically three other techniques for identifying the optimal moment for starting the acquisition. The most lengthy, but accurate, is based on the preventive calculation of the circulating time by means of a bolus test (3.4 cc of contrast medium i.v. is sufficient), and the monitoring of the vessel until the arrival of the contrast agent. The second method is more automatic; it is based on computerized algorithms that calculate signal intensity over a sampling volume positioned inside the vessel and an automatic 3D acquisition start up, once a specific concentration of contrast medium has been reached inside the sampling volume (Smart Prep). Finally, there are semiautomatic techniques where the operator visually monitors the vessel until the arrival of the contrast medium, activating the acquisition in an interactive manner.

The calculation of the transit time can be made using several sequences in Gradient Echo or a sequence that is very sensitive to contrast mediums such as fast turbo-FLASH, SPGR-ET, and others. Acquiring images in a repetitive manner over known times allows to easily identify the arrival of the bolus of contrast medium and its evolution in time.

Once the transit time has been calculated, the next CEMRA scanning is started taking into account some variables, eventually with the aid of correction formulas such as:

delay time = (time to peak intensity in the bolus test)/2) + (calculated length of acquisition/2)

where the delay time is the time between the starting of contrast injection and the starting of acquisition so as to achieve an optimal filling of K-space [3]. This procedure requires extensive experience on the equipment available.

It guarantees a good result at the cost of a greater effort of execution, and with respect to the automatic methods is surely preferable in patients with turbulent flow, as in the case of wide aneurysms or in presence of intimal flaps, phenomena that may lead to system detection errors of the optimal intravascular concentration of the contrast medium.

In the case of automatic detection of the contrast medium for the study of the thoracic aorta, it is suggested to position the sampling volume at the level of the aortic arc using a short axis of the vessel, as in Figure 9.3a. This method, which has the advantage of optimizing the scanning starting moment toward a better SNR, is burdened by a certain number of failures in detecting the arrival of the contrast medium, even if it guarantees excellent image quality when well optimized.

The use of an interactive system seems to facilitate the task of the operator, who must however be somewhat expert to understand when the moment of optimal increase of signal intensity arrives and set off the real acquisition sequence.

The injection of the contrast medium, which presupposes an injector, is generally performed with a speed ranging from 2-4 ml/sec, according to the MRI scanner available. The dose of contrast medium is generally between 0.2 and 0.3 mmol/kg.

The 3D sequence can be synchronized with the ECG to eliminate the artifacts from pulsating flow, determining an improvement of the image at the cost of some additional work. This option requires, however, an optimal triggering with the ECG signal during the entire acquisition time.

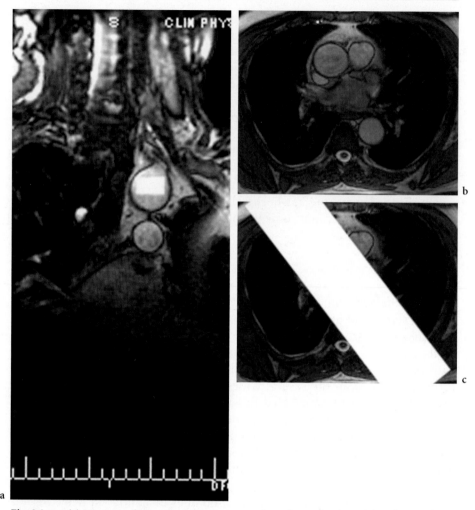

Fig. 9.3 a-c. (a) Images in short axis of the aortic arc, where the tracker is positioned to guide the automatic starting of the 3D CEMRA acquisition according to the smart prep procedure; (b) Axial image at level of the ascending aorta used as a scout for the positioning of the 3D CEMRA volume (white rectangle in Figure c)

In order to visualize the entire vessel from the aortic root to the diaphragmatic aorta the operator positions the acquisition volume in a parasagittal position taking an axial image as reference (Fig. 9.3b, c). The thickness of partitions is 3-3.2 mm. The acquisition is performed with breath-holding, generally in mild expiration, and the entire aorta up to the diaphragmatic area and the first tract of the epiaortic vessels are visualized in the volume obtained, providing important detail if the involvement of the vessels in the pathological process needs to be evaluated.

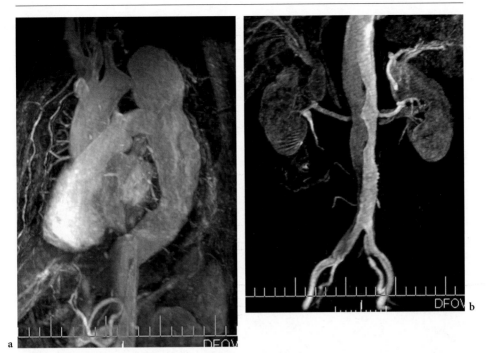

Fig. 9.4 a, b. Acquisition in two consecutive stations to acquire with a single bolus the thoracic aorta (a), and the abdominal aorta (b) with the 3D CEMRA technique

With the 3D methods available today, it is possible to study the thoracic and the abdominal aorta, the iliac aa. and femoral aa. during a single injection of contrast medium, by using methods of sequential acquisition with 2-3 stations (Fig. 9.4a, b). Whenever the choice is for a multi-station acquisition, the contrast medium bolus (e.g. 0.2 mmol/kg, 2 ml/sec) can be followed by a maintenance of 0.1 mmol/kg (0.6 ml/sec).

9.4 Data processing

It is suggested that the vessel dimension be evaluated in two-dimensional images (static or even better dynamic), taking care of locating the major local axis to avoid errors of measurement as can happen, for example, with axial images. For this reason it is advisable to utilize parasagittal images for the antero-posterior dimensions, and orthogonal planes to the major local axis for both the anterior-posterior and the lateral-lateral dimensions. The dimensions usually reported are those of the aortic root, the ascending aorta, the aortic arc, the isthmic region, and the descending aorta at the level of the diaphragm.

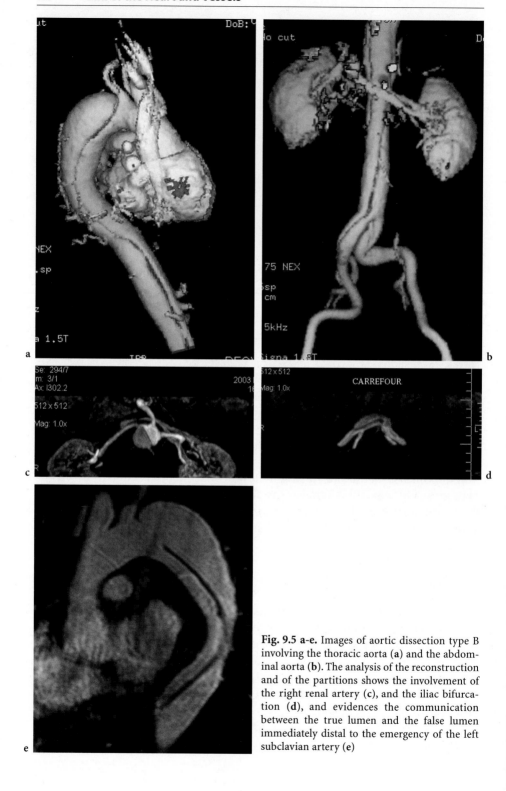

Fig. 9.5 a-e. Images of aortic dissection type B involving the thoracic aorta (**a**) and the abdominal aorta (**b**). The analysis of the reconstruction and of the partitions shows the involvement of the right renal artery (**c**), and the iliac bifurcation (**d**), and evidences the communication between the true lumen and the false lumen immediately distal to the emergency of the left subclavian artery (**e**)

While there is no need of postprocessing for static and dynamic images, the images obtained by CEMRA require a precise reconstruction and evidencing job of the vessel's entire luminogram (Fig. 9.5a, b). Sometimes, as in the case of dissection, it can be just as useful to visualize the single partitions and to perform a Multiplanar Volume Reconstruction (MPVR) in order to visualize the involvement of the large collaterals and the communication sites between the true and false lumen (Fig. 9.5c, d).

9.5 Acquired pathologies of the thoracic aorta

9.5.1 Aneurysms of the aorta

This disease is associated with the aging of the population and is in numerical expansion. To give a practical definition of what an aneurysm is, we can say there is an aneurysm when the vessel diameter has stretched by a factor of 1.5 compared to its expected dimension [4]. The etiology and physiopathology of the aneurysmatic disease is not completely understood. The correlation with atherosclerotic processes is an important association but does not have a direct causal relation. Several factors have been hypothesized: congenital factors such as the degeneration of the tunica media in the syndrome of Marfan (alterations of the extra-cellular elastic fibers), and genetic factors that justify the familiar incidence of thoracic and abdominal aneurysm. In general, we can state that atherosclerotic processes are more frequently associated with aneurysms of the descending aorta and less with those of the ascending aorta where degenerative (such as Marfan) and infective diseases (as lues) prevail. While research continues along its path toward understanding the etiopathological aspects, some physiopathological aspects are quite clear and form the basis for a correct diagnostic pathway. The size of the aneurysm is the only documented risk factor for rupture (16% for a diameter between 4 and 5.9 cm, that increases to 31% for dimensions equal to, or higher than, 6 cm). For this reason the aneurysm must be accurately measured for its internal, external, anterior-posterior, and lateral-lateral dimensions. Other relevant measurements are the longitudinal extension of the aneurysm, the dimensions of the proximal and the distal neck, and the distance from epiaortic vessels, which heavily condition the therapeutic procedure to be chosen, determining whether – for example – an endoprosthesic therapy can be adopted or not. The presence and severity of the aortic valvulopathy that is eventually associated to dilatation or dissection of the ascending aorta covers a key role in a future surgical intervention. Altogether, MRI has demonstrated to be, with its various acquisition techniques, an optimal and repeatable method for such diagnostic purposes (Fig. 9.6a-d).

In addition, it has recently been demonstrated that minor vessels such as spinal arteries, in particular the Adamkiewicz artery, can be visualized in a

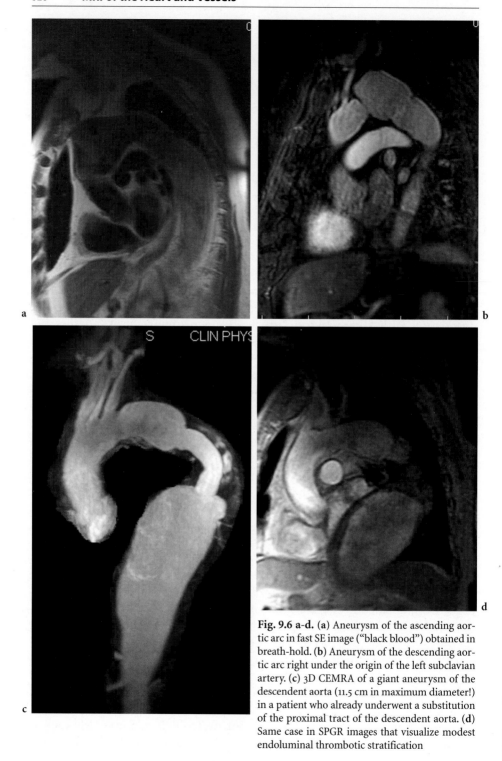

Fig. 9.6 a-d. (a) Aneurysm of the ascending aortic arc in fast SE image ("black blood") obtained in breath-hold. (b) Aneurysm of the descending aortic arc right under the origin of the left subclavian artery. (c) 3D CEMRA of a giant aneurysm of the descendent aorta (11.5 cm in maximum diameter!) in a patient who already underwent a substitution of the proximal tract of the descendent aorta. (d) Same case in SPGR images that visualize modest endoluminal thrombotic stratification

diagnostic manner. Data on this issue, however, are limited to small cohorts of patients and this task is sometimes hindered by the wide anatomical variability of the spinal vessels and in particular of the artery of Adamkiewicz [6].

9.5.2 Aortic dissection

This pathology is potentially life threatening to the patient and therefore requires an immediate and exhaustive cognitive effort that goes beyond the simple diagnostic confirmation. The involvement of the ascending aorta, or its non-involvement in the dissection process (respectively Type A and B according to the Stanford classification) must be evaluated with maximum accuracy because the involvement of the aortic arc and of the ascending aorta foresees a definitely worse prognosis and requires an immediate intervention of corrective surgery (Fig. 9.7a, b). The same accuracy applies to the localization of entrance and re-entry sites, and the involvement of the large arterial collaterals at the level of both the aortic arc and the abdomen (celiac trunk, renal arteries, mesenteric vessels, iliac vessels). It is recommended to have precise information on the diameters of the aorta (external and internal), the degree of flow supply to the false lumen (an important diagnostic index), the involvement of the aortic valve, and so on.

As we have said earlier, MRI has a diagnostic accuracy equal to that of multilayer CT and may be employed in alternative when the patient's conditions allow so [1].

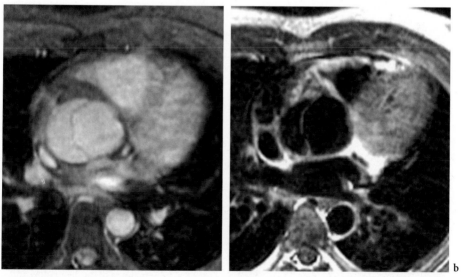

a   b

Fig. 9.7 a, b. Images of axial projection of aortic dissection type A. The intimal flap is evident both in the SPGR "white blood" image (**a**) and in "black blood" SE image (**b**); in both of them the communication between true lumen and false lumen is evident

Although it has been stated that the diagnosis of dissection can be performed in a few minutes with dynamic images alone (SPGR, SSFP, etc.), there is no doubt that phenomena such as perivascolar hemorrhage, pleural or pericardial effusion, as well as the presence of thrombotic material in the true and false lumens are better described by Fast SE T1-weighted and eventually T2-weighted images. The quantification of flow in the false lumen (an objective not easy to achieve) can be done by PC sequences, which add a high degree of accuracy toward the correct formulation of prognosis [5].

If instead the large aortic collaterals are involved, the exam should be completed with a CEMRA acquisition (Figs. 9.4a, b, 9.5a-e).

An accurate combination of such sequences obviously requires a compliant patient and an overall scanning time of over 30 minutes.

9.5.3 Aortic intramural hematoma and ulcer of the aortic wall

Aortic intramural hematoma is defined as an aortic dissection with no communication with the lumen. This condition presupposes a process of auto limitation of bleeding without continuity between the true lumen of the vessel and the hematic collection (Fig. 9.8). According to some authors it should be considered as a variation of the dissecting aneurysm that may ensue spontaneously as a complication of an ulcerating process or trauma. In reality, the evolution of this pathology is unclear as it has the tendency to rupture in the acute phase and stabilize or even regress during chronic phases. MRI offers the advantage of allowing to define, within certain limits, the age of the hematoma

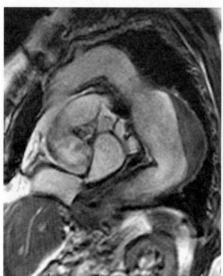

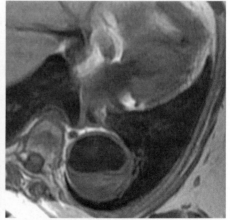

Fig. 9.8 a, b. Hematoma of the descending aorta. (a) Image obtained by a SSFP (FIESTA) sequence through a parasagittal plane. (b) Image obtained by a fast "black blood" SE sequence on an axial plane through the hematoma

a

by exploiting the information obtainable through T1- and T2-weighted images in regards to the presence of oxyhemoglobin (0-7 days), or methemoglobin (sub-acute phase (7-28 days)) or hemosiderin (in older hematomas).

CEMRA has a marginal importance but is an unavoidable completion of the study, which provides indications on the residual lumen and on the general 3D profile of the vessel.

The diagnosis of penetrating ulcer of aorta is based on the visualization of a "plus" in the aortic profile, almost always in the descending tract of the vessel. It is generally an occasional finding but may require a particular effort in understanding the patient's symptoms. The atherosclerotic process that is often widespread among these patients shows a tendency to evolve locally, destroying the elastic lamina, causing the local accumulation of blood as a hematoma, the local phenomena of dissection, and eventually the formation of perivascular pseudo-aneurysms. The static (Fast SE T1) and dynamic (SPGR of SSFP) imaging sequences associated to CEMRA images provide an excellent arsenal for defining the site and the extension of the ulcerating process in 3D (Fig. 9.9a-d).

In order for the physician to detect future evolutionary tendencies of these pathologies and engage in a more aggressive therapeutic approach, patients must undergo a regular follow-up.

9.5.4 Traumas of the aorta

Although MRI, intended as an association of static, dynamic and CEMRA images, provides a detailed characterization of the aortic trauma, the complexity of the method and the length of the exam, added to a frequent general compromising of the traumatized patient, suggest to rely on techniques such as TEE and, especially, multi-slice CT for the diagnosis in the acute phase.

Yet, it must be said that MRI has excellent sensitivity and specificity (practically 100%) in describing the site of the lesion (usually immediately distal to the isthmus), its extension, the presence of a periadvential hemorrhagic phenomena, and the presence of pericardial and/or pleural effusion – the latter being an indirect sign of an evolutionary tendency of the lesion. In the sub-acute patient, these characteristics obviously make MRI comparable to other techniques (Fig. 9.10).

9.5.5 Follow-up of aortic disease

Because MRI is highly reproducible, it is ideal for the follow-up of aortic pathologies. The frequency at which the exam should be repeated depends on the dimensions of the vessel, on the tendency of the pathology to evolve, and on agreements with the interventional cardiologist/radiologist or the surgeon. If the dimension of the vessel is over 5 cm the test is repeated every 6

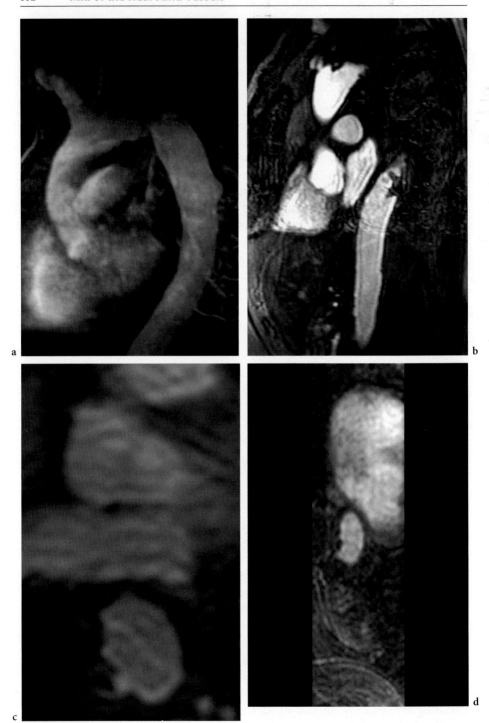

Fig. 9.9 a-d. (a) In these images CEMRA evidences a plus at the level of the descending aorta profile, caused by the presence of an ulcerated plaque that is evidenced in detail in the partitions (b) and in the orthogonal reconstruction of the plaque itself (c, d)

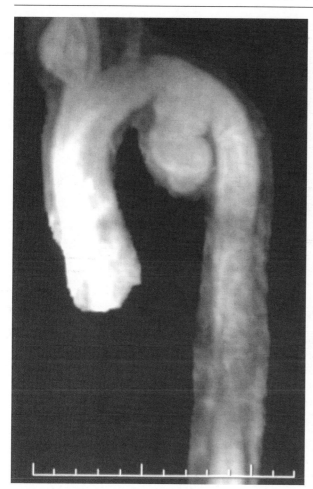

Fig. 9.10. CEMRA image of traumatic aneurysm of the aortic arc caused by a pointy object. The distal segments of the descending aorta are scarcely evident due to movement artifacts, which have been reduced by heavy postprocessing but with a clear reduction of the SCR

months, every 12 months if the vessel size is smaller. Obviously these indications are purely for reference and must be optimized for every single patient.

The monitoring of patients who have undergone surgical placement of vascular prosthesis or intravascular stents, generally requests the first check-up during the first weeks following surgery and then at three, six, and twelve months, and after that once a year. In the case of endoprostheses, the frequency of check-up rate is the same, but for precaution the first control is fixed at 4 weeks after insertion of the device. In this latter case, it is apparent that the endoprosthesis must be made of a material that does not interfere with MR images. Particular importance is given to the position of the stent, the patency of the epi-aortic vessels, the presence of endo-leaks or the exclusion of the aneurysmatic sac. Compared to multi-slice CT, MRI results superior in evidencing complications such as the presence of thrombi, while multi-slice CT seems better in the fine demarcation of the proximal and distal edges of the endoprosthesis [8].

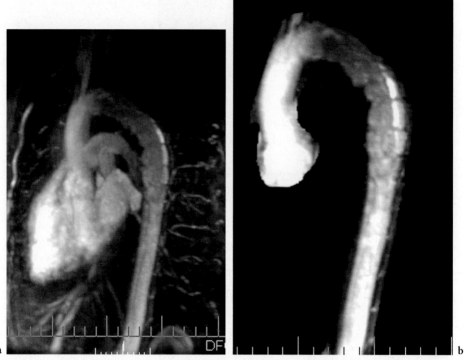

Fig. 9.11 a, b. Images of a MRI-compatible endovascolar prosthesis (nitinol) obtained with the CEMRA technique. The image well evidences the metallic design of the stent and the consequent loss of signal due to the presence of the stent itself

In the case of vascular prostheses, the operator searches the patency of the prosthesis, the presence of complications arising after the procedure (as perhaps a peri-prosthesis haematic leak), the correct functioning of the concomitant valvular prosthesis if implanted, or of the native valve if reconstructed, the dimensions of the native vessels upstream and downstream from the prosthesis, and so on.

Also in this case, the association of static T1- and T2-weighted techniques, IR, and CEMRA is desirable for a complete description of the underlying physiopathological phenomena (Fig. 9.11a, b).

9.5.6 Aortitis

It is often a subtle process in which the artheritic process involving the aorta results in a complex clinical picture. Indipendently from the fact the underlying process be of unknown nature, of immunological nature (e.g. Takayasu, Behçet, giant cells aortitis, Horton, etc.), or of secondary nature due to infective processes (syphilis), MR has demonstrated an excellent diagnostic accuracy in detecting vessel wall thickness, thrombotic deposits on the inside of the vessel, and oedema of the vessel wall itself. The possibility MRI offers for accurately defining the hystopathological status, makes it a very refined and recommended technique, apparently superior to other non-invasive techniques.

The different MRI techniques are in this case absolutely integrating. The SE weighted images with or without contrast media, and perhaps T2-weighted in axial projection are necessary for a correct histopathological definition, while dynamic images (SPGR, SSFP) and even more so CEMRA are extremely useful for highlighting stenosing processes that often accompany such pathologies.

As the occasional regional location of these processes can make research of diagnostic details inconclusive, it is useful to integrate the information obtained by MRI and MRA with those obtained through Positron Emission Tomography (PET) [9] (Fig. 9.12). This integration allows to address diagnostic efforts more appropriately, and greatly increases diagnostic accuracy (Fig. 9.12a-c).

9.6 Limits of the technique

The limits are mostly linked to the patient's collaboration, as small movements or the inability to stay in apnea can cause motion or breathing artifacts (especially in the case of paravalvular segments and in the ascending aorta) that make the exam useless no matter whether static, dynamic or CEMRA techniques are used. Likewise applies to ECG triggering, which presupposes a good ECG graphic signal also during apnea (16-20 sec).

Furthermore, another relevant limitation concerns the necessity of synchronizing in an optimal manner the timings between the injection of the contrast medium and the beginning of the acquisition. It must be mentioned that in CEMRA acquisitions, a partition thickness of 3-3.2 mm is still diagnostic for the aorta, but is unsatisfactory for secondary vessels (mammary arteries, the artery of Adamkiewicz, renal arteries, etc.) that require on occasion ad hoc studies with a better spatial resolution.

9.7 Conclusions

MRI and MRA techniques offer excellent diagnostic accuracy, great potential in defining fine aspects of the pathology being studied, accuracy and practically no hazard. Therefore, it is not surprising that despite several organizational obstacles, an increasing number of patients with aortic disease are being studied with these methods which today give access to very important diagnostic references.

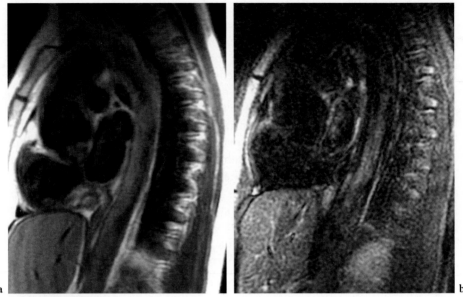

a

b

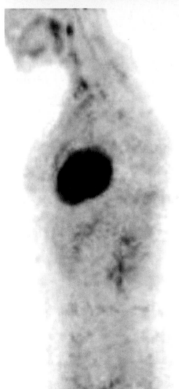

c

Fig. 9.12 a-c. Images in para-sagittal plane of aortitis of Takayasu. The images (**a**) evidence wall thickness of the aortic wall astride of the diaphragm; in the IR image (**b**) the flogistic process is enhanced as a hyperintense band-like signal at the same level of the thickness; (**c**) comparison with PET with FDG

References

1. Erbel R, Alfonso F, Boileau C et al (2001) Task force on aortic dissection, European Society of Cardiology. Diagnosis and management of aortic dissection. Eur Heart J 22: 1642-1681
2. Prince MR Gadolinium enhanced MR aortography (1994) Radiology 191:155-164
3. Pereles FS, McCarthy RM Baskaran V et al (2002) Thoracic aortic dissection and aneurysm: evaluation with non enhanced true FISP MR angiography in less than 4 minutes. Radiology 223:270-274
4. Fattori R (2003) MRI and MRA of thoracic Aorta in Cardiovascular MRI & MRA C. B. Higgins and Albert De Roos Edts. Lippincott Williams & Wilkins, Philadelphia, pp 71-392
5. Bernard Y, Zimmermann H, Chocron S, Litzler JF, Kastler B, Etievent JP, Meneveau N, Schiele F, Bassand JP (2001) False lumen patency as a predictor of late outcome in aortic dissection. Am J Cardiol 87:1378-8132
6. Lee JJ, Chang Y, Tirman PJ, Ryum HK, Lee SK, Kim YS, Kang DS (2001) Optimizing of gadolinium-enhanced MR angiography by manipulation of acquisition and scan delay times. J Eur Radiol 11:754-766
7. Yamada N, Okita Y, Minatoya K, Tagusari O, Ando M, Takamiya M, Kitamura S (2000) Preoperative demonstration of the Adamkiewicz artery by magnetic resonance angiography in patients with descending or thoracoabdominal aortic aneurysms. Eur J Cardiothorac Surg 18:104-111
8. Merkle EM, Klein S, Wisianowsky C, Boll DT, Fleiter TR, Pamler R, Gorich J, Brambs HJ. Magnetic Resonance Imaging versus multislice computed tomography of thoracic endografts (2002) J Endovasc Ther 9, suppl 2:112-113
9. Meller J, Grabbe E, Becker W, Vosshenrich R (2003) Value of F-18 FDG hybrid camera PET and MRI in early Takayasu aortitis. Eur Radiol 13:400-405

10 Renal arteries

Mirco Cosottini, Maria Chiara Michelassi, Guido Lazzarotti

10.1 Introduction

The kidney vascular district can be affected by several pathologies: steno-occlusive disease, artero-venous fistula, aneurysm, and dissecting disease. Most of these diseases can lead to a progressive decrease in kidney perfusion, entailing renovascular disease, which can appear under two different clinical pictures: renovascular hypertension and vascular nephropathy. The most common causes of these conditions are atherosclerotic stenosis and, secondly, fibrodysplasia of the renal artery.

Arterial hypertension represents one of the most important health problems in developed countries. About 1.5% of the population in western countries is affected by arterial hypertension [1]. From an etiological point of view, hypertension is essential in 90-95% of cases, and is secondary to a specific etiological cause in the other 5-10% [2], specifically: 2-3% to renal parenchymal disease and 1-4% to stenosis of the renal artery; the latter represents a relatively rare cause for hypertension but is potentially the most curable form. The surgical correction or endovascular treatment of stenoses of the renal artery prevents or limits complications such as hypertension and kidney failure; the screening method for those patients with clinical suspicion of renovascular hypertension should be non-invasive and not requiring exposure to radiation or procedural risks for the patient.

The vascular system can be explored accurately with invasive techniques; good results can also be achieved with non-invasive methods such as Echo-color Doppler and angio-Computed Tomography (CT) but they are not as completely satisfying as those obtained by digital angiography. The continuing technological evolution of the new MR angiographic techniques has allowed to overcome at least some obstacles in the diagnostics of the vascular system. Magnetic Resonance Angiography (MRA) in fact allows to obtain vascular images with a wide Field Of View (FOV), with or without the aid of contrast agents.

Within the setting of instrumental techniques for evaluating renal arteries, the technological improvement of ultrasound equipment has opened the way to the study of blood flow in the renal arteries allowing to obtain accurate and repeatable velocimetric indices, which are important elements for the diagnostic evaluation. So far, this technique is among the most promising in the field of diagnostics of renovascular diseases because of its non-invasiveness and affordable cost, although it still burdened by some unsolved problems. Just to cite an example, simple cases of obesity or meteorism can make the study of some indices like systolic peak velocity or indices derived from velocities particularly difficult. Echo-color Doppler is not suitable for the study of accessory renal arteries: as 75-100% go undetected [3]; moreover the accuracy of the technique depends on the operator's expertise and qualified skills. A further progress in the identification of renal arteries is provided by contrast ultrasonography where the presence of microbubbles amplifies the amplitude of the Doppler signal, which allows to sample the signal also in below-optimal conditions. Moreover, the use of contrast mediums offers the possibility of identifying accessory vessels that may escape routine surveys because of their small dimensions.

Thanks to volumetric acquisitions with mono- or multi-layer equipment, rapidity of performance, and to insensitivity to turbulences, spiral CT can yield high-quality vascular images that can be reconstructed in two- and three-dimensional angiograms. Among the advantages of CT, noteworthy are its ability to identify calcifications [4], poststenotic ectasias, and parenchymographic abnormalities with the same accuracy of conventional angiography. Spiral CT, however, is not suitable for routine screening as it employs ionizing radiation, it often requires administration of a contrast medium to patients with reduced kidney function, is expensive and has long reconstruction times.

The diagnostic gold standard in the study of renal arteries is represented by Digital Subtraction Angiography (DSA) [5]. The technique is performed in local anesthesia through transfemoral arterial catheterism, producing a panoramic aortography that allows the operator to vision the abdominal aorta and its main branchings. Moreover, it allows to detect eventual accessory renal arteries. Although it has high specificity and sensitivity, this exam presents a degree of risk, not to mention the risk deriving from the administration of a iodinated contrast medium, which would compromise an already weakened renal function.

The exam is completed with a selective study of the renal arteries and with the measurement of pressure values downstream the stenosis and in the abdominal aorta. The aim is to show the hemodynamic significance of the stenosis as assessed by the presence of a pressure gradient >20% between the aorta and renal artery.

MRA [6-9] is capable of visualizing the vascular structures selectively by utilizing either flow related techniques (Time Of Flight, TOF, Phase Contrast, PC) or sequences capable of detecting the presence of a contrast medium inside the vessels (ultrafast MRA with contrast bolus "CEMRA").

10.2 MRA techniques

10.2.1 Time Of Flight MRA (TOF-MRA)

Time Of Flight MRA is a Gradient Echo sequence that is characterized by a TR much smaller than T1 of stationary tissues, which leads to saturation of motionless spins [6]. This phenomenon, known as flow-related enhancement is the basis of this type of acquisition: the refreshed flow that constantly enters into a section receives few radio frequency pulses and, therefore, has a higher signal than stationary tissue, which instead receives a much greater number of pulses and quickly reaches saturation. When flow is constant, a higher signal can be obtained by using an additional gradient (flow compensation) which rephases the protons. Otherwise, when flow is turbulent there is a loss of proton phase coherence with a consequent fall in signal (flow void).

To obtain diagnostically valid images by TOF MRA, the sections of interest need to be perpendicular to the direction of the vessels so that the operator can exploit the flow enhancement effect to the most. It is also important to select the shortest echo time to minimize flow voids, and an adequate size of voxel. In fact, within a small voxel it is easier to have dephasing phenomena among spins with different velocity than within a small voxel, where otherwise a significant reduction of Signal-to-Noise Ratio (SNR) occurs.

Using spatial saturation bands, only the vessels with a preestablished flow direction can be visualized, thereby discriminating arteries from veins, or more in general producing selective angiograms. This technique, however, does not give an optimal suppression of stationary tissues and often gives motion artifacts, elements that limit the possibility of multiplanar reconstruction. Yet, the greatest drawback of TOF that discourages its use remains the 'in-plane' effect whereby vessels coursing parallel to the acquisition plane tend to saturate as stationary tissues do; this occurs because the protons moving in the direction of the plane are subject to multiple radio frequency pulses that do not allow the recovery of longitudinal magnetization.

10.2.2 Phase Contrast MRA (PC-MRA)

When spins in motion are subjected to a magnetic field gradient, they experience a shift of phase relative to static spins [6-8].

PC-MRA uses the speed-induced phase shift to separate flowing blood from stationary tissue. The vector of transversal magnetization induced by a radio frequency pulse on a system of spins can be represented with an amplitude and a direction or phase. The loss of phase coherence is mainly linked to in-homogeneity of the static magnetic field.

The application of a gradient determines an additional change in phase to the system of spins. The application of a positive gradient provokes an increase in resonance frequency and a change of phase. When the gradient interrupts its activity there is a return to the normal precessing frequency, but the change of phase remains.

PC sequences are built in a way to produce two images: the first image is obtained by applying a positive gradient to the spin system, determining a phase accumulation; the second image is obtained by applying the same gradient (as for intensity and time length) but with an opposite direction, determining a loss of phase. The difference between the two images determines a phase accumulation equal to zero in the stationary tissue, while in the dynamic tissues the phase accumulation is given by:

$$\Delta\phi = \gamma v \Delta M_1$$

where γ is the gyromagnetic constant, v the velocity of the moving spins and ΔM_1 is the change of the gradient's first-degree moment.

Therefore, in function of the phase accumulation of the moving spins we can calculate the spin velocity in a system of reference. In function of the sign of the velocity in relation to the phase encoding, the intensity of the pixel can be conventionally identified with black or white pixels so as to establish the direction of flow. The intensity of the pixel is instead a function of velocity.

From the above equation we may see that the maximum phase difference that can be obtained between two spin systems is of 180° for a given ΔM_1, whose value depends on the amplitude and duration of the gradient. From this follows that the maximum velocity measurable will be the one that determines a 180° difference in phase. This velocity is known as Velocity Encoding (VENC) and is the highest velocity measurable by the sequence, beyond which the flow goes towards aliasing, i.e. an artifact that does not allow the measurement of blood flow velocity.

Normally, the VENC can be established by the operator by modifying the shape of the gradient. As the formula indicates, if ΔM_1 is large, small flow velocity changes determine great differences in phase; conversely, if ΔM_1 is small, a large velocity change will be needed to obtain the same difference of phase. In this manner, we can measure different blood flow velocities, such as that of artery flow (fast) or venous flow (slow), by simply changing the VENC and thus using a high VENC for fast flow and a low VENC for slow flow. The PC sequences used in clinical practice are the 2D PC, and the 3D cine-PC. As we infer from the principles intrinsic to the technique itself, it is possible to perform a quantitative analysis inside the vessel if the scanning is done orthogonal to the direction of flow.

The 2D PC techniques produce velocity maps of the average velocity inside the voxels. This velocity is a temporal average of instantaneous velocities and is determined by the acquisition length, which is equal to the acquisition time for non-synchronized sequences. While this method can be sufficient for measuring venous flow, pulsing artery flow requires a multiple measurement in several moments of the cardiac cycle. For this reason the 2D PC technique has been substituted by the combined technique of 2D PC with cine, which allows to acquire a velocity map over time in the transverse section of a vessel.

Because the accuracy of flow analysis is strongly influenced by the shape of the flow wave, it is necessary to have the best temporal resolution possible.

In the cine-PC technique, acquisition time is linked to the number of phase encodings for each heartbeat; therefore the duration of the acquisition is determined by heart frequency and by the number of phases. Hence, a sequence acquired with a 256×256 matrix has an average duration of 8-9 minutes. The length of acquisition does not allow to perform the test in breath-hold; therefore, motion artifacts induce an overestimation of the vessel diameter [10].

The limited spatial and temporal resolution of cine-PC can be overcome by implementing fast sequences with the segmentation of K-space. Fast sequences utilize a short TR (5-10 msec), and differently from cine-PC, acquire more phase encodings per cardiac cycle (views per segment); therefore the acquisition time is reduced by a factor equal to the number of views per segment (usually 4-8 for a cardiac sequence between 60-129 bpm) [11].

The calculation of flow is made multiplying the mean velocity inside the pixel times the surface of the pixel. If the image is obtained in a plane orthogonal to the vessel we can have an accurate measure of the flow in function of time. The 3D PC sequences are obtained positioning the acquisition plane in coronal position and adopting as a scout an axial image through renal vessels. Typical acquisition parameters are TR 28 msec, TE 8.1 msec, matrix 128×256, FOV 24×17 cm, thickness 2 mm, 28 partitions, inferior saturation band, VENC 50 cm/sec, acquisition time 3-6 min.

The 2D fast PC scanning synchronized with the heart beat is performed on a plane perpendicular to the renal vessel, about 1 cm from the ostium or 1 cm downstream the stenosis (with TR depending on the R-R interval), TE 3.6 msec, matrix 128×256, FOV 24×17 cm, thk 5 mm, flow compensation, phase difference, view per segment 4, n. phases 30, VENC 155 cm/sec, acquisition time 18-25 sec in function of heart rate. In vitro and in vivo studies have demonstrated that an accurate measurement of flow is only possible on breath-held acquisitions [10].

The 2D fast PC sequences are later reconstructed using an independent workstation in order to obtain graphics representing the shape of the velocity and flow wave in function of time by means of a program of automatic detection of the area of the renal arterial vessel (Fig. 10.1).

Flow maps seem to overcome the limit of many techniques in predicting the hemodynamic significance of a lesion and may be employed as a complement to the morphological image of the renal artery.

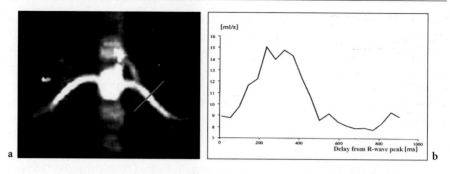

Fig. 10.1 a, b. Collapsed image on the axial plane of a 3D PC sequence of the normal renal arteries. (a) the white line indicates the positioning of the 2D fast PC sequence set perpendicular to the axis of the renal vessel for a quantitative measure of velocity and blood flow. The slope of average flow wave (b) in function of the time achieved: there is an evident early systolic peak at 234 msec and a middle-systolic peak at 310 msec, followed by a diastolic plateau. The average value of the arterial flow is 652,39 ml/min

10.2.3 Contrast Enhanced MRA (CEMRA)

The 3D CEMRA substantially differs from the previous sequences for the fact that it uses a contrast agent which makes the technique relatively independent from flow [7, 12]. A gadolinium-based contrast agent injected i.v. determines the shortening of blood T1, which in turn translates into hyperintensity of the flow signal in relation to the surrounding tissues.

The first 3D contrast enhanced acquisitions that were used with conventional gradients had a scanning time in the order of 3-5 minutes, were performed in free-breathing and did not give an adequate resolution, especially for small-sized vessels.

The introduction of high performance gradients has allowed us to sample the volumes of interest in few seconds so that acquisitions in apnea could be made, with the result of a much better image quality (without artifacts due to breathing). Optimization of image quality is now achieved reducing TR to 3-7 msec and TE to 1-3 msec, and using a flip angle between 30°-50°. Space resolution is improved through elevated matrixes, increasing the number of partitions and applying interpolation algorithms in the direction of layer and frequency. To maintain the acquisition time sufficiently low, a rectangular FOV is used; the variable band is increased, and the Half-Fourier Transform is applied [9].

The visualization of the vascular structures is further optimized when the contrast medium inside the district of interest is at its maximum concentration at the moment the central portion of K-space is being acquired. The acquisition of the central part of the K-space depends on the construction of the sequence. In sequential acquisitions, where the K-space is filled from the periphery in a sequential manner, the information on contrast resolution will be located in the central portion (1/3 of total space); with the centrical sequences in which the covering of K-space starts from the central data, the information on the contrast are the first to be gathered. Once the acquisition method of the sequence is acknowledged, it is relatively easy to calculate the delay necessary to make the contrast bolus peak match the acquisition of the center of K-space. In particular if the system has a sequential acquisition of K-space as in most cases, the scanning delay will be SD = CT – 1/3 ST, where ST is the sequence scanning time. The only unknown is the contrast Circulation Time (CT), calculated using the bolus test. The bolus test is performed by injecting minimum amounts of contrast medium (1-2 ml) and evaluating the maximum enhancement inside the vessels under exam [13] through the execution of a fast T1-weighted sequence such as SPGR conducted on an axial plane passing at the level of the renal arteries, repeated for a total of 50 sec with the following parameters: TR 22 msec, TE 2,6 msec. FA 60° matrix 256×128, FOV 40×28, layer thickness 20 mm, NEX 1. To date, there are automatic methods for detecting the arrival of the contrast bolus by which the operator positions the sampling volume on the vascular district of interest; the sequences turn on automatically the moment the contrast bolus arrives so that the center of the K-space is filled at contrast peak concentration (Smart-Prep). There are interactive fluoroscopic methods where the operator must detect the arrival of the bolus by a real time monitoring sequence and start the 3D acquisition when the optimal increase in signal intensity is reached.

The CEMRA is a 3D fast SPRG sequence performed on the coronal plane. Typical acquisition parameters are: TR 5.5 msec, TE 1.6 msec, FA 30°, matrix 128-160×256-320, FOV 35-38 cm, phase FOV, thk 1.6 mm, 38 partitions, zero filling in the direction of layer and frequency, NEX 0.5-1, selective pulse for fat saturation, acquisition time 19-22 sec.

In addition to the technique above, a dynamic multiphase time-resolved contrast-enhanced MRA acquisition technique has also been developed; the method allows to repeat the acquisition of the volume of interest over time so to obtain images before, during, and after artery peak enhancement [14, 15]. This technique is based on the 3D fast SPGR scannings, that are so short that they can be repeated during the respiratory apnea, allowing the operator to follow the path of the contrast medium both inside the arterial and venous vascular district and obtain images in the early arterial phase, in the arterial phase with maximum enhancement of the main renal arterial vessels, in the parenchymographic phase with low enhancement of the venous vessels, in the early venous phase and in the late venous phase with maximum enhancement of the venous system [15]. The consecutive acquisition of sets of images helps overcome the relevant problem of perfect timing with the arrival of the contrast medium inside the vascular district being studied and allows to obtain a better visualization of the distal portion of the renal arteries and of the intrarenal vessels. Using this technique, the venous contamination no longer affects the arterial visualization, allowing the operator to easily see stenosing pathologies of the distal tracts that develop with fibromuscular dysplasia. Moreover, the multiphase technique allows the study of the venous vascular district through the subtraction of images obtained in the arterial phase from the images with perfect venous enhancement.

The multiphase techniques are 3D Fast SPGR sequences performed on the coronal plane with the parameters: TR 3.2 msec, TE 1.1 msec, FA 30°, matrix 128-160×256, FOV 35-38 cm, phase FOV, thk 1.8-2.5 mm, 30-35 partitions, zero filling in the direction of layer and frequency, NEX 1, selective pulse of fat saturation, acquisition time 28 sec (4 sets of 3D data each lasting 7 seconds).

The 3D images obtained using both the single phase technique and the dynamic multiphase one have to be reconstructed on independent work stations with multiplanar methods utilizing the Maximum Intensity Projection (MIP) algorithm with the option of obtaining images oriented on any plane.

10.3 Technical features

The protocol for the study of renal arteries foresees the acquisition of scout images obtained by a coronal GRE sequence in coronal plane, so the following three-dimensional PC sequence is positioned on the axial plane. Furthermore, a 2D fast PC sequence can be acquired for the quantitative evaluation of the hemodynamics. Finally, a 3D fast SPGR with contrast bolus (0,2 mmol/kg of contrast agent in bolus at the speed of 2 ml/sec) is performed in apnea in coronal plane.

The typical technical characteristics of the equipment for performing such sequences are: magnet 1-1.5T, gradient intensity >30 mT/m/msec and rise time <200 μs, specific phased-array coil for abdomen, and an automatic injector MR compatible.

10.4 Clinical applications

10.4.1 Stenosing pathologies

The most frequent cause for stenosis of the renal artery (66% of cases) is the atheromasic plaque located at the origin of the artery itself [1]. The second most frequent type of stenosing affection is fibromuscular dysplasia. Atherosclerosis and fibromuscular dysplasia account for 90% of the stenoses of the renal artery; in the remaining cases the etiology can be reconducted to congenital abnormalities (malformations and artero-venous fistulas), neurofibromatosis (in children), aneurysms of the renal artery stretching the artery itself, atheritis and extrinsic obstructions (muscular structures such as the pillars of the diaphragm, sympathetic ganglia, etc.) [2].

The atheromasic stenosis is observed prevalently in males and the incidence rises with age and in patients affected by diabetes mellitus. Generally, the plaque is eccentric with an overlapping thrombosis, and in 80% of patients is associated to atherosclerotic injuries in other districts. In 1/3 of cases it is bilateral. The atherosclerotic lesion may evolve towards complete occlusion, which inevitably leads to kidney failure.

However, the stenosing plaque of a renal artery is not necessarily cause for hypertension; in fact the plaque is frequently found among elderly persons without hypertension and in many subjects with a hypertension that is not due directly to the plaque itself.

The second most frequent stenosing pathology of the renal artery is the fibromuscular dysplasia. This is a group of heterogeneous lesions of unknown pathogenesis, characterized by a fibrous or fibromuscular thickening of the intima, media, or adventitia. Such lesions are thereby classified as intimal, medial, and adventitial hyperplasia, of which the medial lesion is the most frequent. Differently from artheriosclerosis, muscular fibrodysplasia mainly affects young women, in average about 30 years of age [16]. From an anatomopathologic view the pathology may consist of a single well-defined stenosis, or of a number of narrowings of the medium or distal portions of the renal artery, at times involving the segmental branches and becoming bilateral. Fibromuscular dysplasia interests the renal arteries bilaterally in 2/3 of patients. In addition, it is associated to a progression toward complete closing with a frequency varying between 16-66% of cases [16]. Fibromuscular dysplasia can be distinguished from artherosclerosis on arteriographic images in which the vessel appears with an irregular profile of wider segments alternated to narrowed ones ("bead-thread").

The physiopathological mechanism responsible for renovascular hypertension is linked to hypoperfusion, chronic ischemia that settles in the kidney supplied by the stenotic artery, and to the consequent activation of the renin-angiotensin system (the homeostatic mechanism that works to maintain adequate glomerular filtration). Renin causes an increase in arterial pressure directly through the vaso-constricting action of angiotensin II and indirectly through the suprarenal production of aldosterone, which stimulates sodium tubular uptake and consequently water uptake. In the initial phases of the disease the increase in pressure values is uniquely mediated by the hemodynamic effects of ischemia. With the evolving of the disease, if the factor responsible for hypertension is not removed and this condition is kept stable, the hypertensive state induces the development of arteriolar injuries in the systemic vessels and in the controlateral renal artery that worsens or maintains the hypertensive status [16].

The diagnosis of renovascular hypertension is based on clinical and laboratory findings listed by the Working Group on Renovascular Hypertension [2] and on the demonstration of the presence of a stenosis in the renal artery, either indirectly through abnormalities of renal function or directly through the visualizations of the vessel's caliber. In clinical practice there are several tests that aim to uncover alterations in renal function consequent to the presence of a stenosis of the renal artery; among these are the Captopril test that allows to evaluate to what degree the pressure increase depends on the renin plasmatic levels and the dosage of renin from the renal vein, and the renal sequential scintigraphy with the Captopril provocative test. In consideration of its invasiveness and the high number of false positive results, the dosage of renin from the renal vein is seldom performed.

MRA is considered, especially after the introduction of CEMRA, a powerful tool for evaluating renal arteries directly [9] (Fig. 10.2). As with digital angiography, CEMRA is a luminography, and as such provides exclusively morphological data. Data documented by a recent meta-analysis indicate that CEMRA has a 97% sensitivity and a 93% specificity in the grading of the renal artery stenosis, which are higher values than those that can be obtained by flow based MRA techniques, which respectively yield a sensitivity and specificity of 94 and 85%. Moreover, CEMRA has an 82% sensitivity and a 95% specificity in detecting accessory arteries [17] (Fig. 10.3).

However, it has a tendency to overestimate the stensosis, as has been documented in several other vascular districts. The causes of this are the limited spatial resolution as compared to digital angiography, which remains the gold standard, and artifacts of bad timing of the contrast bolus (blurring and ringing), and an intravoxel dephasing component that also affects CEMRA. Another factor contributing to the overestimation of stenosis can come from

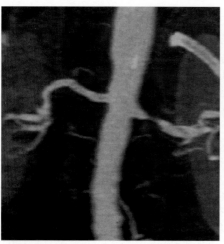
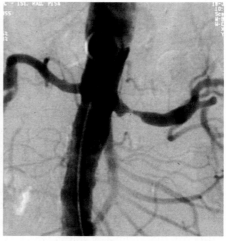

a   b

Fig. 10.2 a, b. Patient with para-ostial stenosis of the left renal artery. Multiplanar reconstruction of the renal arteries evaluated by CEMRA (**a**), that allows the physician to identify the grade of stenosis of the renal artery with a good overlapping of the result, as compared to the digital angiographic method of reference (**b**). Noticeable, also a good visualization of the peripheral branches of the renal arteries can be obtained

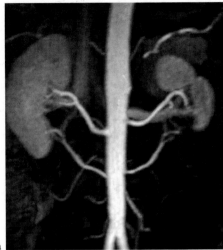

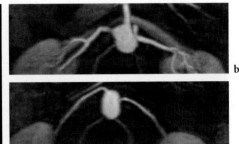

Fig. 10.3 a-c. Compared with other non-invasive methods, CEMRA has demonstrated to be useful in the detection of the accessory renal arteries, thanks to its landscape view. Coronal (a) and axial (b, c) reconstruction that give an optimal view of both the principal renal and the accessory districts

image postprocessing methods. If, indeed, the set of acquired images is not perfectly void of venous overlapping, it may well happen that during reconstruction the vein be included with the renal artery in the voxels on which the MIP algorithm is being applied. In such cases the presence of a stenosis is overestimated (Fig. 10.4). Hence, by overestimating the stenoses, CEMRA may lead to unjustified digital angiographic procedures – notwithstanding its high diagnostic accuracy. In order to avoid these errors of overestimation, these purely morphological studies can be completed by MR techniques, which provide hemodynamic information on flow inside the vessel.

The techniques providing hemodynamic information are those sensitive to flow; among these, the 3D PC that shows directly the flow alteration inside the renal artery through the absence of signal in the angiogram obtained: the grading of the stenosis can be made according to the presence and length of signal loss [18]. A stenosis over 60% causes a segmentary loss of signal (signal void) more or less extended in function of its severity, until flow signal completely disappears, while with stenosis under 60% there is no signal loss downstream.

The quantitative and qualitative analysis of the curves obtained with cine-PC is another additional method for evaluating hemodynamic abnormalities in the stenosis of the renal arteries and limits the overestimation of morphological techniques [19] (Fig. 10.5). Hemodynamic parameters such as the reduction of the mean flow and reduction and delay of flow at systolic peak, have a 90% sensitivity and a 94% specificity in detecting stenoses of the renal arteries.

The combination of morphological and functional studies has been reported by several authors as an efficient method for evaluating the renal vascular district [15, 19, 20]. Literature reports studies that evaluate the varia-

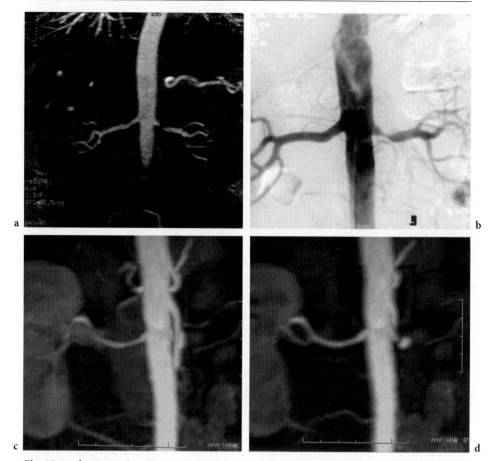

Fig. 10.4 a-d. CEMRA has demonstrated to be a technique with an elevated concordance with digital angiography in the evaluation of stenosis of the renal artery, despite its tendency to overestimate the stenosis. In this example, the stenosis visualized with CEMRA (**a**) referencing to the paraostial tract of the left renal artery is overestimated compared to the grading made by digital angiography (**b**). One factor contributing to overestimation, which is not caused by factors inherent to the methods, derives from a mistaken reconstruction of the set of 3D data on behalf of the MIP algorithm, in occurrence of venous overlapping. Panel (**c**) shows a stenosis >50% of the proximal segment of the superior branch of the right renal artery. The MIP reconstruction has been done including the renal vein, which is partially filled by the contrast agent. In (**d**) the stenosis is no longer visible because the MIP was performed taking care of not including the renal vein in the volume of reconstruction, thus allowing the visualization of the normal renal vessel

tion of specificity and accuracy, combining the various techniques of angio-MRI. Integrating the algorithms obtained by 3D TOF with those obtained by 3D PC, the specificity and accuracy in the evaluation of renal artery stenoses of over 50% increase respectively to 90 and 92% [21]. More recently the combination of CEMRA and 3D PC has demonstrated an increase in sensitivity up to 100% in detecting a stenosis of the renal artery over of 50% [22]. For

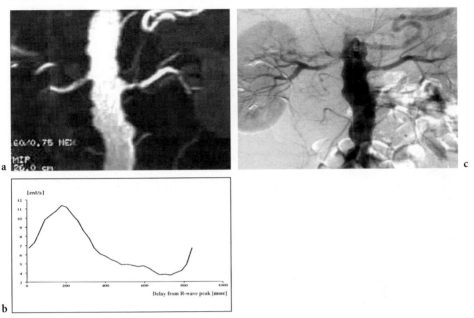

Fig. 10.5 a-c. The tendency of CEMRA to overestimation can be reduced by its integration to MRA flow-based methods, such as the 3D-PC or the 2D fast PC, which determine an increase in the diagnostic accuracy of the MRA as a non-invasive technique. Above is an example of aid provided by hemodynamic data in the diagnosis of a non-significant stenosis. MRA (**a**) with contrast bolus of the left renal artery demonstrates the presence of a paraostial stenosis to which the observing radiologist must still assign the degree of significance. The flow graph (**b**) in function of time, obtained downstream from the stenosis: no alterations of the morphology can be appreciated in the graph for the average flow (497,48 ml/min), or the average and maximum velocity, which result overlapping to the results of the non stenotic artery. The hemodynamic analysis obtained with 2D fast PC technique is indicative of a non-significant stenosis. Digital angiography (**c**) confirms the presence of a modest narrowing of the left renal artery. In this case, the use of the angio-MR PC has added useful information to a doubtful morphological MRA result

these reasons, in the diagnostic protocols of renal arteries it is advisable to couple the CEMRA acquisition to at least the hemodynamic information obtainable with 3D PC. Sometimes the hemodynamic findings may be obtained through the quantitative evaluation of flow and velocity with the Fast PC. Yet, it remains that in several studies, breath-held CEMRA has demonstrated to be more sensitive and more specific in the study of renal arteries than flow-sensitive techniques [23, 24].

In relation to what has been said on the physical principles of MRA sequences, the techniques based on flow have a limited role in case of dysplasia of the renal artery. The alterations of the vessel wall in fibrodysplasia may or may not cause a significant stenosis of the vessel wall, therefore in analogy to what can be detected by Echo-color Doppler, PC techniques may not detect an alteration of hemodynamics whenever a fibrodysplastic wall alteration

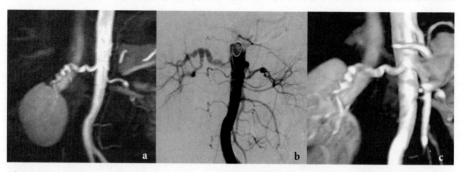

Fig. 10.6 a-c. CEMRA is based on a shortening of the T1 of blood induced by the paramagnetic contrast agent and shows little trace of the intravoxel dephasing effect, which allows a good evaluation of the wall profile of the renal vessels and demonstrates its usefulness in the evaluation of the fibrodysplasia. (a) The typical "bead-thread" aspect of the medium distal region of the right renal artery, and the aneurysmatic stenosis of the predicotomic tract of the left renal artery in a patient with fibro-dysplasia valued by CEMRA, which corresponds to the clinical picture produced by digital angiography (b). Three-dimensional reconstruction (c) of the 3D set of data of CEMRA

does not provoke a stenosis of over 60%. On the contrary CEMRA, like DSA, evidences the "bead-thread" aspect also when there is no hemodynamically significant stenosis (Fig. 10.6). If we consider that fibrodysplasia prevalently affects the distal tracts of the renal arteries – a district difficult to evaluate with MRA flow-based techniques – we may presume that, thanks to the capacity of detecting wall profile changes, CEMRA covers an important role as a non-invasive method for this pathology. Yet, to date, there are no systematic studies regarding the diagnostic accuracy of CEMRA in fibrodysplasia reported in literature.

10.4.2 Non-stenosing pathologies

Aneurysms of the renal artery affect 1% of the population and are rarely symptomatic, if not for the high-pressure values found in 70% of cases. Most aneurysms are found by chance in patients who undergo angiography. From an etiological point of view they can be caused by atherosclerosis, fibromuscular dysplasia, congenital abnormalities, traumas, and poliarteritis nodosa. Therapeutic intervention is indicated for aneurysms over 1.5 cm in diameter and symptomatic aneurysms associated with hypertension. The use of magnetic resonance in the evaluation of both aneurysmatic pathology and vascular abnormalities has assumed an important role in the presurgical evaluation of these patients. The detection of aneurysms of the renal artery by PC techniques yields variable results – in relation to the size of the aneurysm – of sensitivity, specificity, and accuracy [12, 25]. With CEMRA, which is relatively affected by dephasing phenomena induced by turbulence, the aneurys-

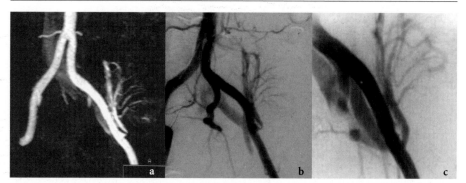

Fig. 10.7 a-c. Anastomosis at the level of the external iliac left artery in a patient who has undergone a renal transplant. CEMRA (**a**) shows a significant stenosis in proximity of the anastomosis, consequence of a vascular complication of the transplant; the finding was confirmed by invasive angiography (**b**). With an accurate evaluation of MRA it is possible to visualize an early clouding of the iliac vein and of the lower cavity upstream from the anastomosis, without the further opacification of either the downstream segment of the anastomosis of the left iliac vein, or of the controlateral iliac venous axis. The digital angiography (**c**) shows that the finding evidenced by CEMRA is due to the presence of an iatrogenic artero venous fistula

matic sac is usually completely filled by contrast agent, with a presumed diagnostic gain. As masking effects of the aneurysmatic lesion have been reported in MIP reconstruction, it is also advisable to perform an evaluation of the single partitions.

Artero-venous fistulas between the renal artery and vein are rarely congenital and are often caused by percutaneous biopsies. The evaluation of this pathology by CEMRA has not been reported in relevant cohorts of patients; yet in those few cases reported, the evaluation has not been easy, since the lack of temporal resolution does not allow a direct visualization of the fistula. The pathology can be hypothesized in the occurrence of early opacification of the renal vein during the arterial phase of the angiogram, however the rapidity of the renal circulation that often causes venous overlapping makes this sign poorly reliable (Fig. 10.7). Probably the time resolved CEMRA will be able to provide more accurate evaluations.

10.4.3 Kidney transplant

The transplanted renal artery is usually anastomised to the internal iliac artery when the transplant is performed from a living donor; while it is anastomised between the renal artery of the transplanted kidney and the common or external iliac artery of the receiver when the transplant is from a cadaver. The incidence of complications arising after the kidney transplant is 15%, and from a clinical point of view it is important to distinguish the vascular complications from those caused by rejection in view of the different therapeutical implications. Thanks to use of non-iodinated contrast agents and the large field of view, MRI can be considered a powerful tool in the evaluation of the vascular situation of the transplanted kidney especially if the kidney function is partially compromised (Fig. 10.7) The most useful sequences foresee the combination of CEMRA, and postcontrast GRE T1-weighted images [26]; this allows the evaluation of both eventual stenoses of the renal artery and defects of renal perfusion linked to renal ischemia, cortical necrosis, or hemorrhage of the transplanted organ.

In the evaluation of a stenosis of the transplanted artery, free-breathing high resolution CEMRA (since the iliac fossa in which the transplanted kidney is usually positioned, is hardly affected by respiratory motion) has shown to be a useful non-invasive screening technique as compared to digital angiography, with a sensitivity and specificity respectively of 100% and 75% in detecting stenosis exceeding 50% [27]. One of the main problems in the evaluation of a stenosis of a transplanted artery concerns a possible overestimation caused by the presence of metal clips in the transplant area, which can induce artifacts.

References

1. Novicz AC (1994) Atherosclerotic ischemic nefropathy. Epidemiology and clinical considerations. Urol Clin North Am 21:195-200
2. Working Group on Renovascolar Hypertension (1987) Final report of the Working group on renovascolar hypertension. Arch Intern Med 147:820-829
3. Van Der Hulst VP, Van Baaten J, Kool LS et al (1996) Renal artery stenosis: endovascular flow wire study for validation of Doppler us. Radiology 200:165-168
4. Siegel CL, Ellis JH, Korobkin M et al (1994) CT-detected renal arterial calcification: correlation with renal artery stenosis on angiography. Am J Roentgenol 163:867-872
5. Simonetti G, Bonomo L, Cornalba GP, De Caro G, Falappa PC et al (1993). L'angioplastica renale percutanea transluminale. Esperienza italiana in 13 centri. Radiol Med 86:503-508
6. Debatin JF, Spritzetr CE, Grist TM et al (1991) Imaging of the renal arteries. Value of MR angiography. Am J Roentgenol 157:981-990
7. Snidow JJ, Johnson MS, Harris VJ et al (1996) Three dimensional gadolinium-enhanced MR angiography for aortoiliac inflow assessment plus renal artery screening in a single breath-hold. Radiology 198:725-732
8. Richter CS, Krestin GP, Eichemberger AC, Schopke W, Fuchs WA (1993) Assessment of renal artery stenosis by phase contrast magnetic resonance angiography. Eur Radiol 3:493-498
9. Debatin JF, Hany TF (1998) MR-based assessment of vascular morphology and function. Eur Radiol 8:528-539
10. Debatin JF, Ting RH, Wegmuller H, Sommer FG, Fredrickson JO, Brosnan TJ, Bowman BS, Myers BD, Herfkens RJ, Pelc NJ (1994) Renal artery blood flow: quantification with phase contrast imaging with and without breath-holding. Radiology 190:371-378
11. Leug DA, Debatin JF (1998) Ultrafast magnetic resonance imaging of the vascular system in ultrafast MRI. Springer Berlin
12. Holland GA, Dougherty L, Carpenter JP et al (1996) Breath-hold ultrafast three-dimensional gadolinium-enhanced MR angiography of the aorta and the renal and other viscer-

al abdominal arteries. Am J Roentgenol 166:971-981

13. Hany TF, Mc Kinnon GC, Leung DA, Pfammatter T, Debatin JF (1997) Optimization of contrast timing for breath-hold three-dimensional MR angiography. Magn Reson Imaging 7:551-556

14. Van Hoe L, De Jaegere T, Bosmans H, Stockx L, Vanbeckevoort D, Oyen R, Fagard R, Marchal G (2000) Breath-hold contrast-enhanced three-dimensional MR angiography of the abdomen: time-resolved imaging versus single-phase imaging. Radiology 214:149-156

15. Schoenberg SO, Bock M, Knopp MV, Essig M, Laub G, Hawighorst H, Zuna I, Kallinowski F, van Kaick G (1999) Renal arteries: optimization of three-dimensional gadolinium-enhanced MR angiography with bolus-timing-independent fast multiphase acquisition in a single breath hold. Radiology 211:667-679

16. Schreiber ML, Pohl MA, Novick AC (1984) The natural history of atherosclerotic and fibrous renal artery disease. Urol Clin North Am 11:383-392

17. Tan KT, Van Beek EJ, Brown PW, Van Delden OM, Tijssen J, Ramsay LE (2002) Magnetic resonance angiography for diagnosis of renal artery stenosis: a meta-analysis. Clin Radiol 57:617-624

18. Wasser MN, Westenberg J, van de Hulst VP, van Baalen J, van Bockel JH, van Erkel AR, Pattynama PMT (1997) Hemodynamic significance of renal artery stenosis: digital subtraction angiography versus systolically gated three-dimensional phase-contrast MR angiography. Radiology 202:333-338

19. Schoenberg SO, Knopp MV, Bock M, Kallinowski F, Just A, Essig M, Hawighorst H, Schad L, van Kaick G (1997) Renal artery stenosis: grading of hemodynamic changes with cine phase-contrast MR blood flow measurements. Radiology 203:45-53

20. Dong Q, Schoenberg SO, Carlos RC, Neimatallah M, Cho KJ, Williams DM, Kazanjian SN, Prince MR (1999) Diagnosis of renal vascular disease with MR angiography. Radiographics 19:1535-1554

21. Loubeyre P, Trolliet P, Cahen R, Grozel F, Labeeuw M, Minh VA (1996) MR angiography of renal artery stenosis: value of the combination of three-dimensional time-of-flight and three-dimensional phase-contrast MR angiography sequences. Am J Roentgenol 167:489-494

22. Hahn U, Miller S, Nagele T, Schick F, Erdtmann B, Duda S, Claussen CD (1999) Renal MR angiography at 1.0 T: three-dimensional (3D) phase-contrast techniques versus Gadolinium-enhanced 3D fast low-angle shot breath-hold imaging. Am J Roentgenol 172:1501-1508

23. De Cobelli F, Venturini M, Vanzulli A, Sironi S, Salvioni M, Angeli E, Scifo P, Garancini MP, Quartagno R, Bianchi G, Del Maschio A (2000) Renal arterial stenosis: prospective comparison of color Doppler US and breath-hold, three-dimensional, dynamic, gadolinium-enhanced MR angiography. Radiology 214:373-380

24. Thornton MJ, Thornton F, O'Callaghan J, Varghese JG, O'Brien E, Walshe J, Lee MJ (1999) Evaluation of dynamic gadolinium-enhanced breath-hold MR angiography in the diagnosis of renal artery stenosis. AJR 173:1279-1283

25. Takebayashi S, Ohno T, Tanaka K, Kubota Y, Matsubara S (1994) MR angiography of renal vascular malformation. J Comput Assist Tomogr 18:596-600

26. Wiesner W, Pfammatter T, Krestin GP, Debatin JF (1998) MRI and MRA of kidney transplants-evaluation of vessels and perfusion. Fortschr Roentgenstr 169:290-296

27. Chan YL, Leung CB, Yu SC, Yeung DK, Li PK (2001) Comparison of non breath-hold high resolution gadolinium-enhanced MRA with digital subtraction angiography in the evaluation on allograft renal artery stenosis. Clin Radiol 56:127-132

11   Abdominal aorta

Virna Zampa, Marzio Perri, Simona Ortori

11.1 The technique

11.1.1 Ultrafast technique with contrast bolus

Magnetic Resonance Angiography (MRA) with ultrafast techniques with contrast bolus such as Contrast Enhanced Magnetic Resonance Angiography (CEMRA) represent the elected technique for MR studies of the great vessels, and in particular of the abdominal aorta. The introduction of this technique has allowed to overcome major obstacles in this study, particularly the long acquisition times and artifacts of the Time Of Flight (TOF) and Phase Contrast (PC) techniques, which are at present seldom employed in the study of the abdominal aorta.

Thanks to MRA's intrinsic capacity for examining wide regions of interest in a single breath-hold, this technique has appeared, right from its first applications, particularly adequate for the study of the great arterial abdominal vessels, as it permits to obtain images with high diagnostic value with the visualization of the entire aortic artery, iliac arteries and main collateral branches in short time spans.

From a morphological standpoint, the information obtained is comparable to that of an angio-Computed Tomography (CT), while the multiplanarity, tridimensionality, and especially the non-invasiveness of this technique make MRA preferable to Digital Subtraction Angiography (DSA) [1-2].

11.1.1.1 Patient preparation

In the study of the abdominal aorta by CEMRA, the patient is previously provided with a brachial venous access and put in a dorsal position, possibly with arms under the head or gathered over the chest. The patient is invited to remain motionless during the exam, and in the case of breath-held sequences the patient is asked to hyperventilate and then stay in apnea for about 20-30 seconds.

The choice of the coil is linked to the patient's body structure: above all phased-array coils are preferred for their excellent Signal-to-Noise Ratio (SNR), while the body coil is preferred for patients with a hefty body structure. Cardiac gating, or more simply peripheral and respiratory gating is also advised. In the case of patients with intestinal bloat, it is best to administer glucagon intravenously to reduce the artifacts linked to bowel peristalsis [3].

11.1.1.2 Data acquisition

Images are generally acquired on the coronal plane. In rare cases, when there is the need to have an aimed evaluation of the celiac trunk, or of the superior mesenteric a. and of its branches, a specifically oriented acquisition may be requested.

The volume of the 3D acquisition must cover the entire abdominal aorta and the iliac arteries with the upper limit above the origin of the celiac trunk, under the heart, in order to reduce artifacts linked to cardiac movement; for this purpose a wide FOV (40-48 cm) is generally employed.

To verify the complete coverage of the volume of interest and the absence of aliasing, it is best to perform also a 3D acquisition before contrast agent injection; this acquisition can then be used later as a mask for the elaboration of subtraction images.

When the acquisition is performed with fat signal saturation, image subtraction is not necessary.

The exact synchronization between the administration of a bolus and the sequence represents a pivotal point for obtaining high quality images; as a matter of fact, acquisitions that occur too early or too late compromise the quality of the test causing, respectively, a low signal intensity of the artery district, or an overlapping of the venous structures and the enhancement of stationary tissues (Fig. 11.1). Furthermore, the synchronization between administration of the bolus and the start of the sequence is fundamental so that the maximum intravascular concentration of the contrast agent is reached during the filling of the central portion of K-space. Indeed, it is known that the data relative to the signal intensity and to contrast resolution are stored at the center of K-space, while the information on the spatial resolution of the image is stored at its periphery.

Therefore, it is necessary for the operator to be familiar with the kind of filling of K-space the machine is equipped with (sequential, central, or elliptic) and choose the most appropriate. If the filling is sequential, from the bottom upwards, the filling of the central lines occurs in the middle of the acquisition; the centrical filling begins from the center outward to the peripheral regions so that the central lines are acquired early; the elliptic filling performs a centrical filling and continues in the peripheral area, providing images with high spatial resolution and with an intrinsic suppression of the veins; this method is chosen for the studies of those districts

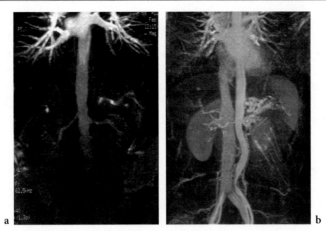

a   b

Fig. 11.1 a, b. Importance of the correct synchronization of the test in function of the administration of the contrast agent in the study of the abdominal aorta with CEMRA. Acquisitions made at a premature phase (**a**) detect a low signal intensity at the level of the arterial vascular compartment with scarce representation of the abdominal aorta and its collaterals. Acquisitions made in a late phase (**b**) evidence overlapping venous structures (inferior vena cava, iliac vessels, renal veins) that obstacle an optimal visualization of the abdominal aorta

that present problems of venous overlapping, as in the area of inferior limbs.

The synchronization between the acquisition and the moment of maximum concentration of the contrast medium inside the vessels within the volume of interest can be achieved in several ways [4-5]. The most empiric one (*best guess*) presumes a standard circulation time, and a scanning delay time that is applied accordingly (in the case of the abdominal aorta, a scanning delay of 30 seconds) [6]. This method is easy to execute but presents a high degree of approximation linked to the interpersonal variability of the circulation time, caused by a number of factors (age, hydration status, conditions of cardiovascular apparatus, etc.).

A more accurate method is that utilizing a preliminary bolus for establishing the time of circulation (bolus test). See Chapter 2 for methodological details.

At present, companies offer signal-intensity tracking systems that detect the arrival of the contrast medium in real time and allow the operator to optimize the start of the acquisition. The fluoroscopic trigger for example allows a real time detection of the arrival of the contrast, leaving the operator the task of starting the acquisition at the most appropriate moment; otherwise there are also automatic signal-intensity detection systems that start the acquisition automatically (Smart Prep) once the threshold value of concentration has been reached in a sampling volume positioned in the vessel of interest [7-8].

By means of an automatic injector (preferred over manual), 0.05-0.3 mmol/kg of contrast medium are administered at an infusion rate of 2-3 ml/sec.

In selected cases, it can be useful to complete the study with axial acquisitions SE T1-, T2-weighted and IR with fat suppression; indeed these techniques allow an accurate analysis of the vascular wall and of the endoluminal thrombosis. In fact when there is the suspicion of a complicated or inflammatory aneurysm, such acquisitions have a very high diagnostic significance. In order to have a better evaluation of the wall, Fast SE "black blood" acquisitions can also be used (see Chapter 9).

11.1.1.3 Data postprocessing

The raw data of the 3D acquisitions are bound to an off-line processing workstation through the use of dedicated software that yield 2 and 3D images in relatively short times, and with valuable additional information. In particular, although 3D MIP (Maximum Intensity Projection) reconstructions are highly diagnostic, the employment of Multiplanar Volume Reconstructions (MPVR) performed at the level of the origin of the main branches of aorta or of iliac aa. can further increase the value of the exam. The availability of software that can elaborate surface and volume reconstructions (Surface and Volume Rendering) has allowed to create extremely suggestive 3D images; yet, the high iconographic value of these images does not always truly match the increase of diagnostic information.

Thanks to the recent application of virtual angioscopy, it is now also possible to "surf" inside the lumen of the aorta and its main collateral branches obtaining endoscopic-like images with 3D visualization of the internal vessel surface.

During the reconstruction, undesired structures can be erased from the images by digital subtraction of unnecessary data and by increase of contrast resolution. In reality, the application of this technique is particularly troublesome for studies inside the abdomen, as acquisitions in respiratory apnea generate inevitable discrepancies between the two acquisitions responsible for artifacts and the following subtraction phase [9, 10]. Generally, the fat signal saturation is used with a minimum time increase, with a significant trade-off in terms of signal and contrast/noise ratio.

11.1.2 Phase Contrast MRA (PC-MRA)

The information provided by CEMRA can be further enriched by acquisitions with cardio-synchronized 3D PC images, and especially with 2D PC. These allow to plot flow and velocity on time curves that produce precise quantitative evaluation of vascular hemodynamics [3] (see Chapter 10).

In reality, although this technique has found important applications in the study on stenosing pathology of the kidney artery, its application in the evaluation of the abdominal aorta remains, to date, quite limited.

11.2 Clinical applications

11.2.1 Atherosclerotic and inflammatory aneurysms

Most aneurysms in the abdominal aorta are of atherosclerotic origin and are usually located below the origin of renal arteries. They usually have a fusiform shape and, in rare cases, have a saccular morphology. A correct presurgical evaluation foresees the exact measurement of the vascular diameter in the point of maximum dilation of the vessel and of the superior neck, and the precise definition of the longitudinal extension of the aneurysm. Another important parameter is the measure of the caliber of the patent lumen in cases of thrombotic wall deposit (Fig. 11.2).

Multiplanar reconstruction allows to make very precise measurements and is extremely useful in the planning of a future surgical intervention [11].

The dimensional characterization of the aneurysm requires that the measures performed on CEMRA images be integrated with those of the conventional images that allow a better acknowledgment of the external dimensions of the vessel. It is important to underline that the prognosis of the aneurysm depends more on the total dimensions of the lesion rather than on the dimensions of the patent lumen, and that the measurements must be taken along a plane perpendicular to the vessel's local major axis and not on pure axial images. In addition, serial investigations must be performed over time to assess the lesion's growth rate, which is a decisive factor for evaluating the risk of rupture.

Presurgical evaluation also requires an evaluation of the spatial relations among the aneurysm, renal arteries, visceral aa. and iliac aa. and of the presence of a concomitant steno-occlusive disease of such vessels (Fig. 11.3). Data concerning the presence of renal accessory arteries (which require a revascularization when the diameter is over 2mm), kidney anomalies, peri-aneurysm

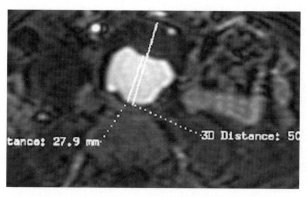

Fig. 11.2. Measurement of the diameter of an aneurysm and of the patent lumen. Such measurements must be performed on images perpendicular to the longitudinal coursing of the aneurysm

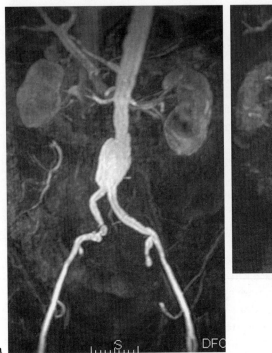
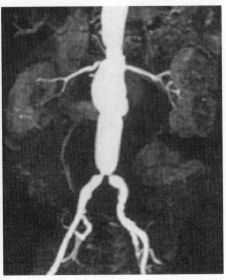

Fig. 11.3 a, b. Aneurysm of the abdominal aorta: CEMRA acquisition, MIP reconstruction. The exam documents the site, extension, and relationships of the aneurysm with the renal arteries in an optimal manner. (a) Aneurysm distal to renal arteries. (b) Aneurysm involving the origin of renal arteries and of iliac arteries

inflammatory tissue and wall calcifications are indispensable to plan the proper intervention. A correct evaluation of the presence and extension of calcifications requires a CT exam (Fig. 11.4).

As to general considerations on the prognostic index, recent studies document that the risk of rupture is approx 1% for aneurysms with a diameter of less than 5 cm, 1.4 % for aneurysms between 5 and 6 cm, and 14-22% for diameters over 6 cm [12]. Another feature of aneurysms that conditions the therapeutic choice is the presence of calcifications within the wall that can obstacle clamping and suturing and impair the mechanical support provided to an endoprosthesis [2, 3].

In view of a percutaneous treatment of the aneurysm with the positioning of an endoluminal prosthesis, the complete study of the iliac-femoral vessels is particularly useful, since eventual tortuous courses or stenoses can compromise the technical outcome of the operation. Other critical factors are the length of the neck and its inclination with respect to the more cranial tract of the vessel, the presence of thrombosis, and calcifications at the level of the neck where the prosthesis should be anchored.

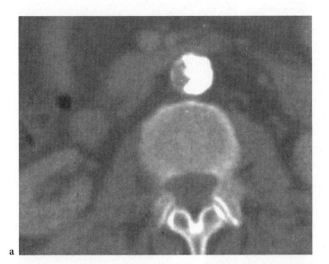

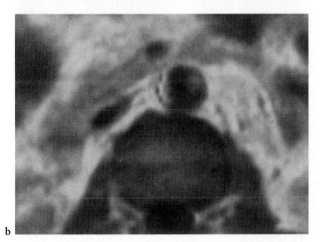

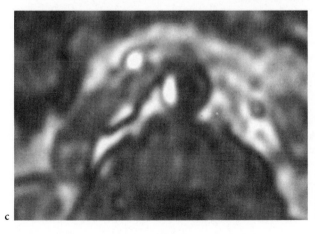

Fig. 11.4. The CT scan (**a**) demonstrates the presence of a wide calcified plaque in the abdominal aorta. At MRI such calcification is hardly visible in SE T1-weighted images (**b**). The use of cine-GRE acquisitions allows to define the size of the patent lumen and the calcified plaque, which appears markedly hypointense (**c**)

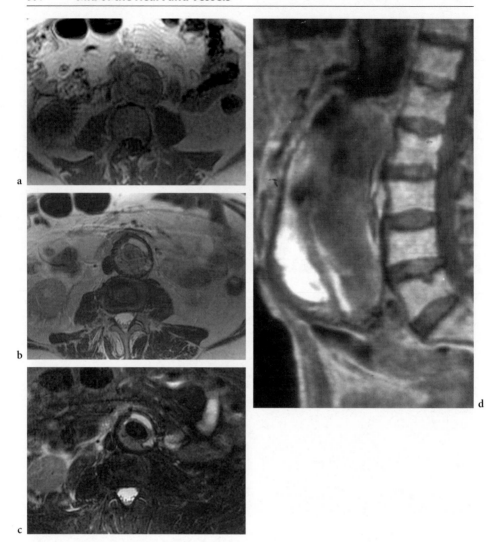

Fig. 11.5 a-d. Axial GRE T1-weighted image (**a**) of endoluminar wall thrombosis: the structure appears in-homogeneous yet hypointense and hardly distinguishable from blood which shows an intermediate intensity signal due to slow flow. The same image in T2 (**b**) and FSE-IR (**c**) better evidences the patent lumen; in the context of the thrombotic material the image evidences a liquid-like stratum, located on the anterior plane, which is indicative of a recent dissection inside the thrombus. Conversely, the non-complicated wall thrombosis shows a hypointense signal. Image (**c**) also evidences the oedema of the peri-aortic tissues extended to the left renal recess and its relationship to the incipient rupture, which was later confirmed by surgery. In a different case the SE T1-weighted sagittal image (**d**) demonstrates a voluminous aneurysmatic formation of the abdominal aorta, which shows anteriorly the markedly hyperintense signal due to the presence of met-hemoglobin within the hematoma in sub-acute phase

MRA findings integrate those provided by conventional sequences, and are absolutely indispensable in occurence of this disease as they allow to characterize and date the thrombotic component, evidence complications in the formation of the aneurysm and the eventual involvement of the para-vascular space (Fig. 11.5). A low signal intensity in T1- and T2-weighted images suggests a non-recent fibrotic thrombosis; the inhomogeneous aspect of the thrombus is often in relation to bleeding and dissection of the thrombus which can be dated according to semiological criteria that allow to identify the different catabolites of hemoglobin (Table 11.1).

The use of Gradient Echo (GRE) sequences can increase the sensitivity in locating wall calcifications, which however remains much below the sensitivity given by CT.

Five to twentythree percent of all aneurysms are inflammatory of the abdominal aorta. With the term "inflammatory" we refer to several histopathological findings: thickening and fragmenting of the elastic lamina, loss of smooth muscle cells from the media, presence of dense neovascularized connective tissue surrounding the aortic wall and seeping of lymphocytes, plasma cells, and histocites; furthermore, there may be adherences to visceral organs (duodenum, ureters) [13]. The opinions on the etiology of inflammatory aneurysms differ. Some authors attribute it to an immunolog-

Table 11.1. MR Signal characteristics of Hemoglobin catabolites

Hemoglobin (Hb) catabolites	T1	T2
Oxy-Hb hyper acute phase (0-12 hours)	hypo	hyper
Deoxy-Hb acute phase (12-72 hours)	hypo	hypo
Intracellular met-Hb early sub-acute phase (3-5 days)	hyper	hypo
Intracellular met-Hb late sub-acute phase (7-15 days)	hyper	hyper
Hemosiderin cronic phase (15 days)	hypo	hypo

The signal characteristics of hemorrhage depend on the onset and the intensity of bleeding.

At 1.5T, the acute hematoma has an intensity similar to that of muscle in T1, and hypointensity in T2 owing to the presence of intracellular deoxy-Hemoglobin – a feature that is even more marked in GRE images.

The sub-acute hematoma shows a hypointense rim produced by hemosiderin, high peripheral adipose-like intensity, and a small internal nucleus that represents the retracted coagulum. In T2, the central nucleus increases the signal compared to the peripheral area and the peripheral rim maintains a low signal. As the internal coagulum matures, its dimensions decrease and the injury becomes homogeneously hyperintense in T1 and T2 (due to further formation of extra cellular met-Hb), and appears as surrounded by a hypointense ring.

In the case of effusion, the hemorrhage cannot establish an organized pattern: the blood mixes with the serous liquids and becomes visible only after the hemorrhage has already become profuse without, however, manifesting the characteristic features of an intraparenchimal hematoma.

ical mechanism: antibody reaction to atherosclerotic material, or aspecific immunological factors towards which the atheromasic and dilated aorta wall would become permeable; other authors believe there is a relationship with retroperitoneal fibrosis.

The correct diagnostic picture of this pathology has important implications on the therapeutic level, since the surgical treatment of aneurysms that have not been diagnosed correctly is burdened by a high mortality and morbidity rate compared to the noncomplicated aneurysmatic pathology. Opinions concerning presurgical steroid therapy are contrasting: although the therapy does reduce the inflammatory reaction, there also seems to be an increased risk of rupture.

In MR images, the aneurysmatic inflammatory reaction can be recognized by the elevated signal intensity in T2-weighted images, which can be better appreciated by fat suppression, and by the marked enhancement following the administration of a contrast agent.

11.2.2 Dissection

The involvement of the abdominal aorta in a process of wall dissection is, in the vast majority of cases, a progression of a descending process originating from the thoracic aorta (see Chapter 9).

When there is a suspicion of aortic dissection, the study by CEMRA involves the entire aorta, thoracic and abdominal, and can either be performed with a single contrast bolus using multi-station techniques (generally two), or performed in separate studies for the two districts. Technically, the multi-station technique performed in a single session foresees the use of a mobile table and the simultaneous use of a surface coil or phased array for one location, and of the body coil for the other.

Recently, the whole-body angiographic technique has been introduced; such technique visualizes the entire artery tree of the body with a consequential acquisition utilizing a mobile coil that moves over the patient.

The CEMRA study allows to evidence and approximately evaluate the differences in flow of both lumens, if present, and eventually identify the true lumen. In reality, the differentiation between the true and false lumen is not always easy and often cannot be determined on the basis of difference in signal intensity alone. Frequently, the two lumens are distinguished according to their disposition as the true lumen is often compressed and located backward and to the left [3, 14].

Usually, CEMRA allows to establish the relationships between the true lumen and the emergence of the splanchnic, iliac, renal arteries, and to evaluate the perfusion of the abdominal organs (Fig. 11.6).

The use of appropriate reconstruction algorithms (MIP and MPVR) implements the informative contents of the exam with an excellent documentation

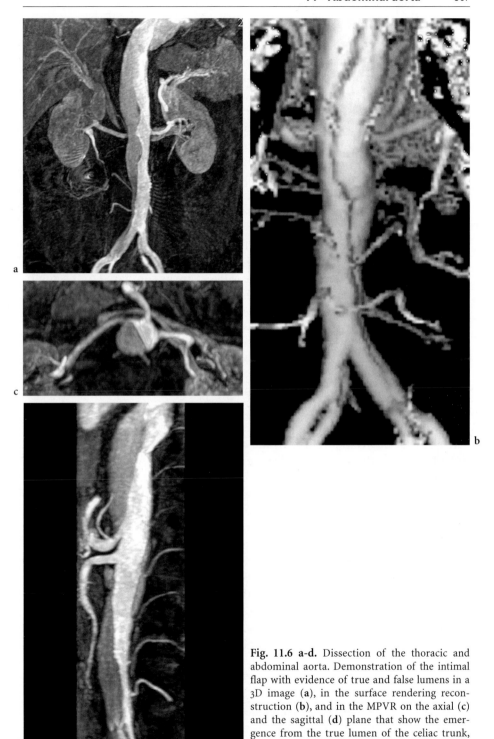

Fig. 11.6 a-d. Dissection of the thoracic and abdominal aorta. Demonstration of the intimal flap with evidence of true and false lumens in a 3D image (**a**), in the surface rendering reconstruction (**b**), and in the MPVR on the axial (**c**) and the sagittal (**d**) plane that show the emergence from the true lumen of the celiac trunk, superior mesenteric a. and left renal a.

on the cranial-caudal extension of the dissection, location of the intimal flap, and the demonstration of the possible involvement of lateral branches.

Using the MPVR images, it is also possible to differentiate a type B dissection where thrombotic material has collected inside the false or the true lumen from an aneurysm with intraluminal thrombosis based on morphological characteristics: indeed, the interface between flow and the thrombus appears sharp and, usually, has a spiraling aspect. In some cases endoscopic reconstruction can provide a better definition of the anatomical details with high values of sensitivity in identifying of the true and false lumen and their relationship with the epi-aortic, splanchnic and renal vessels. The virtual endoscopic images can provide an immediate perception of the dissection, visualizing location and extension of the intimal flap and of the two lumens.

Lastly, thanks to the employment of 2D cardio-synchronized PC sequences, it is possible to perform a direct quantification of the blood flow inside the two lumens.

With no doubt, the main limit to the MRA exam as compared to the angio-CT, is linked to the scarce sensitivity in detecting calcifications in the aortic wall, or in the dissected intimal flap. On the other hand, MRA presents an important advantage of not employing nephro-toxic contrast agents an element which must not be underestimated for the high concomitance of patients with altered kidney function or involvement of renal arteries.

11.2.3 Steno-occlusion

The steno-occlusive pathology of the abdominal aorta finds its main etiological factor in atherosclerotic disease. The site typically affected is located below the renal artery with frequent extension to the iliac arteries and in its most severe cases, to the femoral arteries (Fig. 11.7). The syndrome of Takayasu, other non-specific kinds of arteritis, and congenital malformations represent other causes (definitely more rare) of aortic steno-occlusion. As it is known, atherosclerotic disease can determine wall alterations (atherosclerotic plaques of large dimensions or complicated by thrombosis) that can cause severe reductions of the lumen caliber of the aorta. Diabetes, and cigarette smoke can dramatically worsen the picture.

The Leriche's syndrome is a disease of the infrarenal aorta and common iliac arteries that sometimes becomes complicated with the complete occlusion of these vessels. The symptomatology of this syndrome is characterized by the absence of femoral pulses, by gluteal claudication, impotency, and when the picture persists over time by hypotrophy of muscular masses of the lower limbs.

In the case of Leriche's syndrome complicated by occlusion, MRA can document stenoses and irregularities in the abdomen wall and the bifurcation providing useful information on the degree, site and extension of the obstruc-

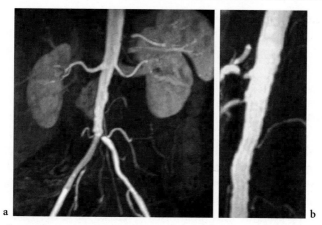

a   b

Fig. 11.7 a, b. The CEMRA test with MIP documents the atheromasic engagement of the abdominal aorta with medium-severe stenoses at the origin of the left common iliac a., which is well visible in the coronal image (**a**), and engagement of the celiac trunk, which is visible in the reconstruction obtained on sagittal plane (**b**)

tive disease; in addition MRA allows to visualize possible compensative collateral circles and vessels of the distal vascular run-off (Fig. 11.8). CEMRA can diagnose vascular occlusions correctly with sensitivity and specificity values of 100% at the level of the juxta-renal aorta, and of 100 and 98% at the levels of the common iliac aa. The protocol for the MR study on patients with aortic steno-occlusive disease also foresees the employment of late T1-weighted axial acquisitions that not only allow to document the presence and the location of the atherosclerotic plaques, but also to unveil the possible etiology of the inflammatory obstruction (e.g. arteritis of Takayasu) showing a characteristic, pathologic, late peri-aortic contrast enhancement. For what concerns

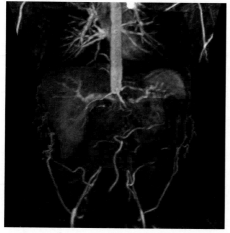

Fig. 11.8. Leriche's syndrome: CEMRA, MIP and reconstruction on axial plane. The abdominal aorta appears completely occluded immediately after the origin of the renal aa. More distally, the iliac axes are visible in proximity to the bifurcation through collateral circulation

the characterization of the wall thrombosis, the use of T1- and T2-weighted basal acquisitions allows to discriminate organized (low signal intensity both in T1 and T2), disorganized (high signal in T1 and T2), and mixed thrombotic material.

11.2.4 Control of vascular stents/prostheses

The role of MRA and in particular of CEMRA in the control of vascular stents and prostheses used in revascularization interventions and in the treatment of the steno-occlusive and aneurysmatic pathology of the abdominal aorta is still to be clearly defined. The artifacts of magnetic susceptibility generated by the ordinary metallic endoprotheses (Fig. 11.9) and the risk of complications linked to a dislocation or deformation of the prosthesic device during MRI exam have with no doubt contributed to delaying the large-scale application of angio-MR methodologies in the follow-up of patients who have undergone stenting procedures.

Nonetheless, the recent introduction of prostheses made of MR-compatible materials (e.g. nitinol) has demonstrated the degree of safety and reliability of CEMRA in evaluating the positioning of aortic prostheses (Fig. 11.9), particularly in the more complicated cases in which an invasive procedure with DSA would be unfeasible [15-17].

The visualization of stents and graft-stents is indeed linked to the geometry and metallic composition of the device: nitinol stents do not provoke significant distortions of angio-MR signal and are, therefore, well identified in SE-T1 and FSE-T2 acquisitions and do not disturb the CEMRA image; conversely, steel stents cause a total lack of signal because of the artifact by magnetic susceptibility that makes the direct visualization of the device and of the flow inside it impossible. In the case of nitinol stents, which can be visualised by MRA, the use of particularly short echo times (TE <2 msec) for 3D-Fast SPGR acquisitions, further reduces magnetic susceptibility artifacts, with a significant increase of the diagnostic confidence values of the CEMRA exam.

The protocol for the MRI study on the control of prostheses and stents positioned at the level of the abdominal aorta foresees axial acquisitions SE T1-weighted and FSE T2-weighted images obtained at the level of the abdominal aorta and of the iliac arteries, a CEMRA study of the aortic-iliac district performed in double arterial and venous acquisition, and lastly a late SE T1-weighted axial image.

The use of axial sequences performed before and after the administration of contrast agent allows to evaluate retroperitoneal peri-aortic tissues and to have a correct diagnostic picture of any future complications (periprosthesic hematoma, abscess, thrombosis, pseudoaneurysm). The CEMRA studies feature high sensitivity values in the evaluation of the patency and in the docu-

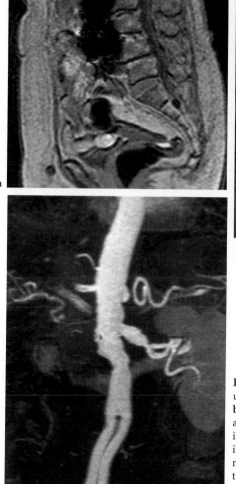

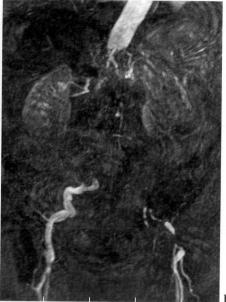

Fig. 11.9 a-c. Follow-up on aortic prostheses using CEMRA. Steel aortobisiliac prosthesis (**a**, **b**): the complete lack of signal, prevents the visualization of the prosthesic device and of the flow inside it. Aortobisiliac prosthesis in MR-compatible material (**c**): the lack of artifacts due to magnetic susceptibility allows an optimal visualization and demonstration of the regular patency of the device. The image also documents the patency of the bypass between the aorta and the left renal a.

mentation of deformations of the prosthesis; in addition they provide a complete visualization of the entire aorto-iliac axes and collaterals. CEMRA is also accurate in the demonstration of eventual periprosthesic supply (endoleaks). The endoleak, defined as flow inside the aneurysmatic sac outside the lumen of the endoprothesis, represents the major limit to the technical success during endoluminal treatment of the aortic aneurysms.

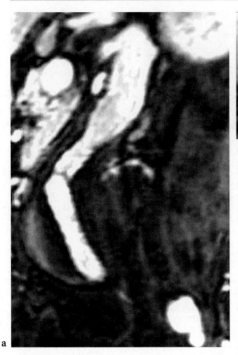

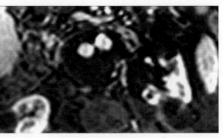

Fig. 11.10 a, b. Patient with endoprosthesis for aortic aneurysm. Type 2 endoleak. The lumbar branch supplying the aneurysmatic sac can be recognized in the sagittal (a) and axial (b) reconstruction

According to White's classification, endoleaks are distinguished in four different types: type 1 is caused by a defect in the proximal (1a) or distal (1b) anchorages; type 2 has the sac supplied by collateral branches of the aorta (Fig 11.10); type 3 is caused by defects of the prosthesis or by incomplete anchoring (sealing) between the components of modular prostheses; and lastly, type 4 is linked to the microporosity of the prosthesis.

Recent studies documented in literature have underlined the particularly high sensitivity values of angio-CT and CEMRA, which are virtually similar in the demonstration of proximal migration retraction or disconnections of the prosthesis wall, typical in endoleaks of type 1 and 3; such studies also report higher sensitivity on behalf of the CEMRA technique as compared to the CT techniques in the documentation of small type 2 endoleaks [18]. The employment of late T1-dependant acquisitions provokes a further increase in diagnostic confidence values.

With no doubt, the major drawbacks of this methodology, compared to angio-CT, are linked to the less-than-optimal visualization of the prostheses in terms of morphology and structure, which is accompanied by a sometimes difficult definition of the proximal and distal anchorages. In addition, the CT exam provides a better evaluation of the aneurismal sac, allowing to document more precisely any morphological or volume changes of the sac. Conversely, angio-MR offers remarkable advantages linked to the absence of ionizing radiations and nephro-toxic contrast mediums.

Thanks to the ever growing availability of MR-compatible prostheses, the scarce invasiveness of the methodology, and the high sensitivity in evaluating the patency parameter and in reporting eventual complications, it is likely that CEMRA may be inserted in the follow-up of patients who have undergone stenting procedures [19]. To date, however, the standards of all follow-up protocols foresee evaluation by echo-Doppler and angio-CT exams.

11.2.5 Retroperitoneal fibrosis

This is an insidious pathologic process characterized by the proliferation of fibrous tissue on the posterior side of the retroperitoneus, which tends to envelope vessels and ureters. Although approximately two thirds of cases are idiopathic, there is a recognized association between some drugs (methysergide), mechanical trauma (pulsating aneurysm, surgical intervention), autoimmune diseases (mediastinic fibrosis, arteritis) and primitive or metastatic tumors.

Characteristically, such tissue involves the peri-aortic soft tissue that is delimited antero-laterally by the peritoneum, saving the posterior vascular wall and extending bilaterally; the unilateral aspect must be considered as an evolutionary phase of the process. Usually the fibrotic tissue is found in the lumbar region extending to the aortic bifurcation embracing the aorta and vena cava without dislocating them; frequently the iliac vessels are involved, as are the ureters that are attracted medially and compressed by the fibrosis with consequent hydronephrosis. The lateral extension, which is often asymmetrical, reaches the external edge of the psoas muscle while more widespread forms may involve the root of the mesenteric a. and the bordering organs or go beyond the diaphragm hiatus and reach the chest where the process become visible under the form of mediastinic fibrosis. The extension can reach the pelvic area determining contraction of the rectus-sigma. Histologically, there are different possibilities that vary from an inflammatory tissue in florid phase to a fibrotic hyaline acellular tissue reaction.

In agreement with different histological pictures, MRI findings also vary: a low intensity of the T1 and T2 signal reflects a mature and quiescent fibrosis stage , formed by collagen and few cells, while hyperintensity in T2 indicates a florid phase with hypercellularity and vascularization of the diseased tissue. Likewise, the detection of the contrast agent will depend on the stage of the pathological process (Fig. 11.11). The study of angio-MR documents any aortic-iliac dilatations or narrowing and, whenever appropriate, an MR urography of the urinary excretory tract is performed.

The added value of MRI compared to other imaging techniques is represented in this specific case by the capacity of distinguishing active forms from chronic ones on the basis of the signal characteristics and of contrast media

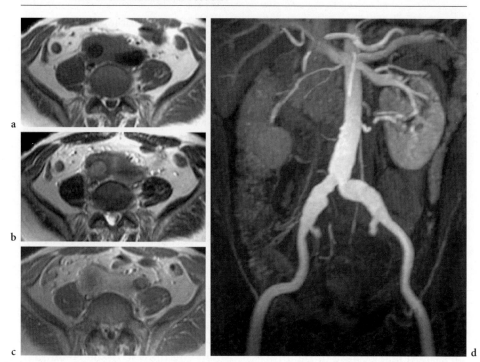

Fig. 11.11 a-d. Retroperitoneal fibrosis. SE T1 (**a**) and SE T2 (**b**) acquisitions allow us to identify the retroperitoneal fibrous tissue with low signal intensity in T1 and T2, which envelopes the median vascular structures. After the contrast (**c**) there is an appreciable enhancement of signal from the tissue wrapping the iliac aa. CEMRA (**d**) documents the ectasia of the abdominal aorta in the pre-carrefour region and the aneurysmatic dilatation of the common iliac arteries

dynamic uptake which are, among other things, useful for the follow-up and evaluation of the response to treatment.

An important element in differential diagnosis with tumors of the retroperitoneus is the absence of anterior dislocation of the large vessels associated with the morphology and signal of the lesion.

References

1. Glockner JF (2001) Three-dimensional gadolinium-enhanced MR angiography: applications for abdominal imaging. Radiographics 21:357-370
2. Prince MR, Grist TM, Debatin JF (2003) 3D contrast MR angiography, 3rd ed. Springer-Verlag, New York, pp. 111-124
3. Arlart PI, Gerlach A (2003) Abdominal aorta and its branches. In: Prince MR, Grist TM, Debatin JF (eds) 3D Contrast MR angiography. Springer-Verlag, New York, pp. 207-344
4. Carroll TJ, Grist TM (2002) Technical developments in MRA. Radiol Clin N Am 40:921-951
5. Hany TF, McKinnon GC, Leung DA, Pfammatter T, Debatin JF (1997) Optimization of contrast timing for breath-hold three-dimensional MR angiography. J Magn Reson Imaging 7:551-556

6. Prince MR, Chabra SG, Watts R et al (2002) Contrast material travel times in patients undergoing peripheral MR angiography. Radiology 224:55-61

7. Foo TK, Saranathan M, Prince MR, Chenevert TL (1997) Automated detection of bolus arrival and initiation of data acquisition in fast, three-dimensional gadolinium-enhanced MR angiography. Radiology 203:275-280

8. Riederer SJ, Bernstein MA, Breen JF et al (2000) Three-dimensional contrast-enhanced MR angiography with real-time fluoroscopic triggering: design specifications and technical reliability in 330 patient studies. Radiology 215:584-593

9. Watanabe Y, Dohke M, Okumura A et al (2000) Dynamic subtraction contrast-enhanced MR angiography; technique, clinical applications, and pitfalls. Radiographics 20:135-152

10. Rofsky NM (1998) MR angiography of the aortoiliac and femoropopliteal vessels. Magn Reson Imaging Clin N Am 6:371-384

11. Van Hoe L, De Jaegere T, Bosmans H et al (2000) Breath-hold contrast-enhanced three-dimensional MR angiography of the abdomen: time-resolved imaging versus single-phase imaging. Radiology 214:149-156

12. Brown PM, Zelt DT, Sobolev B (2003) The risk of rupture in untreated aneurysms: the impact of size, gender, and expansion rate. J Vasc Surg 37:280-284

13. Nitecki SS, Hallet JW Jr, Stanson AW et al (1996) Inflammatory abdominal aortic aneurisms: a case-control study. J Vasc Surg 23:860-868

14. Corti R, Osende JI, Fuster V et al (2001) Artery dissection and arterial thrombus aging: the role of noninvasive magnetic resonance imaging. Circulation 103:2420-2421

15. Thurnher S, Cejna M (2002) Imaging of aortic stent-grafts and endoleaks. Radiol Clin North Am 40:799-833

16. Shellock FG, Shellock VJ (1999) Metallic stents: evaluation of MR imaging safety. Am J Roentgenol 173:543-547

17. Hilfiker PR, Quick HH, Pfammatter T, Schmidt M, Debatin JF (1999) Three-dimensional MR angiography of a nitinol-based abdominal aortic stent graft: assessment of heating and imaging characteristics. Eur Radiol 9:1775-1780

18. Hilfiker PR, Pfammatter T, Lachat M (1999) Depiction of an endoleak after abdominal aortic stent-grafting with contrast-enhanced three-dimensional MR angiography. Am J Roentgenol 172:558-562

19. Haulon S, Lions C, McFadden EP et al (2001) Prospective evaluation of magnetic resonance imaging after endovascular treatment of infrarenal aortic aneurysms. Eur J Vasc Endovasc Surg 22:62-69

12   Peripheral arterial system

Virna Zampa, Irene Bargellini

12.1 Introduction

The studies of arterial pathologies of the lower limb mostly concern steno occlusive pathologies, either of atherosclerotic nature or deriving from other causes (Syndrome of Buerger); less frequently studies can be requested to determine vascular alterations caused by other pathologies, such as vascular lesions of the soft tissue, vascular obstructions ab extrinsico, or studies of the vascular architecture of the neoplasias.

When there is a clinical suspicion of peripheral vascular obstructive pathology, it is preferable on a first approach to perform simple non-invasive tests (Echo-color Doppler and Plethysmography) to detect the vascular location involved and point out its hemodynamic significance.

Today, the technological advances allow to study the vascularization of the lower limbs by means of the multi-slice Computed Tomography (CT), providing adequate images of the whole peripheral arterial tree, from the abdominal aorta down to the arteries of the foot, in less than one minute of scanning. Nevertheless, this diagnostic procedure requires higher doses of ionizing radiation, and large amounts of iodinated contrast agent.

Considerable progress has also been seen in the last few years for Magnetic Resonance Angiography (MRA): the introduction of the phase array coil and ultrafast sequences allows the study of the peripheral arteries using moderate quantities of paramagnetic contrast agent. The method still needs further technical methodological refinements and rigorous studies to evaluate its real diagnostic accuracy, but it is likely to become the chosen, second level non-invasive, diagnostic method for patients with pathology of peripheral arterial obstruction, limiting the role of Digital Subtraction Angiography (DSA) to the preintervention phase.

Although DSA represents the method of reference for assessing the exact morphological vascular involvement, which is indispensable for a correct therapeutic planning (medical, interventional or surgical), it is invasive and not free from risks, therefore it is to be used on adequately selected patients, when revascularization treatment is foreseen.

The techniques and the means of execution for the MRA are numerous, however, at present the three-dimensional MRA with administration of contrast bolus (3D, contrast enhanced MRA – CEMRA) represents the method of choice to obtain images of highly diagnostic accuracy [1].

12.2 Technique

12.2.1 Patient preparation

The patient is placed face up on the scanner moving-bed, with arms above the head or over the chest, and the lower limbs positioned in such a way so as to reduce the antero-posterior extension of the volume to be examined, keeping in mind the most anterior and posterior point of the coursing of the peripheral arteries (common femoral artery at the level of the head of the femur and the popliteal a. in the homonymous cavity). The antero-posterior extension of the volume of interest can be limited by simply having the patient fold the limb in such a way that the knee is placed slightly higher than the plane passing the femur head [2]. The patient is put under respiratory monitoring and, on occurrence, also peripheral pulse or cardiac triggering for a better quality of images.

The study of the lower limbs usually implies the evaluation of the subrenal aorta, the femoral-iliac vessels, and arteries of the leg. To cover the entire area of interest, the body coil and phased-array are used in sequence, positioned along the longitudinal axis of the patient; when possible, the operator should opt for the use of coils specifically-designed for lower limbs [3] that increase the diagnostic quality of the images.

The most recent angio "surf" technique employs a "phased-array" coil, designed for the study of the vascular system and visualizes within a single session the entire vascular system of the body (total body MRA) [4], through the automated movement of the coil along the longitudinal axis of the patient. The contrast agent is injected intravenously with an automatic injector, generally through a vein in the upper limb; the injector is set for an injection of contrast agent (maximum dose 0.3 mmol/kg) and the subsequent cleansing with physiological solution (about 20 cc). The sequences used most frequently for MRA are the 3D CEMRA and the bidimensional Time Of Flight (2D TOF). Although several sequences have been used for the examination of the lower limbs (3D TOF with contrast medium [5], 2D/3D phase-contrast MRA [6]), the most recent metanalyses show a higher diagnostic accuracy for CEMRA as compared to other techniques [7].

12.2.2 Time Of Flight Angio-MR (TOF-MRA)

In the past, 2D TOF was the preferred sequence for the study of the peripheral vascularization with MR (Fig. 12.1). The typical parameters of acquisition

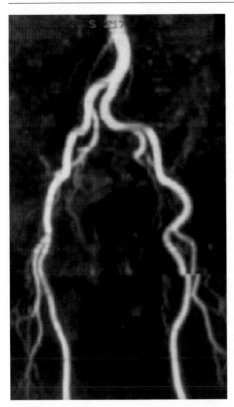

Fig. 12.1. Example of a study of the iliac vessels by cardio-synchronized TOF technique. Although these are good quality images, there are noticeable staircase artifacts that damage the quality and hinder the interpretation of the image

for this method are: TR/TE = 30-45/6.9 msec, flip angle = 60°, FOV = 240-320 mm, matrix = 256×128. The images are acquired perpendicular to the flow of the vessel to minimize the transit time of the proton inside the layer and exploit the effect of the flow to the most, thereby reducing the artifacts and increasing the contrast between vessels and stationary tissue. Generally, the thickness of the layer with overlapping is 4 mm.

To increase the quality of the images, the acquisitions are taken during the systolic phase, when the velocity of the flow is at its highest; this minimizes the artifacts associated with the pulsations of the vessels, and the change in the velocity of the flow during the cardiac cycle, as well as the effect of the retrograde-flow [8]. To obtain selective images of the arteries, saturation bands are applied distally to the sections in order to null the signal coming from the veins. If available, sequential saturation (the band moves in concomitance with the layer studied) is used with a gap of 10 mm, 5 mm at the level of the foot. It is important to choose the correct distance between the band and the volume to be examined, since their overlapping determines a hyperintense line in the picture (horizontal bar artifact), while their excessive distance does not cancel out the venous flow in an adequate manner. The TOF sequence has intrinsic limits that reduce its practicability: long times of acquisition, rather often insufficient quality of the images, overestimation of the extension and grade of the stenosis, presence of artifacts. The most frequent artifacts are flow-void and ghosting; the latter are caused by pulsation and by the consistent systolic-diastolic excursion of the velocity of the peripheral flow. Both are significantly reduced by cardiac triggering.

The flow void is determined by the saturation of the protons inside the layer (tortuous vessels, excessive layer thickness, slow flow) and by the turbulence of the flow that accelerate the loss of the phase coherence (typically in poststenotic site). The absence of signal can be caused by the saturation bands of the venous flow if the selected gap is insufficient, or in case of back flow (diastolic phase, collateral circles). Recent studies have found minor sensibility and specificity for the 2D TOF (70-80%) in comparison to the CEMRA (90-100%) in the evaluation of the peripheral vascular pathology [7].

12.2.3 Contrast Enhanced MRA (CEMRA)

Three-dimensional CEMRA represents the real technological advance in the study of the peripheral arterial tree. It gives images of high spatial- and contrast-resolution, with substantially the same quality of traditional angiography [9].

The use of short TR assures the saturation of the stationary tissue; by slightly extending the acquisition it is possible to saturate the signal from fat and significantly increase the Signal-to-Noise Ratio (SNR).

After a scout image (axial 2D TOF at intervals of 20-30 cm along the whole limb, sagittal in median position or tri-planar of the different anatomical stations), the coronal 3D acquisitions are positioned to include the abdominal aorta, up to the arteries of the foot (3/4 stations) (Fig. 12.2) [10].

The typical parameters are: TR <7 msec, TE <2.5 msec, flip angle = 30°-40°, matrix 512×192×24 rebuilt to 512×512×48 through the zero "padding", FOV = 38-48 cm.

The increase of contrast resolution requires the digital subtraction of the images, similarly to the studies of other anatomical areas. This implies the acquisition of a set of mask images.

Please refer to chapter 2 for the synchronization of scanning/contrast bolus, and to chapter 3 for image postprocessing.

Despite the sophisticated options available, establishing the exact delay in scanning the most peripheral arteries can be more complicated than for other districts, sometimes due to the excessive dilution of the contrast agent, or to hemodynamic differences in the two limbs (Fig. 12.3).

The method of approaching the exam depends on the equipment that is available. If the examining bed is fixed, the 2D TOF sequence can be used for the study of the leg vessels because of their less turbulent flow, followed by the

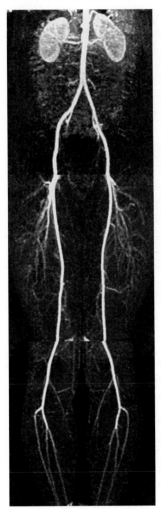

Fig. 12.2. Example of multi-station technique (bolus-chase MRA) of the abdominal aorta and of the arterial tree of the inferior limbs (40 cm FOV, TR/TE 3.7/0.9 msec, matrix 24×256×128, 1 NEX, zip 2, acquisition time <20 seconds, per station). Images on the coronal plane elaborated with subtraction. One single bolus of contrast agent allows a complete visualization of the whole peripheral arterial tree in 3 stations

3D CEMRA of the aorto-iliac and femoral region, synchronized by means of "bolus triggering" [11].

If the equipment has a moving-bed, the acquisition of the different stations is associated to the injection of the contrast medium. This method ("bolus-chase" or "floating table" MRA) can be performed with fast or slow infusion of the contrast agent.

The technique of rapid infusion (1-2 ml/sec) implies a total acquisition time of less than 60 sec, hence it is necessary to have ultra-rapid sequences with short TR (3-8 msecs) and a fast moving bed, in consideration of the fact that the contrast agent moves from one station to the next in about 5-6 seconds [12]. The possibility of acquiring an elliptic K-space, especially in the

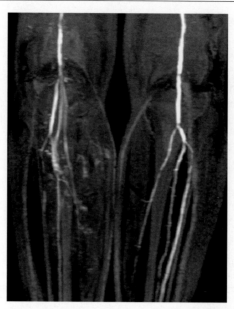

Fig. 12.3. Study of the arteries of the inferior limbs in a diabetic patient. 3D CEMRA on coronal plane. Different hemodynamic flow in the two limbs: on the right, the visualization of the leg artery is inadequate due to a suboptimal concentration of contrast agent. On the right, image detects an atypical origin of the posterior tibial a. from the poplitea and the higher origin of the anterior tibial a. The tibial aa. are occluded at the medium-proximal third with the peroneal artery patent although pluri-stenotic. On the left, the popliteal a. appears pluristenotic; downstream there is an evident complete channeling of the anterior tibial a. alone with a sub-occlusion at the third medium of the posterior tibial a. and of the peroneal a.

distal stations, increases the spatial resolution and limits the overlapping of venous structures.

If ultra-rapid sequences and/or the fast moving-bed are not available, the contrast medium is injected slowly (0,3-0,5 ml/secs) using a longer TR (>8 msecs). In this case the concentration of contrast agent inside the vessel is less, but the use of the longer TR determines a minor saturation of the signal from the blood and, therefore, a greater intensity of the vascular signal. The image subtraction performed off-line eliminates the signal from the stationary tissues; the contrast agent, which is extracted from the extra cellular space, determines a poor visualization of the venous structures [13]. This technique has a longer acquisition time, which leads to problems of the length of the apnea in the abdominal area. Nevertheless, it has been proven that the quality of the image is adequate if the patient breath-holds for at least 75% of the time of acquisition.

Several techniques for reducing the time of the examination have been proposed.

12.2.3.1 Shoot and Scoot

After the acquisition of the mask, the central data of K-space from which contrast resolution depends are acquired in the arterial phase; to this follows an acquisition centered on the peripheral portion of K-space that dominates the spatial resolution of the image. The data is then elaborated again combining the central and peripheral portion of K-space and subtracting the mask [14].

12.2.3.2 Moving the bed manually

Manual movement of the bed can be faster than automatic movement and is performed by some operators to achieve efficient results in a short time, even if the method can represent an intrinsic variability.

Recently, manufacturers have introduced moving-beds with tabletops in continuous motion, similar to those working in the spiral CT; however, the continuous movement of the bed can determine movement and reconstruction artifacts, an issue which has yet to be solved [2].

12.2.3.3 Wakitrak

The method consists in the application of parallel imaging techniques (SENSE, SMASH) (approx 10 sec) with phased-array coil for the study of the abdomen and the pelvis, followed by a rapid (approx 10 sec) low-resolution coronal acquisition at the level of the thighs – both procedures with minimum venous enhancement. Finally, legs and ankles are acquired on the sagittal plane in about 70 seconds, with high-resolution sequence and elliptic K-space, using a phased-array coil [2].

12.2.3.4 Time-resolved (multiphase) MRA

With this method synchronization with contrast bolus is no longer necessary, since the arterial phase of the passage of the contrast is visualized every few seconds. Using the 3D TRICKS sequence (Time-Resolved Imaging of Contrast KineticS) it is possible to visualize the progression of the contrast medium along the arterial tree [15]. The acquisition (which lasts about 7 seconds) is repeated several times to catch the phase of arterial enhancement and follow the dynamics of the flow (Fig. 12.4).

The contrast agent is administered in fractioned boli with increasing doses at every anatomical station in order to reduce the accumulative effects of the contrast agent in the tissues and in the venous structures (Fig. 12.5).

This method is useful for evaluating circulation velocity and the differ-

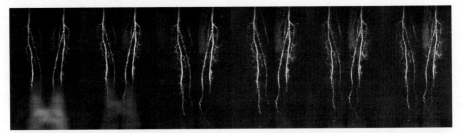

Fig. 12.4. Three-dimensional MRA using TRICKS (Time-Resolved Imaging of Contrast Kinetics) pulse sequence. In this case 6 consecutive acquisitions (starting from the left panel) of the arteries of lower limbs have been obtained. The method allows to visualize the progressive filling of the arterial vessels

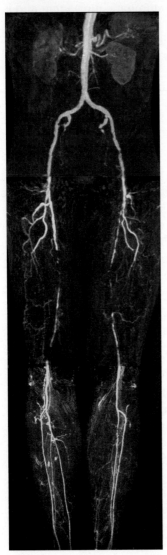

Fig. 12.5. Collateral vascularizations that, starting from the deep femoral, rechannel the downstream vessel in patient with a bilateral occlusion of the superficial femoral a. and atheromasic involvement of all the leg arteries

ences of flow in a limb compared to the controlateral, and gives information similar to that provided by DSA concerning the presence and the direction of the flow of the collateral circles, which are not obtainable with the static MRA images.

12.2.3.5 Time-resolved and bolus-chase MRA

In this method the time-resolved 3D TRICKS is performed at the ankle and foot level, followed by a bolus-chase MRA from the abdomen to the calf.

12.3 Clinical applications

The clinical applications of MRA in the study of peripheral vascularization are more or less the same as those of the DSA.

12.3.1 Atherosclerosis

The atherosclerotic pathology represents the first and most important indication toward the study of the peripheral arterial vessels. The atherosclerotic pathology, either in its steno-obstructive manifestation (Fig. 12.5), or in its ectasic one (Fig. 12.6) finds in MRA an ideal method of study for the simultaneous and three-dimensional evaluation of a large anatomical region.

This pathology involves mostly the proximal district (aorta and iliac-femoral arteries) whereas it is more common in the distal site (particularly below the popliteal a.) in patients with diabetes.

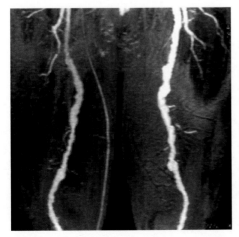

Fig. 12.6. Atheromasic involvement of both the superficial femoral aa. with multiple atheromasic plaques and diffused bilateral ecstasies

12.3.1.1 Steno-obstructive pathology

MRA provides valid information on the degree, area, and extension of the steno-obstructive pathology; its diagnostic accuracy has been increased by CEMRA, reaching sensibility and specificity equal to 90-100% when evaluating the steno-obstructions [7]. Studies made on diabetic patients show that the accuracy of the CEMRA is even superior to that of DSA for visualizing peripheral arteries [16].

Collateral circles of compensation can be easily located, but so far it has not been possible to evaluate the velocity of flow, particularly in presence of vascular obstructions or an evident difference in the speed of the flow between the two limbs. Time-resolved MRA can partially overcome this limit.

The diagnostic accuracy of CEMRA is significantly reduced at the arterial districts, which are distal to the popliteal a., the area where the vessels are very small and the collateral circles are often difficult to recognize and very difficult to diagnose [17].

Furthermore, a tendency to overestimate the steno-obstructions has been demonstrated in the aortic-iliac-femoral arteries as well as in the most distal arteries such as the tibial arteries [18].

12.3.1.2 Aneurysmatic pathology

MRA represents an alternative, sophisticated, diagnostic instrument (Fig. 12.7) for the study of arterial aneurysms of the inferior limbs, even if it gives incomplete information about the wall of the vessels and, particularly, on possible intimal calcifications.

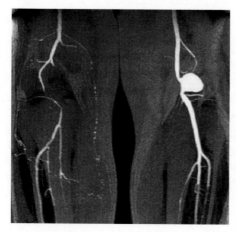

Fig. 12.7. Patient who has already undergone a femoral-popliteal bypass to intervene on an aneurysm of the right popliteal a. The MRA study shows the occlusion of the bypass and consequent rechanneling of the trifurcation of the leg by collateral circles. On the left, an aneurysmatic formation of the popliteal a. with a good channeling of the downstream arteries

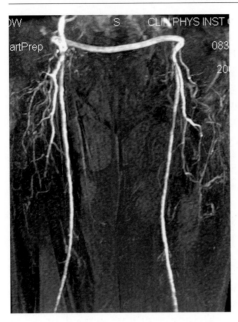

Fig. 12.8. Patient who has undergone a femoral-femoral bypass for an occlusion of the left iliac a. The MRA exam demonstrates a good channeling of the bypass and both superficial femoral aa.

12.3.2 Surgical arterial bypass

The follow-up of surgical bypass represents a further application of MRA, as a fast, accurate and reproducible non-invasive method (Fig. 12.8). Published studies demonstrate values of sensibility and specificity of 90-100 % when evaluating the patency of the arterial distal bypass [19]. However, there are important limits that have not yet been overcome completely, such as the presence of the metal clip, collateral circles, artero-venous fistulas or pseudo-aneurysms in proximal or distal sites to the bypass.

12.3.3 Vascular lesions of the soft tissue and vascularization of tumoral lesions

Notwithstanding the numerous and complicated classifications proposed by many authors, when studying the vascular malformations of the soft tissues it is fundamental to distinguish forms of high or low flow when studying the vascular malformations of the soft tissues. This distinction is the basis for any correct therapeutic planning, since high flow is susceptible to embolizing treatments and slow flow is susceptible to percutaneous or surgical treatments. Today CEMRA associated to the use of surface coils allows to obtain specific information on the hemodynamics of the vascular lesions of the soft tissues, avoiding invasive procedures, unless strictly required for therapeutic reasons.

In these circumstances, the acquisition is repeated at least three times to capture the arterial, venous and late phases, thereby obtaining information relative to the vessels and the parenchymal component. In particular the demonstration of arterial feeders is suggestive of the high-flow forms (Fig. 12.9). Another elegant demostration is the display of the artero-venous malformations, however the hyperkinetic circle simultaneously yields images of venous and arterial structures, which makes it difficult to establish the direction of the flow. The use of time-resolved MRA could provide, also in this pathology, additional diagnostic elements.

Sometimes MRA can be used to evaluate the vascularization of muscular-skeletal tumors. This information can give indicative elements on the aggressiveness of the lesion towards a better planning of the surgical operation. It is important to determine the extension of the lesion and the relationship with the surrounding tissues, a possible infiltration, or compression of the vessels, and the existence of significant arterial afferent vessels (Fig. 12.10). The latter are particularly important in the case of hypervascularized bony lesions, (typically, metastasis of the medullar carcinoma of the thyroid or from neuro-endocrine tumors) that can be subjected to embolizing treatments. The reaction to the treatment can be evaluated with conventional MRI and MRA exams.

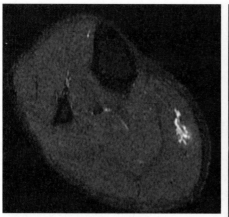
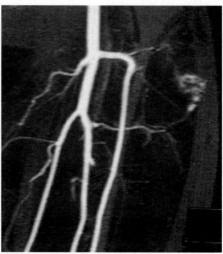

Fig. 12.9 a, b. Small intramuscular vascular snake-like lesion, hyperintense in the FSE-IR sequence with fat suppression (**a**). The MPVR reconstruction of CEMRA in arterial phase (**b**) shows two feeders pertaining to the peroneal a. and anterior tibial a. indicating a high flow lesion

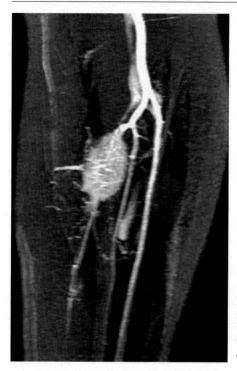

Fig. 12.10. MRA study of a left tibial osteosarcoma. An evident intense vascularization of the tumoral lesion fed by a hypertophic feeder pertaining to the posterior tibial a. with rapid filling of venous vessels

12.3.4 Obstructive pathology due to external compression

The steno-obstructive vascular pathology can also be caused by factors external to the vascular lumen. In such a case, MR takes on the double function of evaluating the vascular lumen through MRA, and of identifying the extrinsic pathology by means of the classical sequences [20].

12.4 Advantages

The advantage of MRA over DSA is that it is non-invasive and, therefore, better tolerated by the patient. The whole exam, including the processing of the images, is quick and generally easier to interpret, not only for the radiologist, but also for the surgeon.

This method is effective, safe, and reproducible.

The use of paramagnetic contrast agents allows to perform the exam also on patients who are not suitable for iodinated contrast agents (patients with renal insufficiency, multiple myeloma, or allergic patients). The amount of contrast agent required to visualize the whole arterial tree system is low; this represents an advantage over CT and DSA, which employ a quantity of contrast of about 100-200 ml, with a higher risk of volumetric overload, particularly in cardiac patients.

Furthermore, MRA offers the evident advantage of not using ionizing radiation, an important factor when young patients are involved.

12.5 Limits

Compared to other techniques of vascular imaging, MRA involves some difficulties, as listed below.

12.5.1 Timing

The synchronization between the acquisition and the arrival of the contrast agent (Fig. 12.11) is a crucial factor influencing image quality. A delayed acquisition determines the overlapping of the venous structures and a poor vascular opacity because of the dilution of the contrast agent; an anticipated acquisition determines missed or non-optimal visualization of the vascular lumen.

The correct synchronization of the sequence becomes particularly complex when the time of flow differs significantly in the two limbs, or when an occlusion causes a slow opacity of the downstream flow through multiple and complex lateral flows.

Such problems can in part be avoided using time-resolved MRA or with a slow infusion of contrast agent.

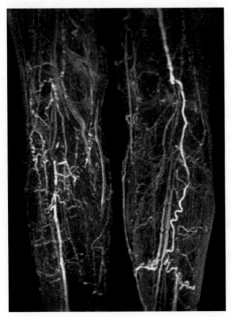

Fig. 12.11. Multi-station MRA study in a diabetic patient: wrong timing with venous overlapping. At the level of the legs there is a bilateral occlusion at the medium-proximal third of both popliteal aa. with evident collateral circulation. The images show a significant reduction of the diagnostic quality due to the overlapping of the superficial and deeper venous system

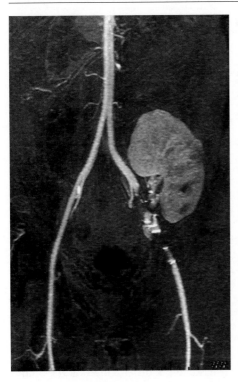

Fig. 12.12. Iliac-femoral MRA in patient who underwent a kidney transplant: artifacts due to metallic material. The presence of metallic clips in the area of the vascular anastomosis determines an artifact due to the magnetic susceptibility with absence of signal, which makes the direct evaluation of the patency of the left iliac a. and of the renal a. and vein impossible

12.5.2 Artifacts

The artifacts in MRA can arise from several sources. Among them, we recall the artifacts caused by motion, which however are not frequent if adequate instructions are given to the patient and if ultrafast sequences are used.

Other artifacts caused by the presence of metallic structures (surgical clips or vascular stents) are unavoidable; in these cases images show a characteristic area with an absence of signal (Fig. 12.12) due to magnetic susceptibility, which can be minimized by reducing the TE or by increasing the flip-angle. The impossibility of studying a great part of vascular stents by MRA represent the limit of this method with the exception of those in nitinol or platinum that do not interfere with the local magnetic field: in fact, it can only provide indirect information on the patency of a stent, such as the filling of the downstream vascular lumen [21].

12.5.3 Visualizing the vascular lumen alone

MRA visualizes only the canalized lumen of a vessel, with insufficient information on the wall of the vessel itself (Fig. 12.13). To measure the whole diameter of the aneurysm and visualize the parietal thrombosis we must, therefore, perform an additional axial sequence (T1 or TOF). Moreover, calcified intimal plaques

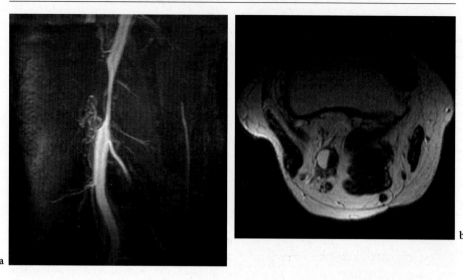

Fig. 12.13 a, b. MRA and conventional MRI study in a patient with dissection of the popliteal artery. MRA study (**a**), reconstruction on a coronal plane shows an evident reduction of the caliber (approx 90%) of the popliteal artery which could be diagnosed, without the help of conventional images, as a stenosis; indeed, the axial T2 image (**b**) clearly shows the dissection of the vessel and the two lumens

can go undetected, especially if they are thin. Recent studies, aimed at the analysis of the structure of the different components of the atherosclerotic plaque are opening new horizons in the comprehension and therapy of this pathology.

12.5.4 Missed visualization of arteries not included in the volume of study

To reduce the length of MRA sequences, sometimes an inadequate reduction in the number of partitions can lead to the missed visualization of a vessel that was not included in the studied volume, and to the erroneous evaluation of a vascular occlusion.

12.5.5 Missed dynamic visualization

Most MRA sequences are substantially static. This means that some details, acquired with DSA are not appreciated by MRA. In particular, it can be difficult to visualize the existence of collateral flows, and even when they are detected, it is difficult to determine the direction, origin and the distal direction of the flow.

Time-resolved MRA appears to be the only sequence that can evaluate the dynamics of the flow and the eventual differences between the two limbs, but needs further validation.

12.5.6 Localizing a lesion

Angio-MR provides accurate images of the vascular lumen alone, canceling out the signal from the surrounding structures. This implies that once the lesion has been visualized it can be difficult to locate it in relation to the other invisible anatomical structures, depleting the study of fundamental data for the planning of a surgical procedure. This problem can be avoided by obtaining, along with the MRA, coronal T1 images at the same level, or by overlapping the two sequences.

12.6 Conclusions

MRA represents a valid alternative to DSA in the non-invasive evaluation of peripheral vascular pathology [22]. Yet, technological advances are necessary to optimize the performance of the method and to improve the evaluation of the arterial distal branches, particularly the smallest vessels distal to the popliteal a.

Decisive factors for are represented by: dimensions of the voxel, quantity and velocity of the injection of the contrast agent, method of acquisition of the K-space, availability of specific coils and time of acquisition [23].

At present, there are new contrast agents (such as the blood-pool) that, from initial trails, seem to increase the SNR and CNR; they are still under development but appear to be very promising in the diagnosing of peripheral flow [24, 25].

Lastly, the development of ultrafast sequences, catheters and soft guides that can be visualized by MRI are being studied and these techniques could replace DSA for vascular interventional therapy in the future [26].

References

1. Loewe C, Schoder M, Rand T et al (2002) Peripheral vascular occlusive disease: evaluation with contrast-enhanced moving-bed MR angiography versus digital subtraction angiography in 106 patients. Am J Roentgenol 179:1013-1021
2. Prince MR, Grist TM, Debatin JF (2003) 3D contrast MR angiography, 3rd ed. Springer-Verlag, Berlin, pp. 185-215
3. Goyen M, Ruehm SG, Barkhausen J et al (2001) Improved multi-station peripheral MR angiography with a dedicated vascular coil. J Magn Reson Imaging 13:475-480
4. Goyen M, Quick HH, Debatin JF et al (2002) Whole-body three-dimensional MR angiography with a rolling table platform: initial clinical experience. Radiology 224:270-277
5. Engelbrecht MR, Saeed M, Wendland MF et al (1998) Contrast-enhanced 3D-TOF MRA of peripheral vessels: intravascular versus extracellular MR contrast media. J Magn Reson Imaging 8:616-621
6. Steffens JC, Link J, Muller-Hulsbeck S et al (1997) Cardiac-gated 2D phase-contrast MRA of lower extremity occlusive disease. AJR 169:749-754
7. Sharafuddin MJ, Stolpen AH, Sun S et al (2002) High-resolution multiphase contrast-

enhanced three-dimensional MR compared with two-dimensional TOF MR angiography for the identification of pedal vessels. J Vasc Interv Radiol 13:695-702

8. Quinn SF, Sheley RC, Szumowski J, Shimakawa A (1997) Evaluation of the iliac arteries: comparison of two-dimensional TOF MRA with cardiac compensated fast gradient recalled echo and contrast-enhanced three-dimensional TOF MRA. J Magn Reson Imaging 7:197-203

9. Ruehm SG, Goyen M, Barkhausen J et al (2001) Rapid magnetic resonance angiography for detection of atherosclerosis. Lancet 357:1086-1091

10. Huber A, Heuck A, Baur A et al (2000) Dynamic contrast-enhanced MR angiography from the distal aorta to the ankle joint with a step-by-step technique. Am J Roentgenol 175:1291-1298

11. Li W, Zhang M, Sher S, Edelman RR (2000) MR angiography of the vascular tree from the aorta to the foot: combining two-dimensional TOF and three-dimensional contrast-enhanced imaging. J Magn Reson Imaging 12:884-889

12. Prince MR, Chabra SG, Watts R et al (2002) Contrast material travel times in patients undergoing peripheral MR angiography. Radiology 224:55-61

13. Carroll TJ, Korosec FR, Swan JS et al (2001) The effect of injection rate on time-resolved contrast-enhanced peripheral MRA. J Magn Reson Imaging 14:401-410

14. Lee HM, Wang Y (1998) Dynamic K-space filling for bolus chase 3D MR digital subtraction angiography. Magn Reson Med 40:99-104

15. Swan JS, Carroll TJ, Kennell TW et al (2002) Time-resolved three-dimensional contrast-enhanced MR angiography of the peripheral vessels. Radiology 225:43-52

16. Kreitner KF, Kalden P, Neufang A et al (2000) Diabetes and peripheral arterial occlusive disease: prospective comparison of contrast-enhanced three-dimensional MR angiography with conventional digital subtraction angiography. Am J Roentgenol 174:171-179

17. Klein WM, Schlejen PM, Eikelboom BC et al (2003) MR angiography of the lower extremities with a moving-bed infusion-tracking technique. Cardiovasc Intervent Radiol 26:1-8

18. Winterer JT, Schaefer O, Uhrmeister P et al (2002) Contrast enhanced MR angiography in the assessment of relevant stenoses in occlusive disease of the pelvic and lower limb arteries: diagnostic value of a two-step examination protocol in comparison to conventional DSA. Eur J Radiol 41:153-160

19. Dorenbeck U, Seitz J, Volk M et al (2002) Evaluation of arterial bypass grafts of the pelvic and lower extremities with gadolinium-enhanced magnetic resonance angiography: comparison with digital subtraction angiography. Invest Radiol 37:60-64

20. Atilla S, Ilgit ET, Akpek S, Yucel C et al (1998) MR imaging and MR angiography in popliteal artery entrapment syndrome. Eur Radiol 8:1025-1029

21. Link J, Steffens JC, Brossmann J et al (1999) Iliofemoral arterial occlusive disease: contrast-enhanced MR angiography for preinterventional evaluation and follow-up after stent placement. Radiology 212:371-377

22. Goyen M, Reuhm S, Debatin J (2002) MR angiography for assessment of peripheral vascular disease. Radiol Clin North Am 40:835-846

23. Hood MN, Ho VB, Foo TK et al (2002) High-resolution gadolinium-enhanced 3D MRA of the infrapopliteal arteries. Lessons for improving bolus-chase peripheral MRA. Magn Reson Imaging 20:543-549

24. Carroll TJ, Grist TM (2002) Technical developments in MR angiography. Radiol Clin North Am 40:921-951

25. Saeed M, Wendland MF, Higgins CB (2000) Blood pool MR contrast agents for cardiovascular imaging. J Magn Reson Imaging 12:890-898

26. Omary RA, Green J, Finn JP, Li D (2002) Catheter-directed gadolinium-enhanced MR angiography. Radiol Clin North Am 40:953-963